Benign and Neoplastic Conditions of the Esophagus

Editor

NICHOLAS J. SHAHEEN

GASTROENTEROLOGY
CLINICS OF NORTH AMERICA

www.gastro.theclinics.com

March 2013 • Volume 42 • Number 1

ELSEVIER

1600 John F. Kennedy Boulevard • Suite 1800 • Philadelphia, Pennsylvania, 19103-2899
http://www.theclinics.com

GASTROENTEROLOGY CLINICS OF NORTH AMERICA Volume 42, Number 1
March 2013 ISSN 0889-8553, ISBN-13: 978-1-4557-7090-8

Editor: Kerry Holland
Developmental Editor: Donald Mumford

Gastroenterology Clinics of North America (ISSN 0889-8553) is published quarterly by Elsevier Inc., 360 Park Avenue South, New York, NY 10010-1710. Months of issue are March, June, September, and December. Business and Editorial Offices: 1600 John F. Kennedy Blvd., Suite 1800, Philadelphia, PA 19103-2899. Customer Service Office: 6277 Sea Harbor Drive, Orlando, FL 32887-4800. Periodicals postage paid at New York, NY and additional mailing offices. Subscription prices are $305.00 per year (US individuals), $153.00 per year (US students), $508.00 per year (US institutions), $335.00 per year (Canadian individuals), $617.00 per year (Canadian institutions), $423.00 per year (international individuals), $211.00 per year (international students), and $617.00 per year (international institutions). Foreign air speed delivery is included in all *Clinics* subscription prices. All prices are subject to change without notice. **POSTMASTER**: Send address changes to *Gastroenterology Clinics of North America*, Elsevier Health Sciences Division, Subscription Customer Service, 3251 Riverport Lane, Maryland Heights, MO 63043. Telephone: 1-800-654-2452 (U.S. and Canada); 314-447-8871 (outside U.S. and Canada). Fax: 314-447-8029. E-mail: journalscustomerservice-usa@elsevier.com (for print support); journalsonlinesupport-usa@elsevier.com (for online support).

Reprints. For copies of 100 or more, of articles in this publication, please contact the Commercial Reprints Department, Elsevier Inc., 360 Part Avenue South, New York, New York 10010-1710. Tel. (212) 633-3813, Fax: (212) 462-1935, E-mail: reprints@elsevier.com.

Gastroenterology Clinics of North America is also published in Italian by Il Pensiero Scientifico Editore, Rome, Italy; and in Portuguese by Interlivros Edicoes Ltda., Rua Commandante Coelho 1085, 21250 Cordovil, Rio de Janeiro, Brazil.

Gastroenterology Clinics of North America is covered in *MEDLINE/PubMed (Index Medicus)*, *Excerpta Medica*, *Current Contents/Clinical Medicine*, *Science Citation Index*, *ISI/BIOMED*, and *BIOSIS*.

Printed and bound by CPI Group (UK) Ltd, Croydon, CR0 4YY
Transferred to Digital Printing, 2013

Contributors

EDITOR

NICHOLAS J. SHAHEEN, MD, MPH
Professor of Medicine and Epidemiology, Center for Esophageal Diseases and Swallowing, University of North Carolina School of Medicine, Chapel Hill, North Carolina

AUTHORS

TETSUO ARAKAWA, MD
Department of Gastroenterology, Osaka City University Graduate School of Medicine, Osaka, Japan

DAVID ARMSTRONG, MA, MB BChir, FRCP(UK), FACG, AGAF, FRCPC
Professor, Division of Gastroenterology, Department of Medicine, McMaster University, Hamilton, Ontario, Canada

GUY E. BOECKXSTAENS, MD, PhD
Department of Gastroenterology, Translational Research Center for Gastrointestinal Disorders (TARGID), University Hospital of Leuven, Catholic University of Leuven, Leuven, Belgium

DUSTIN A. CARLSON, MD
Chief Medical Resident, Department of Medicine, Feinberg School of Medicine, Northwestern University, Chicago, Illinois

EVAN S. DELLON, MD, MPH
Assistant Professor, Center for Esophageal Diseases and Swallowing, University of North Carolina School of Medicine; Division of Gastroenterology and Hepatology, Department of Medicine, Center for Gastrointestinal Biology and Disease, University of North Carolina School of Medicine, Chapel Hill, North Carolina

MASSIMILIANO DI PIETRO, MD
MRC Cancer Cell Unit, Hutchison MRC, Cambridge, United Kingdom

USHA DUTTA, MBBS, MD, DM, MSc
Clinical Epidemiology, Division of Gastroenterology, Department of Medicine, McMaster University, Hamilton, Ontario, Canada

RONNIE FASS, MD, FACG
Director, Division of Gastroenterology and Hepatology; Head, Esophageal and Swallowing Center, MetroHealth Medical Center, Case Western Reserve University, Cleveland, Ohio

REBECCA C. FITZGERALD, MD
MRC Cancer Cell Unit, Hutchison MRC, Cambridge, United Kingdom

YASUHIRO FUJIWARA, MD
Department of Gastroenterology, Osaka City University Graduate School of Medicine, Osaka, Japan

EMMANUEL C. GOROSPE, MD, MPH
Barrett's Esophagus Unit, Division of Gastroenterology and Hepatology, Mayo Clinic, Rochester, Minnesota

CHRISTOPHER HOM, MD
Division of Gastroenterology, Hepatology and Nutrition, Center for Swallowing and Esophageal Disorders, Vanderbilt University Medical Center, Nashville, Tennessee

PETER J. KAHRILAS, MD, AGAF
Professor, Department of Medicine, Feinberg School of Medicine, Northwestern University, Chicago, Illinois

CADMAN L. LEGGETT, MD
Barrett's Esophagus Unit, Division of Gastroenterology and Hepatology, Mayo Clinic, Rochester, Minnesota

AN J. MOONEN, MD
Department of Gastroenterology, Translational Research Center for Gastrointestinal Disorders (TARGID), University Hospital of Leuven, Catholic University of Leuven, Leuven, Belgium

DYLAN R. NIEMAN, MD, PhD
Research Fellow, Division of Thoracic and Foregut Surgery, Department of Surgery, University of Rochester Medical Center, Rochester, New York

JOHN E. PANDOLFINO, MD, MSCI
Professor of Medicine, Gastroenterology and Hepatology, Department of Medicine, Feinberg School of Medicine, Northwestern University, Chicago, Illinois

JEFFREY H. PETERS, MD, FACS
Professor and Chairman, Division of Thoracic and Foregut Surgery, Department of Surgery, University of Rochester Medical Center, Rochester, New York

SABINE ROMAN, MD, PhD
Associate Professor, Digestive Physiology, Hôpital E Herriot, Hospices Civils de Lyon, Claude Bernard Lyon I University, Lyon, France

MICHAEL F. VAEZI, MD, PhD, MSc (Epi)
Division of Gastroenterology, Hepatology and Nutrition, Center for Swallowing and Esophageal Disorders, Vanderbilt University Medical Center, Nashville, Tennessee

MARCELO F. VELA, MD, MSCR, FACG
Division of Gastroenterology and Hepatology, Associate Professor of Medicine, Director of GI Motility, Michael E. DeBakey VA Medical Center, Baylor College of Medicine, Houston, Texas

NICOLAS VILLA, MD
Division of Gastroenterology and Hepatology, Michael E. DeBakey VA Medical Center, Baylor College of Medicine, Houston, Texas

KENNETH K. WANG, MD, AGAF, FASGE
Director, Barrett's Esophagus Unit, Van Cleve Professor of Gastroenterology Research, Division of Gastroenterology and Hepatology, Mayo Clinic, Rochester, Minnesota

THOMAS J. WATSON, MD, FACS
Chief of Thoracic Surgery, Division of Thoracic and Foregut Surgery; Associate Professor of Surgery, Department of Surgery, University of Rochester School of Medicine and Dentistry, Rochester, New York

CANDICE L. WILSHIRE, MD
Research Fellow, Division of Thoracic and Foregut Surgery, Department of Surgery, University of Rochester School of Medicine and Dentistry, Rochester, New York

Contents

alone or in combination with PPIs; however, novel approaches face significant challenges. The safety and efficacy of current PPIs hamper demonstration of clinical superiority for new acid suppressants, and the multifactorial etiology of reflux disease means that monotherapy using a non-acid suppressant is unlikely to match PPI therapy while combination therapy will be superior only if susceptible patients can be identified reliably. Advances will *come,* not from a 'one size fits all' approach but rather from novel pharmaceuticals allied to novel investigations to permit targeted, personalized reflux therapy.

Antireflux surgery has become a well-established therapy for gastroesophageal reflux disease (GERD) and its complications. The popularization of minimally invasive surgical techniques has brought about a revolution in the use of fundoplication for the long-term management of GERD. A reliable and objective understanding of the outcomes following fundoplication is important for all physicians treating GERD, so that informed decisions can be made regarding the optimal treatment strategy for a given patient. With ongoing study, the appropriate indications for surgical intervention among the array of potential antireflux therapies will continue to be elucidated.

Eosinophilic esophagitis (EoE) is a chronic immune-mediated condition whereby infiltration of eosinophils into the esophageal mucosa leads to symptoms of esophageal dysfunction. EoE is encountered in a substantial proportion of patients undergoing diagnostic upper endoscopy. This review discusses the clinical, endoscopic, and histologic features of EoE and presents the most recent guidelines for its diagnosis. Selected diagnostic dilemmas are described, including distinguishing EoE from gastroesophageal reflux disease and addressing the newly recognized clinical entity of proton-pump inhibitor–responsive esophageal eosinophilia. Also highlighted is evidence to support both pharmacologic and nonpharmacologic treatments, including topical corticosteroids, dietary elimination therapy, and endoscopic dilation.

Barrett's esophagus (BE) and gastroesophageal reflux disease are the strongest risk factors for esophageal adenocarcinoma. To reduce the clinical impact of this disease, endoscopic screening to detect BE has been proposed and nonendoscopic diagnostic techniques are under investigation. Because screening would result in new diagnoses of BE and additional costs related to endoscopic surveillance, novel tools for risk stratification are also warranted. Dysplasia is the gold standard for risk stratification. Molecular biomarkers may provide a more objective and reproducible estimation of the individual risk, and further prospective studies are required as a prelude to introducing biomarkers into routine clinical practice.

Endoscopic therapy for Barrett's esophagus is feasible and likely to decrease the future risk of development of esophageal adenocarcinoma. The most commonly used therapy is radiofrequency ablation, which has been shown to produce reproducible superficial injury in the esophagus. Other thermal therapies include multipolar coagulation, argon plasma coagulation, and thermal laser therapy. The other end of the ablative spectrum includes cryotherapy, which involves freezing tissue to produce mucosal necrosis. Photodynamic therapy has been used to photochemically eliminate abnormal mucosa. Endoscopic therapy has been demonstrated to be effective in high-risk situations such as Barrett's esophagus with high-grade dysplasia.

The treatment of esophageal cancer has evolved considerably in the past decade and depends largely on the extent of disease at the time of presentation. For disease confined to the esophageal mucosa, endoscopic therapy is replacing esophagectomy as the standard of care. For locoregional disease, neoadjuvant chemoradiation followed by esophagectomy is the best strategy for optimizing long-term survival. In the minority of patents who present with metastatic disease, the prognosis is poor. Palliative therapies available for these patients include chemotherapy, radiation, endoscopic therapies to ameliorate obstruction or bleeding, and surgical intervention to optimize nutritional status or to relieve obstruction.

GASTROENTEROLOGY
CLINICS OF NORTH AMERICA

Preface

Benign and Malignant Esophageal Diseases

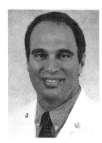

Nicholas J. Shaheen, MD, MPH
Editor

The esophagus is the unsung hero of the chest. In every literary and proverbial setting, the heart gets top billing. For instance, if one behaves with great valor, no one says of him, "That guy showed a lot of esophagus." The lungs are similarly revered. If someone revives a moribund effort, she is said to have "breathed life into the project." Sadly, no one burps life into a project.

Ironic then that the esophagus is the focus of so much medical inquiry and is the seat of some of our most common and devastating maladies. I am honored to introduce this issue of *Gastroenterology Clinics of North America* on benign and malignant diseases of the esophagus. Since this topic was last reviewed 4 years ago, so much has happened in this area. We have seen the epidemic emergence of a major pathophysiologic condition, eosinophilic esophagitis (EoE), which has become the most common source of obstructive dysphagia in some parts of the continent. Revolutions have taken place in the ways that we image the esophagus as well as in the way that we treat neoplastic conditions of the organ. Multiple novel testing modalities have moved from being research tools to being the predominant means of assessing esophageal function.

The most common disorder of the esophagus, gastroesophageal reflux disease (GERD), has also evolved. Whereas the earlier focus of practitioners was on healing the mucosal damage associated with the condition, an increasing awareness has arisen regarding the impact on quality of life associated with ongoing symptoms in the nonerosive patient. Indeed, the battlefield in GERD has shifted from mucosal disease to symptom control, and it is a battle that only the most optimistic would say we are winning.

Despite advances in the care of subjects with esophageal disorders, the epidemic of esophageal adenocarcinoma continues, and this lesion increases in incidence. Our therapies show little impact on survival in this condition, and our attempts at screening and diagnosis for this malady seem to make little dent in the sobering statistics of this

Gastroenterol Clin N Am 42 (2013) xiii–xiv
http://dx.doi.org/10.1016/j.gtc.2012.12.002
0889-8553/13/$ – see front matter © 2013 Published by Elsevier Inc.

gastro.theclinics.com

cancer—approximately 15,000 of the 17,000 people diagnosed with this condition in 2012 will die of it. As the seventh leading cause of cancer death among men in the United States, the terrible toll of esophageal neoplasia is a beacon to those who treat esophageal diseases, and those who study esophageal disorders. We have a moral obligation to do better by these patients.

This issue of *Gastroenterology Clinics of North America* has been designed to highlight landmark shifts in the diagnosis and management of esophageal diseases. In a relatively brief space, our esteemed panel of internationally recognized experts brings the general gastroenterologist, surgeon, or interested primary care provider up to speed on the changes in this rapidly evolving area. What are the best endoscopic and surgical treatments of esophageal neoplasia? What is the most logical way to evaluate someone with suspected extra-esophageal manifestations of GERD? What new therapeutic agents can I anticipate for this disease? How should I incorporate high-resolution manometry and impedance testing into my practice? What is the most efficacious management of incident EoE, and what should I do if it doesn't work? When and how should I screen my patients for esophageal disease? These are not academic questions, but very pragmatic issues that the clinician has a high likelihood of encountering on a daily basis. As such, this volume is designed to be a useful resource in providing your patients with state-of-the-art care for esophageal diseases.

I owe a great debt of thanks to the multidisciplinary team of renowned authors whose work forms the corpus of this volume. I count myself lucky to share a field of interest with such thoughtful, creative, and generous colleagues. Thanks also to Kerry Holland and the staff at Elsevier for their tireless efforts in "herding the cats" to bring this issue together. I hope you enjoy reading the fruits of their labor, and that this work helps you bring better care to your patients.

Nicholas J. Shaheen, MD, MPH
Center for Esophageal Diseases and Swallowing
University of North Carolina School of Medicine
130 Mason Farm Road, Suite 4150
Chapel Hill, NC 27517, USA

E-mail address:
nicholas_shaheen@med.unc.edu

High-Resolution Manometry and Esophageal Pressure Topography
Filling the Gaps of Convention Manometry

Dustin A. Carlson, MD, John E. Pandolfino, MD, MSCI*

KEYWORDS

- Esophageal motility disorders • High-resolution manometry • Achalasia
- Distal esophageal spasm

KEY POINTS

- Diagnostic schemes for conventional manometry and esophageal pressure topography (EPT) rely on measurements of key variables and descriptions of patterns of contractile activity. However, the enhanced assessment of esophageal motility and sphincter function available with EPT has led to the further characterization of clinically relevant phenotypes.
- Differentiation of achalasia into subtypes provides a method to predict the response to treatment.
- A diagnosis of diffuse esophageal spasm represents a unique clinical phenotype when defined by premature esophageal contraction (measured via distal latency) instead of when defined by rapid contraction (measured by contractile front velocity and/or wave progression) alone.
- Defining hypercontractile esophagus with a single swallow with a significantly elevated distal contractile integral, as opposed to using a mean value more than a predetermined 95th percentile, may define a more specific clinical syndrome characterized by chest pain and/or dysphagia.
- EPT correlates of the conventional manometric diagnosis of ineffective esophageal motility include weak and frequent-failed peristalsis; however, the clinical significance of these diagnoses is not completely understood.

Financial support: JEP: Given Imaging (consulting, grant support, speaking), Astra Zeneca (speaking), Sandhill Scientific (consulting).
This work was supported by R01 DK079902 (JEP) from the Public Health Service.
Conflict of interest: John E. Pandolfino: Given Imaging (consulting, educational), Sandhill Scientific (consulting, research).
Department of Medicine, Feinberg School of Medicine, Northwestern University, Suite 3-150, 251 East Huron, Chicago, IL 60611, USA
* Corresponding author. Division of Gastroenterology and Hepatology, Feinberg School of Medicine, Northwestern University, 676 Saint Clair Street, Suite 1400, Chicago, IL 60611-2951.
E-mail address: j-pandolfino@northwestern.edu

Gastroenterol Clin N Am 42 (2013) 1–15
http://dx.doi.org/10.1016/j.gtc.2012.11.001
0889-8553/13/$ – see front matter
gastro.theclinics.com

INTRODUCTION

In 2001, based on a review of the literature to date, Spechler and Castell[1] proposed a classification scheme for esophageal motility disorders incorporating defined conventional manometry (CM) criteria. This description was the state-of-the-art description of manometry at the time. However, the investigators recognized that the clinical significance of any observed manometric findings may be limited because the abnormalities were often reported to occur with poor correlation to symptoms, and therapeutic corrections of manometric findings often did not lead to improvement in symptoms.[2]

A few years after that review, high-resolution manometry (HRM) and esophageal pressure topography (EPT) started to appear on the scene, both in research and clinical practice. HRM is comprised of multiple, closely spaced pressure sensors (usually 1 cm apart) that record pressure without significant gaps in data along the length of the esophagus. This data can be modified using interpolation to generate EPT plots that are color coded, spatiotemporal representations of pressure recordings in the esophagus (Clouse plots). This technology lends itself to an objective assessment of EPT metrics that have been integrated into a new classification scheme for esophageal motility disorders, referred to as the Chicago classification scheme.[3] As clinical and research experience grows with HRM, the Chicago classification scheme has been intermittently updated in an attempt to improve its representation of clinically relevant phenotypes.[4–7] The goal of this review is to compare conventional and HRM classification schemes for esophageal motility disorders and to illustrate how these new clinical phenotypes on EPT have evolved from previous definitions used by Spechler and Castell for CM.

METHODOLOGY: CM AND HRM

The procedure for both types of manometry begins with the placement of the manometry catheter transnasally until the distal pressure sensors cross the esophagogastric junction (EGJ) and enter the stomach. The comparative measurements made with CM and HRM are displayed in **Table 1**.

In CM, a pull-through technique is used to determine the position of the lower esophageal sphincter (LES) pressure by identifying the pressure inversion point and a high-pressure zone. The pressure sensor is then left positioned in the LES, and the basal pressure is recorded over at least 2 minutes with minimal swallowing. Once the baseline recording is complete, LES relaxation is measured during at least 5 wet (5 mL water) swallows with the pressure sensor maintained at the position where the middle of the LES high-pressure zone was recorded. Peristaltic function is typically assessed with pressure sensors spaced anywhere from 3 to 5 cm apart, with a repositioning of the pressure sensors into the body or by simultaneous pressure recording at the LES using a sleeve or single sensor.

In HRM, the distal end of the catheter is passed into the gastric compartment below the LES and hiatal canal, and no pull through is required because the catheter can provide recording from the stomach through the esophagus into the oropharynx. During an HRM study, EPT plots, also known as Clouse plots, are generated by computer software during 10 wet (5 mL water) swallows, and there is no need to perform different steps in the evaluation because all variables can be assessed during the single swallows.[8,9]

Analysis of an EPT study is performed using a stepwise approach that focuses on an algorithm-based scheme that first defines patients based on EGJ relaxation pressures

Table 1
Comparison of CM and HRM metrics

Esophageal Motility Characteristic	CM Measurement	HRM Measurement
LES relaxation		
	LES relaxation with swallow	IRP
Normal[a]	Complete (<8 mm Hg more than gastric pressure)	<15 mm Hg
Peristaltic propagation		
	Wave progression between pressure sensors 8 and 3 cm above the LES	CFV
Normal[a]	2–8 cm/s (UES to LES)	<9 cm/s
	(no corresponding CM metric)	DL
Normal[a]		≥4.5 s
Contractile vigor		
	Mean distal wave maximum amplitude of pressure sensors 8 and 3 cm above the LES	DCI
Normal[a]	30–180 mm Hg	450–5000 mmHg-s-cm

Abbreviations: CFV, contractile front velocity; DCI, distal contractile integral; DL, distal latency; IRP, integrated relaxation pressure; LES, lower esophageal sphincter; UES, upper esophageal sphincter.
[a] Normal values as stated in Refs.[1,6]

and subsequently uses individual swallow patterns defined by EPT metrics to further subclassify patients into specific categories.

- Step 1: Assessment of EGJ pressure morphology at baseline
  - The first step of the analysis process focuses on describing the pressure morphology of the EGJ to determine whether a hiatus hernia is present and where the pressure inversion point is located because this can have dramatic effects on the measures of EGJ function. The baseline end-expiratory pressure and inspiratory augmentation are recorded to assess the integrity of the crural diaphragm as an extrinsic sphincter.
- Step 2: Assessing EGJ relaxation and bolus pressure dynamics through the EGJ
  - Patients are defined as having normal or abnormal EGJ relaxation using the integrated relaxation pressure (IRP). The IRP is the lowest mean EGJ pressure for 4 contiguous or noncontiguous seconds during the deglutitive period. As demonstrated in **Fig. 1**, the IRP has replaced the conventional measures of nadir or end-expiratory LES relaxation pressure on CM because EPT evaluation made it quite clear that the pressure measured through the EGJ during swallowing was heavily reliant on intrabolus pressure and was not a pure measure of LES relaxation.[10,11]
- Step 3: Assess integrity of the peristaltic wave
  - Once the IRP is measured, esophageal peristaltic integrity is characterized to determine if the peristaltic activity is intact, failed, or associated with small (2–5 cm) or large (>5 cm) peristaltic breaks in the 20-mm Hg isobaric contour. This step is performed before any other measurements are made because the subsequent measurements depend on the presence of intact or preserved peristaltic integrity in the distal esophagus. This metric is similar to using

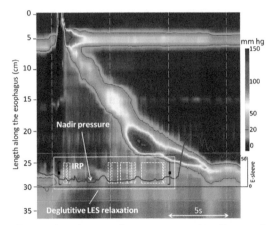

Fig. 1. Assessment of EGJ relaxation. Nadir LES pressure (CM line tracing, *purple*) and IRP (*dotted white boxes* indicating lowest LES pressure segments over 4 noncontiguous seconds) are demonstrated in a normal swallow. IRP 4.8 mm Hg. Nadir LES pressure 0.3 mm Hg more than gastric pressure. The nadir pressure is likely a measurement of intragastric pressure.

a 30-mm Hg threshold at 3 and 8 cm above the proximal border of the LES to define effective swallows.[12] However, the isobaric contour tool provides a more complete assessment of the swallow as demonstrated in **Fig. 2**.

- Step 4: Determine the location of the contractile deceleration point (CDP)
  - The CDP is defined as the inflection point along the contractile wavefront defined by the 30-mm Hg isobaric contour tool where the greatest deceleration occurs and the function of the esophagus converts from a stripping wave to a compartmentalized ampulla to promote emptying of the remaining bolus (**Fig. 3**). This landmark is in close proximity to the proximal border of the LES

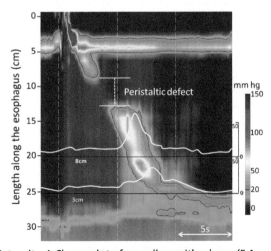

Fig. 2. Peristaltic integrity. A Clouse plot of a swallow with a large (5.1 cm axial length) peristaltic defect in the 20-mm Hg isobaric contour is displayed. CM line tracings at 3 and 8 cm would not normally detect this defect in the transition zone. Black lines indicate the CM recording sites with their position from the LES (eg, 3 cm, as labeled).

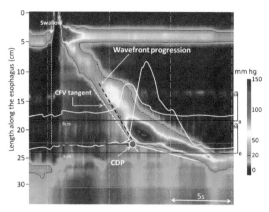

Fig. 3. Propagation of peristalsis. The EPT metrics of CDP, distal latency (DL), contractile front velocity (CFV), and the CM wavefront progression are displayed on a normal swallow. The CDP (*red circle*) is located at the intersection of the CFV tangent (*white dashed line*) and the velocity tangent of the terminal segment of esophageal peristalsis (*solid white line*), which correlates with emptying of the esophageal ampulla. The DL (*purple arrow*) is defined as the time from the initiation of the swallow to the CDP and measures 7 seconds in the swallow. The wavefront progression (*black dashed line*) is determined from CM line tracings (measuring 5.0 cm/s) and is comparable to the CFV (3.4 cm/s) in EPT.

during maximal shortening and is usually associated with maximal concurrent axial contraction of the esophageal body.[13] The CDP should be localized within the third contractile segment defined by Clouse, and there is no method or measure on CM that localizes the CDP.[8]

- Step 5: Assess propagation
  - Propagation and timing of peristalsis is defined by assessing the distal latency to determine whether the swallow is premature and possibly associated with impaired inhibitory function of the esophageal body. It is defined as the interval between upper esophageal relaxation and the CDP, as demonstrated in **Fig. 3**. There is no correlate to this metric in CM.
  - Velocity of the stripping wave is determined by an assessment of the contractile front velocity (CFV). It is defined as the slope of the tangent approximating the 30-mm Hg isobaric contour between the proximal pressure trough and the contractile deceleration point. This measurement is akin to the measurement of velocity using the pressure sensor located 3 and 8 cm above the proximal aspect of the LES on CM. It is interesting that the 3-cm point used on CM closely approximates the CDP; thus, this measure has good correlation with CFV.
- Step 6: Measure contractile vigor
  - Contractile vigor has been revised to objectively measure all of the contractile activity within the domain of the distal smooth muscle esophagus below the transition zone. The transition zone is typically localized approximately 6 cm below the lower border of the Upper esophageal sphincter (UES) and represents the first pressure trough between segments 1 and 2 on the Clouse plot. The metric used to quantify the contractile activity between the transition zone and proximal aspect of the EGJ is termed the *distal contractile integral* (DCI), and it uses the space time domain of the second and third contractile segments to provide a single number that quantifies contractile vigor (**Fig. 4**). The DCI is

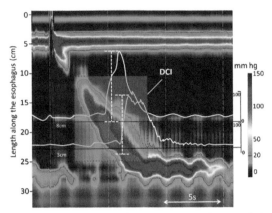

Fig. 4. Contractile vigor. The DCI is the software-generated sum of the esophageal body contractile activity from the transition zone to the distal pressure trough (area within the transparent box). CM assessment of contractile vigor is depicted by the mean of the peak wave amplitudes at 3 and 8 cm from the LES (*white dashed lines*). In the hypertensive swallow, the DCI is 7195 mmHg-s-cm and the mean peak amplitude is 214 mm Hg.

used in place of measuring the mean value of the highest wave amplitude at 3 and 8 cm above the proximal aspect of the LES on CM. The EPT plots also allow a qualitative assessment of the contraction that helps define focal contractile abnormalities and disorders associated with LES after contraction.

- Step 7: Determine whether abnormal pressure patterns are present
  - Abnormal intrabolus pressure is a sign of abnormal mechanics of bolus transit related to either an outflow obstruction in the distal esophagus/EGJ or a poorly compliant esophageal wall. It is measured using the isobaric contour tool that is referenced to atmospheric pressure to identify pressurization patterns. These patterns can be compartmentalized between a propagating peristaltic wavefront and the EGJ or between the 2 sphincters (panesophageal pressurization). There is no correlate for this measure on CM; however, astute clinicians can assess the initial ramp pressure on tracings (**Fig. 5**) or identify isobaric pressure patterns on tracings (**Fig. 6**B).

EPT CORRELATES OF CM DEFINITIONS
Disorders with Abnormal LES Relaxation

Abnormal LES relaxation is the hallmark of achalasia, the best defined of the esophageal motility disorders and the one with the most effective therapies.[1,14] Classically, achalasia also demonstrates a lack of esophageal peristalsis on manometry, although other manometric findings and subclassifications have been described and proposed.

Conventional criteria

The proposed criteria for a diagnosis of classic achalasia by CM criteria included incomplete relaxation of the LES (defined as a mean LES relaxation pressure during swallowing more than 8 mm Hg above gastric pressure) and aperistalsis of the esophageal body (either simultaneous contractions with amplitudes less than 40 mm Hg or no apparent esophageal contraction).[1] *Atypical disorders of LES relaxation* are also described that exclude a diagnosis of classic achalasia with some preserved peristalsis and/or esophageal contractions with amplitudes greater than 40 mm Hg, the latter situation often being referred to as *vigorous achalasia*.

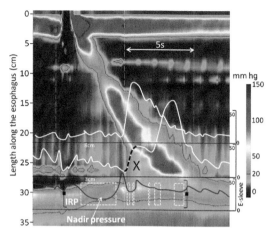

Fig. 5. Compartmentalized pressure. Compartmentalized intrabolus pressure (X) visualized on EPT can also be implicated via assessment of ramp pressure (*black dashed* portion of line tracing at 3 cm from the LES) on CM line tracings. This Clouse plot is an example of a swallow characteristic of EGJ outflow obstruction with abnormal EGJ relaxation (IRP 25.6 mm Hg; nadir LES pressure 28.9) and evidence of intact peristalsis.

Achalasia phenotypes

The classification of achalasia has evolved with the updated revisions of the Chicago classification to reflect different achalasia subtypes that have demonstrated varying symptom profiles and responses to different treatment modalities. The achalasia subtypes are all associated with abnormal EGJ relaxation and are categorized based on the pattern of esophageal body contraction and pressurization: type I, absent peristalsis; type II, achalasia with panesophageal pressurization in 20% or more of swallows; and type III, spastic achalasia (no normal peristalsis and premature contractions in 20% or more of swallows).[6,7] Representative Clouse plots with overlying CM line tracings are displayed in **Fig. 6**. This subclassification of achalasia distinguishes separate clinical phenotypes that are helpful in predicting the response to therapy, and this scheme is supported by 3 separate retrospective studies.[15–17]

The authors' initial study analyzed 99 patients with newly diagnosed achalasia with EPT who underwent balloon dilation, Heller myotomy, and/or Botox injection.[15] Another study analyzed 246 patients with achalasia, 230 with CM, and 16 with EPT, and followed patients after undergoing Heller-Dor myotomy.[16] A third study analyzed 51 patients with EPT, 45 of which underwent pneumatic dilation.[17] In each study, pretreatment symptom assessment suggested that chest pain may be more common in patients with type III (spastic) achalasia. The response to treatment was consistent across all 3 studies, with type II patients having the best and type III patients having the worst response to treatment. The study assessing the response to dilation, myotomy, and/or Botox even suggested that type I patients may have a better response to myotomy (compared with dilation or Botox injection) as the initial treatment.[15] Although prospective treatment trials are needed for further evaluation, these initial studies suggest that achalasia subtypes represent unique clinical phenotypes and may have predictive benefits in treatment planning for patients with achalasia.

EGJ outflow obstruction

EPT analysis also demonstrates a population of patients with abnormal EGJ relaxation with remaining peristaltic activity that fails to meet criteria for a diagnosis of achalasia,

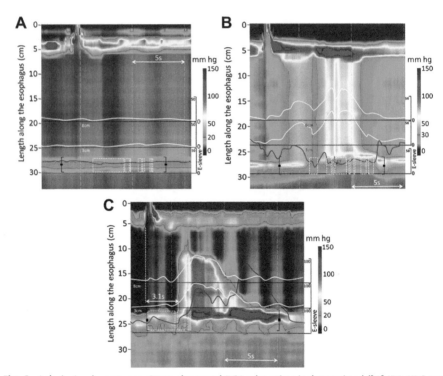

Fig. 6. Achalasia phenotypes. Once abnormal EGJ relaxation is determined ([*A*] IRP 17.6 mm Hg, nadir LES pressure 23.3 mm Hg; [*B*] IRP 26.5 mm Hg, nadir LES pressure 25.3 mm Hg; [*C*] IRP 46.5 mm Hg, nadir LES pressure 42.3 mm Hg), these disorders can be further classified based on their esophageal body contractility patterns. Type I (*A*) classic achalasia is characterized by absent peristalsis. Type II (*B*) achalasia with esophageal compartmentalization demonstrates pressurization spanning the length of the esophagus without intact peristalsis. Panesophageal pressurization can be identified with CM by noting the isobaric pressure tracings, as seen here. Type III (*C*), spastic achalasia, can demonstrate fragments of distal peristalsis and/or premature esophageal contractions, as demonstrated here with a shorter-than-normal latency (*white arrow*) of 3.1 seconds. Elevated wave amplitudes are also present on the CM line tracings, which has previously prompted labeling as vigorous achalasia.

similar to those with *atypical disorders of LES relaxation* in the conventional criteria. This pattern was termed *functional obstruction* in the early Chicago classification schemes.[4–6] However, further analysis of patients with these EPT findings displayed similar characteristics, including an elevated intrabolus pressure, as patients with a known mechanical obstruction, such as postfundoplication. Thus, this entity is now categorized as EGJ outflow obstruction.[7,18] A representative swallow is displayed in **Fig. 5**. Again, these manometric findings seem to reflect a clinical phenotype that frequently presents with dysphagia and/or chest pain, may respond poorly to balloon dilation or Botox injection overall, and may have a favorable outcome in response to treatment with myotomy.[19] Although additional study is needed to further characterize this group, it is possible that patients with this manometric profile may represent undetected inflammatory or infiltrating malignant disorders or may be a variant or earlier form of achalasia. Given this heterogeneous differential diagnosis, it may be helpful if these findings are correlated with either endoscopic ultrasound or other imaging modalities.

Diffuse Esophageal Spasm

Diffuse esophageal spasm (DES) is often implicated as the cause of noncardiac chest pain or dysphagia; however, the manometric criteria for the diagnosis of DES has frequently been questioned. Although differences in the requirements for repetitive, spontaneous, high-amplitude, or rapid contractions have varied in the previous literature, simultaneous esophageal contractions are nearly universally described as manometric criteria for DES and have been proposed to be the essential criteria in the diagnosis of DES.

Conventional criteria

Spechler and Castel[1] proposed that a diagnosis of DES should require (1) simultaneous contractions with more than 10% of wet swallows and (2) a mean simultaneous contraction amplitude of more than 30 mm Hg.[1] They reported that other common, but not required, features may include spontaneous contractions, repetitive contractions, multiple peaked contractions, and intermittent normal peristalsis. They also stated that if the LES pressure is abnormal, the disorder is better classified as an atypical disorder of LES relaxation.

Distal esophageal spasm

Simultaneous contractions were interpreted in the early versions of the Chicago classification as rapid contractions, which were defined by a CFV of more than 8 mm/s.[3,5,6] The CFV, however, has been demonstrated to be susceptible to regional variability in contractile velocity within the swallow and, thus, is a nonspecific finding of unknown significance.[20] The distal latency (DL), however, seems to be a more reliable measure of premature contractions that likely represents a clinical phenotype defined by dysphagia and chest pain.

A study that analyzed 1070 consecutive interpretable EPT studies found 24 patients that exhibited premature contraction (defined by DL <4.5 s) and 67 patients that were found to have rapid contractions alone (defined as CFV >9 m/s) but normal DL.[20] A review of medical records revealed that all 24 of the patients with premature contractions had a dominant symptom of dysphagia or chest pain and were diagnosed and managed as DES (6 patients) or spastic achalasia (18 patients). The 67 patients with rapid contractions with normal latency had a more heterogeneous dominant symptom (56% dysphagia, 34% gastrointestinal reflux disease [GERD], and 10% other) and were ultimately diagnosed and managed with an array of manometric diagnoses (14 normal, 39 weak, 5 hypertensive, 7 EGJ outflow obstruction, and another 2 patients had rapid contraction with normal latency that could potentially have been described as weak peristalsis given the large breaks in the 20-mm Hg isobaric contour plot). Thus, the current version of the Chicago criteria requires 20% or more of the swallows to have a reduced DL (**Fig. 7**A), defined as less than 4.5 s, to meet the criteria for a diagnosis of DES.[7] Patients with 20% or more of the swallows with a rapid CFV (>9 cm/s) but with normal DL (see **Fig. 7**B) are categorized as rapid contraction, which is a diagnosis without a known clinical significance.

Although further study of treatment outcomes using DL as the diagnostic criterion for DES is needed for additional support for the use of DL, this study suggests that the diagnosis of DES based on an abnormal DL defines a more distinct clinical phenotype and, in agreement with Spechler and Castell,[1] is likely an uncommon disorder.

Esophageal Hypercontraction

Another disorder frequently associated with noncardiac chest pain and dysphagia is nutcracker esophagus, a disorder usually defined by an elevated intensity of

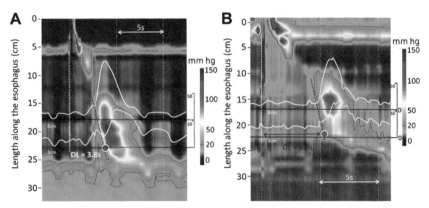

Fig. 7. Distal esophageal spasm. (*A*) DES, when defined by premature contractions (DL <4 seconds), is nearly uniformly associated with chest pain or dysphagia. (*A*) DL 3.8 seconds; CFV 12.1 cm/s. (*B*) Rapid contraction (CFV >9 cm/s) with normal latency (DL 5.3 seconds, CFV 14.1 cm/s) is associated with various clinical symptoms as well as in normal control. The EGJ relaxation is normal in both panels ([*A*] IRP 12.3 mm Hg, [*B*] IRP 0 mm Hg). DL (*purple arrow*). CDP (*red circle*). CFV (*red dashed line*).

esophageal peristaltic contractions. Nutcracker esophagus is the primary disorder of esophageal hypercontractility described by Spechler and Castell[1] and the early versions of the Chicago criteria. However, further evaluation with EPT has again refined this spectrum of esophageal hypercontractile disorders to distinguish borderline motor function from a primary abnormality of peristalsis.

Conventional criteria
Previous studies on nutcracker esophagus with CM have generally defined the disorder by a distal wave amplitude of more than 2 standard deviations more than the normal. However, normal values and the location of high amplitude contractions (eg, diffuse or segmental) have varied. Thus, Spechler and Castell[1] proposed that the diagnostic criteria for nutcracker esophagus be focused on a mean distal esophageal peristaltic wave amplitude more than 180 mm Hg, measured as the average amplitude of the 10 swallows at recording sites 3 and 8 cm above the LES.[1] Increased contraction duration was an inconsistently described characteristic of nutcracker esophagus and, thus, was not required for manometric diagnosis.

Phenotypes of hypercontractile disorders
Although the elevated wave amplitude has persistently been a part of the diagnostic criteria of nutcracker esophagus, its occurrence is not always associated with the characteristic symptoms of dysphagia and chest pain.[21] EPT uses the metric of DCI to measure peristaltic contractile vigor, which accounts for both contractile intensity (akin to wave amplitude) and duration. EPT analysis of normal subjects (N = 75) and patients (N = 400) defined a mean normal (95th percentile) DCI value of less than 5000 mmHg-s-cm, although there was substantial heterogeneity in the group of patients with a mean DCI of 5000 to 8000 mmHg-s-cm (a group classified as *hypertensive peristalsis* or *nutcracker esophagus*).[4] In addition, a mean DCI more than 8000 mmHg-s-cm (defined in the early Chicago classifications as *spastic nutcracker esophagus*) was a rare finding, seemed to exhibit a distinct pattern with repetitive high-amplitude contractions (**Fig. 8**), and was universally associated with dysphagia and/or chest pain.[4–6]

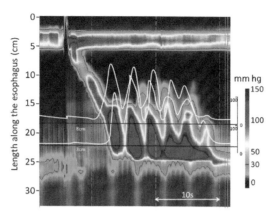

Fig. 8. Jackhammer esophagus. Clouse plot with overlying CM line tracings of a hypertensive swallow with significantly elevated DCI (15,025 mmHg-s-cm), mean wave amplitude (260 mm Hg), and displaying multi-peaked esophageal body contractions.

Further evaluation of EPT studies of 72 asymptomatic controls and 1070 patients led to the refinement of this classification.[22] The examination of individual swallows, as opposed to the *mean* DCI, found that within the control group, subjects often had individual swallows with DCIs more than 5000 mmHg-s-cm (median DCI 2073 mmHg-s-cm, 5th–95th percentile 757–5946); the highest single DCI value seen in the control group was 7732 mmHg-s-cm. On the other hand, 44 patients (4.1%) were found to have at least one swallow with a DCI more than 8000 mmHg-s-cm, the majority (75%) of whom presented with dysphagia and generally had a positive response to a variety of treatments (including antireflux, anticholinergic, and endoscopic Botox injection). Classifying patients based on a *single* swallow with a DCI more than 8000 mmHg-s-cm, a group whose *mean* DCI had an interquartile range of approximately 3900 to 8700, had a high proportion of patients that presented with symptoms of chest pain and dysphagia, thus deterring the use of the previous arbitrarily set use of the *mean* DCI.

Multi-peaked contractions were frequently seen in the patients with a DCI more than 8000 mmHg-s-cm (36 out of 44, 86%); thus, the term *jackhammer esophagus* was coined to describe this pattern. The patients that displayed multi-peaked hypertensive contractions were more likely to have a normal IRP than patients who were hypertensive without multi-peaked contractions. Although the presence or absence of these multi-peaked contractions did not seem to have an association with the symptom profile or to have an association with the response to treatment, this was a retrospective report of an uncontrolled data set with a wide variety of treatments. Further systematic treatment trials classifying patients with hypertensive (DCI >8000 mmHg-s-cm) peristaltic contractions based on the presence or absence of multi-peaked, jackhammerlike contractions may lend additional insight on the clinical phenotype of this manometric pattern.

Based on this study, the current version of the Chicago classification describes the diagnostic criteria for determining hypercontractile (jackhammer) esophagus based on at least one swallow with a DCI more than 8000 mmHg-s-cm (with or without multi-peaked contractions), whereas hypertensive peristalsis (nutcracker esophagus) is defined as a mean DCI more than 5000 mmHg-s-cm but not meeting criteria for hypercontractile esophagus.[7]

Hypocontractile Disorders: Ineffective Esophageal Motility

Spechler and Castell[1] classified a group of disorders with hypocontractile characteristics as ineffective esophageal motility disorders (IEM). These disorders had previously often been referred to as *scleroderma esophagus* and *nonspecific esophageal motility disorders*, although many other disorders other than scleroderma (eg, GERD) may demonstrate similar motility patterns.

Conventional criteria

The CM diagnostic criterion for IEM proposed in the 2001 review was ineffective wet swallows in 30% or more of the swallows. Ineffective swallows could be demonstrated manometrically by any combination of (1) distal esophageal peristaltic wave amplitude of 30 mm Hg or less, (2) simultaneous contractions with amplitudes of 30 mm Hg or less, (3) failed peristalsis (the peristaltic wave does not traverse the length of the distal esophagus), and/or (4) absent peristalsis. These criteria were based on previous findings that similar esophageal CM metrics were associated with impaired bolus transport or ineffective esophageal acid clearance.[1,23] An additional study using impedance-manometry to assess esophageal bolus clearance refined the criteria of IEM, demonstrating that a cutoff of 50% or more of the ineffective swallows improved identification of patients with abnormal esophageal bolus transport and had a trend toward representation of a group of patients more likely to demonstrate dysphagia and/or heartburn.[24,25]

EPT: weak and failed peristalsis

EPT allows one to characterize the contractile activity of the entire esophagus as opposed to separated axial measurements as used in studies using CM. Thus, EPT offers improved detection of breaks in the peristaltic wavefront (**Fig. 9**). Studies using EPT and intraluminal impedance have demonstrated that peristaltic breaks of more than 2 cm in the 20-mm Hg isobaric contour plot may be associated with impaired bolus transport.[26,27] The Chicago criteria describes hypocontractile disorders as *weak peristalsis* and *frequent failed peristalsis*. *Weak peristalsis* is defined by >30% of swallows with small (2–5 cm) peristaltic defects or >20% of swallows with large

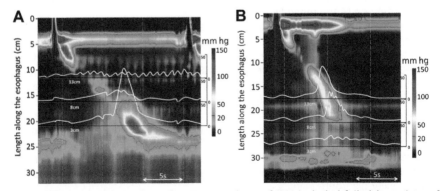

Fig. 9. Ineffective esophageal motility. EPT correlates of IEM included failed (not pictured) and weak (*A, B*) peristalsis. Axial separation of CM pressure sensors limits the assessment of esophageal peristaltic integrity as demonstrated with the Clouse plots with overlying CM line tracings from recording sites at 3, 8, and 13 cm from the LES of a swallow with a large transition zone peristaltic defect (*A*) and another swallow with both proximal and distal defects (*B*). Of note, the DCIs of swallows in (*A*) and (*B*) are 820 and 316 mmHg-s-cm, respectively.

(>5 cm) peristaltic defects.[7] Frequent failed peristalsis is defined by >30%, but <100% of swallows with failed peristalsis.[7] A comparison of EPT characteristics of 75 normal controls and 113 patients with nonobstructive dysphagia demonstrated that weak peristalsis with small and large peristaltic breaks (but not failed peristalsis) were all seen more commonly in the patients than the controls.[27] However, the peristaltic breaks were only seen in approximately one-third of the patients and were also occasionally present in the normal controls.

Although hypocontractile peristalsis could be defined adequately using weak peristalsis and frequent failed peristalsis on EPT, many clinicians and investigators were hesitant to adopt this new terminology and continued to use IEM. This idea was the impetus for a recent study that sought to correlate the CM diagnosis of IEM (a diagnosis not included in the Chicago classification) with EPT findings. They compared individual swallows and manometric classifications (based on a complete 10-swallow study) in terms of CM line tracings (taken at 3 and 8 cm from the LES) and EPT.[12] IEM was defined by the updated CM criteria (>50% ineffective swallows), and EPT studies were analyzed according to the Chicago classification diagnoses of weak peristalsis and frequent-failed peristalsis (defined earlier). EPT abnormalities (individual swallows with peristaltic break or failed swallow; classification of weak or frequent failed peristalsis) were found in more than 25% of swallows deemed normal by CM and more than 35% of studies classified as normal. By removing comparison with EPT studies with proximal pressure trough (transition zone) defects, the agreement in manometric characterization between the two methods increased appreciably. The addition of a CM line tracing at 13 cm from the LES considerably increased the ability of CM line tracings to detect the presence of a transition zone defect (see **Fig. 9**A), which is a defect whose size may have an association with symptoms such as heartburn or dysphagia.[28]

The same study described earlier also suggests that DCI had a strong correlation with mean wave amplitudes at 3 and 8 cm from the LES.[12] Low DCI, a measure not previously included in the Chicago classification, was shown to be a strong predictor of ineffective (DCI <450 mmHg-s-cm) or failed (DCI <50 mmHg-s-cm) peristalsis and, thus, could potentially be incorporated into automated manometry diagnostic software and possibly future revisions of the Chicago classification.

As expected, the additional data of peristaltic integrity generated by EPT are able to increase the characterization of disorders of esophageal hypocontraction, although a correlation could be made between the CM diagnosis of IEM and the combined EPT classifications of weak peristalsis with small or large defects and frequent-failed peristalsis. Nonetheless, the clinical significance of any of these disorders or findings is not completely clear, and further manometric pattern assessment and clinical treatment trials may offer additional insight into their contribution to heartburn and/or dysphagia.

SUMMARY

Increased clinical experience with EPT has helped identify specific patterns that seem to distinguish clinically relevant phenotypes within the classical description of esophageal motility disorders using CM. The Chicago criteria has attempted to bridge the gap between the previous diagnostic experience with CM and the new technology and has primarily focused on using the enhanced information available with HRM to better define abnormal motor function. The objective metrics of esophageal peristaltic and sphincter function available with EPT analysis also facilitate the use of a diagnostic scheme that uses an algorithm-based diagnostic model that can be incorporated into analytic software programs.

Ultimately, as is initially apparent with achalasia subtype designations, it is hoped that further characterization of clinical phenotypes represented by manometric patterns will offer an improved ability to tailor therapy to specific clinical entities and enhance our ability to care for patients with esophageal motility disorders.

REFERENCES

1. Spechler SJ, Castell DO. Classification of oesophageal motility abnormalities. Gut 2001;49(1):145–51.
2. Richter JE, Dalton CB, Bradley LA, et al. Oral nifedipine in the treatment of non-cardiac chest pain in patients with the nutcracker esophagus. Gastroenterology 1987;93(1):21–8.
3. Fox MR, Bredenoord AJ. Oesophageal high-resolution manometry: moving from research into clinical practice. Gut 2008;57(3):405–23.
4. Pandolfino JE, Ghosh SK, Rice J, et al. Classifying esophageal motility by pressure topography characteristics: a study of 400 patients and 75 controls. Am J Gastroenterol 2008;103(1):27–37.
5. Kahrilas PJ, Ghosh SK, Pandolfino JE. Esophageal motility disorders in terms of pressure topography: the Chicago classification. J Clin Gastroenterol 2008;42(5): 627–35.
6. Pandolfino JE, Fox MR, Bredenoord AJ, et al. High-resolution manometry in clinical practice: utilizing pressure topography to classify oesophageal motility abnormalities. Neurogastroenterol Motil 2009;21(8):796–806.
7. Bredenoord AJ, Fox M, Kahrilas PJ, et al. Chicago classification criteria of esophageal motility disorders defined in high resolution esophageal pressure topography. Neurogastroenterol Motil 2012;24(Suppl 1):57–65.
8. Clouse RE, Staiano A. Topography of the esophageal peristaltic pressure wave. Am J Physiol 1991;261(4 Pt 1):G677–84.
9. Clouse RE, Staiano A, Alrakawi A, et al. Application of topographical methods to clinical esophageal manometry. Am J Gastroenterol 2000;95(10):2720–30.
10. Pandolfino JE, Ghosh SK, Zhang Q, et al. Quantifying EGJ morphology and relaxation with high-resolution manometry: a study of 75 asymptomatic volunteers. Am J Physiol Gastrointest Liver Physiol 2006;290(5):G1033–40.
11. Ghosh SK, Pandolfino JE, Rice J, et al. Impaired deglutitive EGJ relaxation in clinical esophageal manometry: a quantitative analysis of 400 patients and 75 controls. Am J Physiol Gastrointest Liver Physiol 2007;293(4):G878–85.
12. Xiao Y, Kahrilas PJ, Kwasny MJ, et al. High-resolution manometry correlates of ineffective esophageal motility. Am J Gastroenterol 2012;107(11):1647–54.
13. Pandolfino JE, Leslie E, Luger D, et al. The contractile deceleration point: an important physiologic landmark on oesophageal pressure topography. Neurogastroenterol Motil 2010;22(4):395–400. e90.
14. Kahrilas PJ. Esophageal motor disorders in terms of high-resolution esophageal pressure topography: what has changed? Am J Gastroenterol 2010;105(5):981–7.
15. Pandolfino JE, Kwiatek MA, Nealis T, et al. Achalasia: a new clinically relevant classification by high-resolution manometry. Gastroenterology 2008;135(5):1526–33.
16. Salvador R, Costantini M, Zaninotto G, et al. The preoperative manometric pattern predicts the outcome of surgical treatment for esophageal achalasia. J Gastrointest Surg 2010;14(11):1635–45.
17. Pratap N, Kalapala R, Darisetty S, et al. Achalasia cardia subtyping by high-resolution manometry predicts the therapeutic outcome of pneumatic balloon dilatation. J Neurogastroenterol Motil 2011;17(1):48–53.

18. Pandolfino JE, Kwiatek MA, Ho K, et al. Unique features of esophagogastric junction pressure topography in hiatus hernia patients with dysphagia. Surgery 2010; 147(1):57–64.

19. Scherer JR, Kwiatek MA, Soper NJ, et al. Functional esophagogastric junction obstruction with intact peristalsis: a heterogeneous syndrome sometimes akin to achalasia. J Gastrointest Surg 2009;13(12):2219–25.

20. Pandolfino JE, Roman S, Carlson DA, et al. Distal esophageal spasm in high-resolution esophageal pressure topography: defining clinical phenotypes. Gastroenterology 2011;141(2):469–75.

21. Agrawal A, Hila A, Tutuian R, et al. Clinical relevance of the nutcracker esophagus: suggested revision of criteria for diagnosis. J Clin Gastroenterol 2006;40(6):504–9.

22. Roman S, Pandolfino JE, Chen J, et al. Phenotypes and clinical context of hypercontractility in high-resolution esophageal pressure topography (EPT). Am J Gastroenterol 2011;107(1):37–45.

23. Turner R, Lipshutz W, Miller W, et al. Esophageal dysfunction in collagen disease. Am J Med Sci 1973;265(3):191–9.

24. Blonski W, Vela M, Safder A, et al. Revised criterion for diagnosis of ineffective esophageal motility is associated with more frequent dysphagia and greater bolus transit abnormalities. Am J Gastroenterol 2008;103(3):699–704.

25. Tutuian R, Castell DO. Clarification of the esophageal function defect in patients with manometric ineffective esophageal motility: studies using combined impedance-manometry. Clin Gastroenterol Hepatol 2004;2(3):230–6.

26. Bulsiewicz WJ, Kahrilas PJ, Kwiatek MA, et al. Esophageal pressure topography criteria indicative of incomplete bolus clearance: a study using high-resolution impedance manometry. Am J Gastroenterol 2009;104(11):2721–8.

27. Roman S, Lin Z, Kwiatek MA, et al. Weak peristalsis in esophageal pressure topography: classification and association with dysphagia. Am J Gastroenterol 2011;106(2):349–56.

28. Pohl D, Ribolsi M, Savarino E, et al. Characteristics of the esophageal low-pressure zone in healthy volunteers and patients with esophageal symptoms: assessment by high-resolution manometry. Am J Gastroenterol 2008;103(10):2544–9.

Impedance-pH Testing

Nicolas Villa, MD, Marcelo F. Vela, MD, MSCR*

KEYWORDS

- Gastroesophageal reflux • Nonacid reflux • Impedance-pH

KEY POINTS

- Impedance-pH monitoring is considered the most accurate and sensitive tool for measuring all types of gastroesophageal reflux, and it enables detailed characterization of reflux episodes.
- Currently available software for automated detection of reflux episodes in impedance-pH tracings is sensitive but not very specific, and manual editing is still recommended (this may change with further software refinement).
- Nonacid reflux can produce symptoms that are indistinguishable from those caused by acid reflux.
- Some of the main clinical uses of impedance-pH monitoring include the assessment of refractory gastroesophageal reflux disease (GERD) symptoms, GERD-related cough, and belching.
- Limitations include patient discomfort, as it is a catheter-based test; limited duration of monitoring (not more than 24 hours); and limited outcomes studies evaluating the treatment of nonacid reflux.

INTRODUCTION

Gastroesophageal reflux disease (GERD) is a common clinical problem.[1] The role of acid in the pathogenesis of GERD is well established, and gastric acid suppression with proton pump inhibitors (PPIs) is the mainstay of medical therapy. The usual approach for patients presenting with classic symptoms of GERD, such as heartburn and acid regurgitation, is to prescribe empiric antisecretory therapy with a PPI. In the current era of rising GERD prevalence[2] and frequent PPI use, there are increasing numbers of patients in whom symptoms persist despite treatment.[3] In some of these patients, the persistent symptoms may be caused by reflux of gastric contents with a pH ≥ 4, commonly referred to as nonacid reflux.[4,5] Nonacid reflux may be further classified as weakly acidic (pH ≥ 4 but <7) or weakly alkaline (pH ≥ 7).[6] In this article, the term nonacid reflux is used to refer to all reflux with pH ≥ 4. Nonacid reflux may also occur in the absence of acid suppression during the postprandial period when gastric

Division of Gastroenterology and Hepatology, Michael E. DeBakey VA Medical Center, Baylor College of Medicine, 2002 Holcombe Boulevard, Houston, TX 77030, USA
* Corresponding author.
E-mail address: mvela@bcm.edu

Gastroenterol Clin N Am 42 (2013) 17–26
http://dx.doi.org/10.1016/j.gtc.2012.11.003
0889-8553/13/$ – see front matter Published by Elsevier Inc.

contents are buffered by food, or in patients with decreased gastric acid output caused by atrophic gastritis.

Ambulatory reflux monitoring quantifies gastroesophageal reflux by measuring esophageal acid exposure and the number or reflux episodes, and it also enables an assessment of the temporal relationship between reflux episodes and reported symptoms. Ambulatory reflux monitoring was based upon esophageal pH monitoring for many years, a technique that relies on drops in esophageal pH to <4.0 to detect acid reflux. Accurate measurement of nonacid reflux is not possible with conventional ambulatory pH monitoring.[7] An important development in the last decade has been the adoption of impedance-pH monitoring, a method that enables measurement of acid as well as nonacid reflux. This article discusses the principles of impedance-pH monitoring, catheter characteristics and placement, interpretation of studies, and the clinical applications of this form of reflux monitoring.

PRINCIPLES OF IMPEDANCE-pH MONITORING

Multichannel intraluminal impedance measurement as a means to detect flow of liquids in the esophagus was first described by Silny in 1991.[8] Intraesophageal impedance, determined by measuring electrical conductivity across a pair of closely spaced electrodes within the esophageal lumen, is dependent on the conductivity of material through which the current travels. By placing a series of conducting electrodes in a catheter that spans the length of the esophagus, changes in impedance can be recorded in response to movement of intraesophageal material in either antegrade or retrograde direction.[9] Because different bolus materials (ie, swallowed food, air, saliva, or refluxed gastric contents) produce a different change in impedance, the technique enables detailed characterization of gastroesophageal reflux episodes, including composition (air, liquid, or mixed), proximal extent, velocity, and clearance time. During impedance-pH monitoring, impedance detects reflux (retrograde bolus movement), whereas pH changes determine its acidity: acid if pH <4, weakly acidic if pH ≥4 but <7, and weakly alkaline if pH ≥7. Examples of acid and nonacid reflux are shown in **Fig. 1**. Currently, impedance-pH monitoring is considered the most accurate and sensitive tool for measuring all types of gastroesophageal reflux.[6] The method has been found to have good reproducibility,[10] and normal values obtained by independent multicenter studies are similar.[11,12]

Impedance-pH Catheter Characteristics and Placement

Impedance-pH is performed with catheters that incorporate a differing number of impedance-measuring segments and pH electrodes in varying configurations. A typical catheter has a single pH electrode to record pH changes 5 cm above the manometrically determined lower esophageal sphincter (similar to conventional pH testing), along with multiple impedance-measuring segments (each composed of 2 metal ring electrodes, usually spaced 2 cm apart) to detect impedance changes along variable lengths of the esophagus and enable detection of reflux into the distal and proximal esophagus (**Fig. 2**).

The methodology for catheter placement is similar to that of conventional pH monitoring. After a 4- to 6-hour fasting period, a local anesthetic is applied, and the catheter is passed transnasally to the desired position, based upon the location of the lower esophageal sphincter. The catheter is then taped to the patient's nose and connected to an impedance-pH monitor that the patient carries on the shoulder or a belt for ambulatory recording. After catheter placement, the patient is discharged with

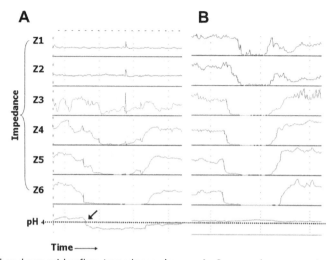

Fig. 1. Acid and nonacid reflux. Impedance changes in 6 measuring segments spanning the esophagus (Z1 to Z6), and pH changes from a single sensor in the distal esophagus are shown in the Y axis. Time is on the X axis. The dotted line marks a pH of 4.0. (*A*) Acid reflux: impedance reflux pattern of sequential drops in impedance starting at the most distal measuring segment and proceeding toward the proximal esophagus. This reflux episode reaches Z3 but does not move further into the more proximal esophagus. The reflux episode that is detected by the impedance changes is associated with a fall in pH to <4.0 (*arrow*), making it an acid reflux episode. (*B*) Nonacid reflux: impedance reflux pattern with drops in impedance that reach the most proximal impedance measuring segment (Z1). During this reflux episode, pH remains >4.0, therefore it is classified as a nonacid reflux episode.

instructions to record meals, body position, and symptoms. The patient returns for catheter removal after 24 hours.

Impedance-pH Interpretation

During assessment of impedance-pH tracings, the impedance channels are used to detect the occurrence of reflux, and pH changes help classify the reflux episodes as acid (pH <4) or nonacid (pH ≥4). The composition of the reflux episode (liquid, gas, or mixed) can be easily ascertained. Liquid-only reflux is defined by sequential drops in impedance beginning in the distal esophagus and progressing upwards toward the proximal esophagus in retrograde direction. Gas reflux is defined by sharp increases in impedance moving in retrograde direction from distal to proximal esophagus. Mixed liquid-gas reflux is defined as gas reflux occurring during or immediately before liquid reflux. Examples of liquid-only and mixed reflux are shown in **Fig. 3**. In addition to acidity and composition, reflux episodes can be further characterized in terms of proximal extent and clearance time.

While impedance-pH monitoring permits detailed characterization of each reflux episode, assessment of impedance-pH tracings for clinical purposes currently focuses primarily on the number of acid and nonacid reflux episodes that contain liquid (liquid only or mixed liquid-gas), along with their relationship to patient symptoms. At the present time, reflux of gas in the absence of liquid is not conventionally reported. Whether measuring gas-only reflux is useful awaits further clinical studies. That said, analysis of the impedance-pH tracing may reveal frequent air intake and expulsion, which may be useful in patients with frequent belching.

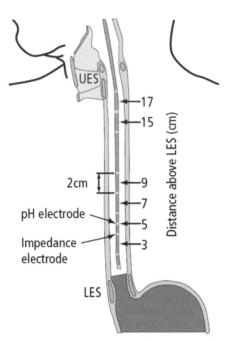

Fig. 2. Impedance-pH monitoring catheter. Impedance-pH catheter with 6 impedance measuring segments (each consisting of 2 impedance electrodes spaced 2 cm apart) and 1 pH electrode. The catheter is placed transnasally and positioned to allow pH monitoring 5 cm above the proximal border of the lower esophageal sphincter (LES), with impedance measurements 3, 5, 7, 9, 15, and 17 cm above the LES. UES, upper esophageal sphincter. (*From* Vaezi MF, Vela MF. The Role of multichannel intraluminal impedance and pH monitoring in the diagnosis of gastroesophageal reflux disease. US Gastroenterology & Hepatology Review 2007;(2):75–7.)

A standard impedance-pH report includes the distal esophageal acid exposure (percentage of time with pH <4 as is done in conventional pH monitoring), the number of reflux episodes (total, acid, and nonacid), and a measure of correlation between reflux and symptoms (usually the symptom index[13] or the symptom association probability[14]). Normal values for 24-hour ambulatory impedance-pH monitoring in untreated healthy subjects are available from a US multicenter trial; this study determined the normal number of total reflux episodes as ≤73, acid reflux episodes ≤59, and nonacid reflux episodes ≤27.[11] One of the advantages of impedance-pH monitoring is an increased yield when studying patients while they continue acid-suppressive therapy with a PPI, as nonacid reflux is frequent in this context and may explain symptoms that are refractory to PPI. However, there are no peer-reviewed publications of normal values for impedance-pH monitoring performed while on PPI. The normal value of ≤48 reflux episodes that is often used for acid-suppressed patients has only been published in abstract form.[15] A multicenter study to determine normal impedance-pH monitoring values in acid-suppressed subjects is currently underway. It is important to mention that while infrequent, the low impedance baseline that may be seen in patients with severe reflux or Barrett's esophagus can make interpretation of impedance-pH tracings more difficult and cumbersome.[16]

Software for automated analysis of the impedance-pH tracing is available from at least 3 companies, but these have not been compared in terms of accuracy and

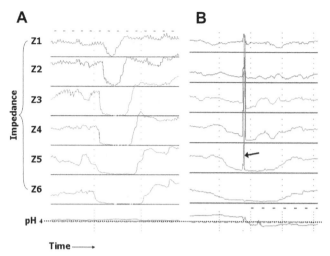

Fig. 3. Liquid and mixed (liquid-gas) reflux. Impedance changes in 6 measuring segments spanning the esophagus (Z1 to Z6), and pH changes from a single sensor in the distal esophagus are shown in the Y axis. Time is on the X axis. The dotted line marks a pH of 4.0. (*A*) Liquid reflux: impedance reflux pattern of sequential drops in impedance starting at the most distal measuring segment and proceeding toward the proximal esophagus. Gas is not detected during this reflux episode. There is no fall in pH to <4.0; therefore this is a nonacid reflux episode containing only liquid. (*B*) Liquid-gas reflux: in addition to the liquid reflux pattern of impedance drops, sharp increases in impedance are also noted in the middle of the reflux episode (*arrow*). This means that the liquid was followed by gas reflux, making this a mixed liquid-gas reflux episode. Since pH falls below 4.0, it is classified as acid reflux.

reliability. However, separate evaluation of 2 of these software options found that they have good sensitivity. Specificity is suboptimal, however, as both tend to overestimate the amount of reflux.[17,18] Therefore, manual editing through visual analysis is required. A commonly used approach is to use the software to initially mark reflux episodes in the impedance-pH tracing, and then review and edit the data manually. It is possible that with further software refinements, fully automated analysis may become available in the future, but this will need to be carefully validated. Compared with analysis of pH monitoring, the required editing of an impedance-pH tracing may be more cumbersome and may take more time.

CLINICAL APPLICATIONS OF IMPEDANCE-pH MONITORING
Clinical Significance of Nonacid Reflux

Because one of the main advantages of impedance-pH monitoring is the ability to measure nonacid reflux, the clinical significance of this phenomenon deserves some discussion. First, it is important to remember that nonacid reflux occurs predominantly in patients who are acid-suppressed with a PPI. In an untreated patient, most reflux episodes will be acid. Exceptions to this are nonacid reflux in patients with decreased acid secretion caused by atrophic gastritis, and nonacid reflux that may occur in untreated patients in the postprandial period, when ingested food can buffer the gastric contents for roughly 1 to 2 hours. Second, it must be kept in mind that reflux with a pH >4 may not always cause symptoms, and some patients who are PPI responders may have some degree of asymptomatic nonacid reflux. Furthermore, damage to the esophageal mucosa from nonacid reflux has not been clearly documented. Therefore, nonacid reflux should be a concern, mainly in patients with ongoing symptoms despite PPI therapy, or in those with frequent postprandial symptoms that are thought to be caused by reflux. Three clinical scenarios in which impedance-pH monitoring is useful (refractory GERD, belching, and reflux-related cough) will be explored in a subsequent section.

An early study in heartburn patients who underwent impedance-pH monitoring before and after 7 days of omeprazole found that PPI therapy did not achieve a significant reduction in the total number of reflux episodes (acid and nonacid reflux combined), causing instead a change in the ratio of acid to nonacid reflux.[4] After PPI therapy, the percentage of acid reflux decreased from 45% to 3%, while nonacid reflux increased from 55% to 97%. Heartburn was more commonly linked to acid reflux but was also produced by nonacid reflux, and regurgitation was unchanged by acid suppression, as it was frequently caused by nonacid reflux in the treated state. This was the first study to demonstrate ongoing nonacid reflux as a potential cause of symptoms in acid-suppressed patients. The observation that nonacid reflux can cause symptoms that are indistinguishable from those that are caused by acid reflux has been confirmed in multiple subsequent studies.[5,19,20] Furthermore, a systematic review that quantified acid and nonacid reflux in studies of GERD patients taking a PPI found that weakly acidic reflux (a form of nonacid reflux) underlies most reflux episodes in these patients and is the main cause of persistent symptoms despite PPI therapy.[21]

The treatment of nonacid reflux is beyond the scope of this article. However, it should be mentioned that nonacid reflux and related symptoms have been successfully managed by treatment approaches that focus on augmenting the function of the antireflux barrier rather than suppressing gastric acid secretion. These approaches include pharmacologic inhibition of transient lower esophageal sphincter relaxations[22] and surgical fundoplication.[23] However, high-quality controlled trials evaluating the role of these treatments for nonacid reflux are not available. While a comprehensive overview of the potential role of impedance-pH monitoring in each of the typical and atypical GERD presentations would be too lengthy, 3 clinical scenarios in which impedance-pH monitoring may be particularly useful are explored below.

Impedance-pH Monitoring in Refractory GERD

As stated earlier, clinicians are faced with an increasing number of patients with symptoms that are attributed to GERD but that do not respond to PPI therapy. In broad terms, there are 3 possible explanations for ongoing symptoms in these patients: (1) PPI failure with persistent acid reflux as the cause for symptoms, (2) successful gastric acid suppression but ongoing reflux of weakly acidic or nonacid material that provokes symptoms, or (3) symptoms not due to reflux, with etiologies that may include other disorders such as eosinophilic esophagitis or a functional presentation like functional heartburn. In patients who fail to respond to acid suppression, impedance-pH monitoring performed while on PPI can identify persistent symptomatic acid or nonacid reflux that will require escalation of therapy. In addition, impedance-pH monitoring in patients refractory to PPIs can be helpful as a means to exclude reflux as the cause of the persistent symptoms. This is important and useful, because in patients in whom GERD is ruled out, diagnostic and treatment efforts can be directed toward other causes. While one reasonable approach to rule out GERD is to perform conventional pH monitoring after discontinuation of PPI, evaluation of patients while on treatment with PPI with a high likelihood of GERD should be performed with impedance-pH monitoring, because in these patients an off-PPI study may reveal GERD but will not clarify the reason for the treatment failure. Conventional pH monitoring in acid-suppressed patients has low yield and a low pretest likelihood of a positive test.[24] The association between symptoms and reflux (acid and nonacid), determined by the symptom index (SI) and symptom association probability (SAP), was reported in two multicenter studies of refractory GERD patients. A study of 144 patients using the SI to evaluate patients refractory to twice-daily PPI therapy found that ongoing symptoms were caused by nonacid reflux in 37% of patients and acid reflux in 11%. In the remaining 52% of patients, there was no association between reflux and symptoms.[5] In another study of 60 patients who were symptomatic despite PPI therapy, the SAP was positive because of nonacid reflux in 17% of patients, acid reflux in 5%, and acid plus nonacid reflux in 15%.[19] Although a discussion of the shortcomings of the SI and SAP is beyond the scope of this article, it is important to note that both of these symptom association analysis tools have well known limitations.[25] Therefore, the SI and SAP should not be used in isolation, always keeping in mind the full clinical context of the patient's symptoms, degree of response to therapy, and endoscopic findings.

Impedance-pH Monitoring in Belching

Because of its ability to detect movement of gas in antegrade and retrograde direction, impedance-pH monitoring has also been used to study belching. In many patients, belching is caused by rapid intake of air into the esophagus followed by expulsion of this air before it reaches the stomach, a phenomenon that has been termed supragrastric belching.[26] Impedance monitoring can distinguish these supragastric belches from gastric belches (ie, those that originate in the stomach). In many patients, this is a behavioral problem, whereby patients develop this habit of injecting air into the esophagus and then quickly expelling it. This is supported by a recent study that used impedance-pH monitoring to evaluate the effect of sleep on excessive belching; in this study, supragastric belches almost ceased completely during the sleep period.[27] This information can potentially identify patients who may benefit from specialized treatment by behavioral therapy or with a speech therapist.[28]

Impedance-pH Monitoring in Cough

GERD has been implicated in the pathogenesis several extraesophageal symptoms, such as laryngitis and chronic cough. Among the extraesophageal presentations, cough may be particularly suited to evaluation with impedance-pH monitoring, because it is not a constant symptom like hoarseness, presenting instead in episodic bursts. Impedance-pH monitoring may be useful when GERD is suspected as a causative factor in coughing, especially when patients do not respond to PPI therapy or when patients have postprandial cough, because, as alluded to earlier, reflux in the postprandial period may be frequently nonacid even without pharmacologic acid suppression. Previous studies demonstrated an association between nonacid reflux and cough in some patients.[29] In fact, in the study of 60 patients with refractory symptoms that were studied using the SAP, the symptoms more frequently associated with nonacid reflux were cough and regurgitation.[19] However, it is important to note that although reflux may induce cough, cough may also trigger reflux, and distinguishing between the two requires objective detection of cough bursts.[30] Recently, the development of ambulatory reflux cough monitoring by combining impedance-pH to measure reflux (acid or nonacid) along with acoustic detection of cough, which eliminates the subjectivity of patient-reported cough, has enabled a more accurate assessment of the relationship between reflux and cough. A recent study using this approach was able to document reflux-induced cough and cough-induced reflux, indicating that most cases of patients with chronic cough are likely multifactorial and that reflux seems to sensitize the neuronal pathways of cough regardless of the etiology.[31] Whether these technical improvements increase the yield of symptom association analysis in patients with cough attributed to reflux requires further study. However, clear documentation that reflux episodes are followed by cough bursts may suggest the need for additional antireflux therapy.

SUMMARY

Currently, esophageal impedance-pH monitoring is considered the most sensitive tool for assessing all types of gastroesophageal reflux (acidic, weakly acidic, and weakly alkaline), their composition, proximal extent, duration, and clearance. Normative data are well established for performing testing off PPI, but peer-reviewed normative data for on-PPI assessment are awaited. While automated analysis software packages are available, manual editing is still advised because of the potential of false positives with the automated software. The main advantage of impedance-pH monitoring over conventional pH monitoring is the ability to detect nonacid reflux (with pH $\geq$4). Nonacid reflux has been shown to produce symptoms that are indistinguishable from those that are caused by acid reflux. In some patients with refractory GERD, the ongoing symptoms that occur despite PPI therapy may be due to nonacid reflux. Therefore, impedance-pH monitoring is useful for the evaluation of GERD symptoms that are refractory to PPIs. In this context, the finding of ongoing reflux can suggest the need for escalation of antireflux therapy, while a negative test may direct the diagnostic and therapeutic efforts elsewhere. While a discussion of all clinical presentations of GERD is beyond the scope of this article, it is important to mention that impedance-pH monitoring appears to be promising for the evaluation of belching and cough. Limitations of the technique include patient discomfort, as it is a catheter-based test, and limited duration of monitoring to only 24-hours.

REFERENCES

1. Peery AF, Dellon ES, Lund J, et al. Burden of gastrointestinal disease in the United States: 2012 update. Gastroenterology 2012;143:1179–87.
2. Dent J, El-Serag HB, Wallander MA, et al. Epidemiology of gastro-oesophageal disease: a systematic review. Gut 2005;54:710–7.
3. Richter JE. How to manage refractory GERD. Nat Clin Pract Gastroenterol Hepatol 2007;4:658–64.
4. Vela MF, Camacho-Lobato L, Srinivasan R, et al. Intraesophageal Impedance and pH measurement of acid and non-acid reflux: effect of omeprazole. Gastroenterology 2001;120:1599–606.
5. Mainie I, Tutuian R, Shay S, et al. Acid and non-acid reflux in patients with persistent symptoms despite acid suppressive therapy: a multicenter study using combined ambulatory impedance-pH monitoring. Gut 2006;55:1398–402.
6. Sifrim D, Castell D, Dent J, et al. Gastro-oesophageal reflux monitoring: review and consensus report on detection and definitions of acid, non-acid, and gas reflux. Gut 2004;53:1024–31.
7. Pandolino JE, Vela MF. Esophageal reflux monitoring. Gastrointest Endosc 2009; 69:917–30.
8. Silny J. Intraluminal multiple electric impedance procedure for measurement of gastrointestinal motility. J Gastrointest Motil 1991;3:151–62.
9. Fass J, Silny J, Braun J, et al. Measuring esophageal motility with a new intraluminal impedance device. First clinical results in reflux patients. Scand J Gastroenterol 1994;29:693–702.

10. Bredenoord AJ, Weusten BL, Timmer R, et al. Reproducibility of multichannel intraluminal electrical impedance monitoring of gastroesophageal reflux. Am J Gastroenterol 2005;100:265–9.

11. Shay S, Tutuian R, Sifrim D, et al. Twenty-four hour ambulatory simultaneous impedance and pH monitoring: a multicenter report of normal values from 60 healthy volunteers. Am J Gastroenterol 2004;99:1037–43.

12. Zerbib F, des Varannes SB, Roman S, et al. Normal values and day-to-day variability of 24-h ambulatory esophageal impedance-pH monitoring in a Belgian-French cohort of healthy subjects. Aliment Pharmacol Ther 2005;22:1011–21.

13. Wiener GJ, Richter JE, Cooper JB, et al. The symptom index: a clinically important parameter of ambulatory 24-hour esophageal pH monitoring. Am J Gastroenterol 1988;86:358–61.

14. Weusten BL, Roelofs JM, Akkermans LM, et al. The symptom association probability: an improved method for symptom analysis of 24-hour esophageal pH data. Gastroenterology 1994;107:1741–5.

15. Tutuian R, Mainie I, Agrawal A, et al. Normal values for ambulatory 24-hour combined impedance-pH monitoring on acid suppressive therapy. Gastroenterology 2006;130(Suppl 2):A171.

16. Heard R, Castell J, Castell DO, et al. Characterization of patients with low baseline impedance on multichannel intraluminal impedance-pH reflux testing. J Clin Gastroenterol 2012;46(7):e55–7.

17. Roman S, Bruley des Varannes S, Pouderoux P, et al. Ambulatory 24-h oesophageal impedance-pH recordings: reliability of automatic analysis for gastro-oesophageal reflux assessment. Neurogastroenterol Motil 2006;18:978–86.

18. Loots CM, van Wijk MP, Blondeau K, et al. Interobserver and intraobserver variability in pH-impedance analysis between 10 experts and automated analysis. J Pediatr 2012;160:441–6.

19. Zerbib F, Roman S, Ropert A, et al. Esophageal pH-impedance monitoring and symptom analysis in GERD: a study in patients off and on therapy. Am J Gastroenterol 2006;101:1956–63.

20. Tutuian R, Vela MF, Hill EG, et al. Characteristics of symptomatic reflux episodes on acid suppressive therapy. Am J Gastroenterol 2008;103:1090–6.

21. Boeckxstaens GE, Smout A. Systematic review: role of acid, weakly acidic and weakly alkaline reflux in gastro-oesophageal reflux disease. Aliment Pharmacol Ther 2010;32:334–43.

22. Vela MF, Tutuian R, Katz PO, et al. Baclofen decreases acid and non-acid postprandial gastro-oesophageal reflux measured by combined multichannel intraluminal impedance and pH. Aliment Pharmacol Ther 2003;17:243–51.

23. Frazzoni M, Conigliaro R, Melotti G. Reflux parameters as modified by laparoscopic fundoplication in 40 patients with heartburn/regurgitation persisting despite PPI therapy: a study using impedance-pH monitoring. Dig Dis Sci 2011;56:1099–106.

24. Charbel S, Khandwala F, Vaezi MF. The role of esophageal monitoring in symptomatic patients on PPI therapy. Am J Gastroenterol 2005;100:283–9.

25. Connor J, Richter J. Increasing yield also increases false positives and best serves to exclude GERD. Am J Gastroenterol 2006;101:460–3.

26. Bredenoord AJ, Weusten BL, Sifrim D, et al. Aerophagia, gastric, and supragastric belching: a study using intraluminal electrical impedance monitoring. Gut 2004;53:1561–5.

27. Karamanolis G, Triantafyllou K, Tsiamoulos Z, et al. Effect of sleep on excessive belching: a 24-hour impedance-pH study. J Clin Gastroenterol 2010;44:332–4.

28. Hemmink GH, Ten Cate L, Bredenoord AJ, et al. Speech therapy in patients with excessive supragastric belching—a pilot study. Neurogastroenterol Motil 2010; 22:24–8.
29. Blondeau K, Dupont LJ, Mertens V, et al. Improved diagnosis of gastro-oesophageal reflux in patients with unexplained chronic cough. Aliment Pharmacol Ther 2007;25:723–32.
30. Blondeau K, Sifrim D, Dupont L, et al. Reflux cough. Curr Gastroenterol Rep 2008; 10:235–9.
31. Smith JA, Decalmer S, Kelsall A, et al. Acoustic cough-reflux associations in chronic cough: potential triggers and mechanisms. Gastroenterology 2010;139: 754–62.

Management of Spastic Disorders of the Esophagus

Sabine Roman, MD, PhD[a], Peter J. Kahrilas, MD[b],*

KEYWORDS

- Distal esophageal spasm • Achalasia • Jackhammer esophagus
- High-resolution manometry • Esophageal motility

KEY POINTS

- Largely as a consequence of refined classification made possible with high-resolution manometry (HRM) and esophageal pressure topography (EPT), the current concept of esophageal spastic disorders has evolved to encompass spastic achalasia, distal esophageal spasm (DES), and jackhammer esophagus.
- These esophageal spastic disorders are conceptually distinct in that spastic achalasia and DES are characterized by a loss of neural inhibition, whereas jackhammer esophagus is associated with hypercontractility, presumably by activation of the cholinergic pathway.
- Because the defining endoscopic features may also occur in the setting of esophagogastric junction (EGJ) obstruction, endoscopic examination is required when esophageal spastic disorders are suspected to evaluate for mechanical obstruction.
- Therapeutic management depends on the presence of EGJ outflow obstruction.
- Extensive myotomy using the POEM technique might have a role in cases of treatment failure.

INTRODUCTION

Although reflux disease is the most common cause of esophageal chest pain, esophageal manometry is often done in the course of its evaluation, and manometric abnormalities indicative of DES are often reported. The identified abnormalities, however, are rarely the cause of chest pain and most investigators would agree that the clinical diagnosis of DES is overused. It was that observation that led to a classic reappraisal of DES by Richter and Castell,[1] conceived during the renaissance of esophageal

This work was supported by Grant No. R01DK56033 from the National Institutes of Health.
Conflict of interest: SR has served as consultant for Given Imaging.
[a] Digestive Physiology, Hôpital E Herriot, Hospices Civils de Lyon, Claude Bernard Lyon I University, Pavillon H, 5 place d'Arsonval, F-69437 Lyon Cedex 03, Lyon, France; [b] Department of Medicine, Feinberg School of Medicine, Northwestern University, 676 Saint Clair Street, 14th Floor, Chicago, IL 60611-2951, USA
* Corresponding author.
E-mail address: p-kahrilas@northwestern.edu

manometry in the early 1980s. Arguing for a more restrictive use of the diagnosis, those investigators proposed 2 required manometric criteria for DES: (1) simultaneous contractions in greater than 10% of wet swallows and (2) intermittent normal peristalsis. Other associated features were also described and some minor modifications were subsequently made, but it was these 2 criteria that became part of the lore of (conventional) manometry.

A lot has changed with respect to esophageal motility testing since 1984. Clinical studies are now commonly done with high-resolution systems using in excess of 30 closely spaced pressure transducers, and esophageal contractile patterns are displayed and analyzed in terms of pressure topography rather than as line tracings. Merging these concepts, current motility studies are more accurately termed, *HRM imaged with EPT*. Although these innovations had their roots in the early 1990s with the pioneering studies of Clouse and colleagues,[2–4] it was not until recently that commercial units became available, facilitating widespread adoption of EPT by the clinical community. The advantages of EPT compared with conventional manometry are several: (1) high-quality studies can be obtained that simultaneously image the entire esophagus, (2) standardized objective metrics have been developed for interpretation,[5–8] and (3) topographic patterns of contractility are easily learned and recognized with great reproducibility.[9,10] EPT also presented challenges, however, not the least of which was the need to reconsider the classification of esophageal motility developed for conventional manometric systems.[11] That classification effort led to improved understanding of achalasia subtypes[12] and hypomotility patterns.[13] Headway has also been made in the domain of hypercontractile conditions, including DES.[14,15] This work led to a conclusion, however, that the 2 essential criteria identified by Richter and Castell were suboptimal for defining DES as imaged in EPT and identified a heterogeneous group of patients, most of whom did not have DES.[14] Hence, the aims of this synopsis are to update the understanding of esophageal spastic disorders in the era of EPT.

WHAT ARE THE SPASTIC DISORDERS OF THE ESOPHAGUS?

Spastic disorders of the esophagus might be conceived of as hyperactive conditions of the esophagus due to contractions of either abnormal propagation (premature contractions) or extreme vigor. In the current iteration of the Chicago classification of esophageal motility disorders,[16] the relevant diagnoses are spastic (type III) achalasia, DES, and hypercontractile (jackhammer) esophagus. Despite differences in pathophysiology, which are discussed, these disorders share many similarities, including their clinical presentation: dysphagia, chest pain, regurgitation, and/or heartburn. The identification of these spastic disorders is based on the contractile pattern observed using HRM with EPT. The current Chicago classification criteria for identification of the spastic disorders are summarized in **Tables 1** and **2**.[16]

Distal Esophageal Spasm and Spastic Achalasia

Definition

DES is an uncommon disorder characterized by an impairment of ganglionic inhibition in the distal esophagus. Using conventional manometry, DES was defined by the presence of simultaneous contractions.[11] Using HRM with EPT, however, the higher-resolution recordings demonstrated that propagation velocity normally varies greatly along the length of the esophagus and finding regions of rapid propagation is common. A consequence of this finding is that the finding of rapidly propagated contractions is nonspecific for esophageal spasm.[14] Alternatively, premature contractions, defined by

Table 1
EPT patterns of spastic disorders

Spastic Disorders	EGJ Relaxation	Esophageal Contractions
Distal esophageal spasm	Normal (mean IRP <15 mm Hg)	≥20% Premature contractions (DL <4.5 s)
Spastic (type III) achalasia	Impaired (mean IRP ≥15 mm Hg)	≥20% Premature contractions (DL <4.5 s)
Jackhammer esophagus	Normal or impaired[a]	At least 1 swallow with DCI >8000 mm Hg · s · cm

EGJ relaxation is assessed using IRP, which corresponds to the 4-s period of the lowest EGJ pressure within the deglutitive window.

[a] EGJ outflow obstruction (defined as mean IRP ≥15 mm Hg in association with some instances of peristalsis) may be associated with hypercontractile swallow.

reduced distal latency (DL), measured as the interval between upper sphincter relaxation and the onset of contraction in the distal esophagus, are more specific for spasm. Physiologically, the DL is likely a manifestation of inhibitory myenteric neuron activity that determines the timing of contraction in the distal esophagus. Premature contractions with normal EGJ relaxation define DES whereas premature contractions with impaired EGJ relaxation are defining criteria for spastic achalasia (also termed, *type III achalasia*).[12]

Table 2
EPT metrics used in the Chicago classification

Abbreviation	Metric	Description	Normal
IRP	Integrated relaxation pressure	Mean EGJ pressure during the 4 s of maximal relaxation (contiguous or noncontiguous) in the 10-s window after UES relaxation	<15 mm Hg
DCI	Distal contractile integral	Amplitude × time × duration (mm Hg · s · cm) of the distal esophageal contraction >20 mm Hg from the proximal pressure through (transition zone) to the EGJ	<5000 mm Hg · s · cm
CDP	Contractile deceleration point	The inflection point along the 30–mm Hg isobaric contour where propagation velocity slows demarcating the tubular esophagus from the phrenic ampulla	—
CFV	Contractile front velocity	Slope of the tangent approximating the 30–mm Hg between the proximal pressure trough (transition zone) and the CDP	<9 cm/s
DL	Distal latency	Interval between UES relaxation and the CDP	>4.5 s

All pressures are referenced to atmospheric pressure except the IRP, which is referenced to gastric pressure.

Impairment of neural inhibition?

DES and spastic achalasia share a common pathophysiology characterized by loss of inhibitory ganglionic neuron function in the distal esophagus. The impairment of inhibitory innervation leads to both premature, rapidly propagated, or simultaneous contractions in the distal esophagus and to incomplete deglutitive EGJ relaxation. Unlike the proximal esophagus, where sequencing of the peristaltic contraction is directly programmed from motor neurons in the medulla, the timing of peristalsis in the distal smooth muscle esophagus is mediated via excitatory (cholinergic) and inhibitory (nitric oxide [NO]) myenteric plexus neurons. Furthermore, a neural gradient exists such that there is an increasing proportion of inhibitory ganglionic neurons progressing distally to the lower esophageal sphincter. The deglutitive response begins with a period of quiescence (deglutitive inhibition) in the distal esophagus that is progressively prolonged approaching the EGJ as a consequence of that neural gradient. Behar and Biancani[17] qualified this period of quiescence as contractile latency and suggested that patients with spasm could be characterized by a reduction in contractile latency. Thus, distal contractile latency, measured from the onset of the pharyngeal swallow to the onset of the contraction in the distal esophagus, was shorter in patients with simultaneous contractions than in those with normal peristaltic propagation. NO is the dominant inhibitory neurotransmitter in the esophageal myenteric plexus.[18] Experimentally scavenging NO with free hemoglobin in control subjects induces simultaneous esophageal contraction and inhibits deglutitive EGJ relaxation.[19] This demonstrates the role of inhibitory innervation in the genesis of DES and impaired EGJ relaxation.

Some structural changes have been observed in the esophageal muscularis propria of patients with DES. These are inconsistent and nonspecific, however. Recent observations by Pehlivanov and colleagues[20] using high-frequency intraluminal ultrasound suggest increased esophageal smooth muscle thickness in DES patients. Even in the absence of esophageal contractions, the muscularis propria in DES patients was thicker than in controls or patients with nonspecific motor disorders. Finally, a study in knockout mice suggested that lack of inhibitory innervation might result in increased muscularis propria thickness.[21]

Jackhammer Esophagus

Definition

The term, *nutcracker esophagus*, was coined in conventional manometry for a novel disorder associated with noncardiac chest pain and characterized by hypertensive but normally propagated peristaltic contractions.[22] Unlike the case of spasm, there were no characteristic fluoroscopic abnormalities. The manometric criterion for nutcracker esophagus were initially an average peristaltic amplitude of greater than 180 mm Hg in the distal esophagus. Subsequently, this threshold value was increased to 220 mm Hg in hopes of improving specificity. With the era of HRM and EPT, peristaltic amplitude was replaced by the distal contractile integral (DCI) as the summary metric of the vigor of the distal esophageal contraction. If the entire distal esophageal contraction is envisioned as a solid with the height of the peaks corresponding to peristaltic amplitude and the footprint corresponding to the length of the involved esophagus and the duration of the contraction, the DCI, expressed as mm Hg · s · cm, is the volume of that solid above a 20–mm Hg minimum. A DCI mean value of 5000 mm Hg (hypertensive peristalsis in the Chicago classification) approximately corresponds to nutcracker esophagus in conventional manometry. Even that value is seen in up to 5% of normal subjects, however, making it inherently nonspecific. Alternatively, an extreme phenotype of hypertensive contractions was described based on the occurrence of at least one contraction with a DCI greater than 8000 mm Hg · s · cm, a value never observed in controls.[15] This was termed, *esophageal hypercontractility* or *the jackhammer esophagus*. Although still somewhat heterogeneous (the pattern is sometimes seen with EGJ outflow obstruction), this extreme phenotype is likely more clinically relevant than hypertensive peristalsis (nutcracker esophagus). Hypercontractility is commonly associated with multipeaked contractions, sometimes resulting in DCI values in excess of 50,000 mm Hg · s · cm.

Excess of cholinergic stimulation?

The pathophysiology of esophageal hypercontractility likely involves an excess of cholinergic drive. Temporal asynchrony between the contractions of circular and longitudinal muscle layers of the muscularis propria have been observed with high-frequency intraluminal ultrasound in patients with nutcracker esophagus.[23] This asynchrony was reversed with atropine.[24] The observations of Loo and colleagues[25] in diabetics with autonomic neuropathy are also an indirect argument for an excess of cholinergic stimulation. Multipeaked contractions occurred more frequently in diabetics with neuropathy than in control subjects or diabetics without neuropathy. Multipeaked contractions became single-peak contraction after atropine injection. Multipeaked contractions are also a common finding in jackhammer esophagus.[15] It remains to be determined if atropine may change the multipeaked pattern in such patients. Finally, as with DES, increased muscle thickness has been observed in patients with nutcracker esophagus[26] and with esophageal hypercontractility (Kahrilas, 2011, unpublished observations).

Esophageal Spastic Disorders: A Consequence of EGJ Obstruction?

Both DES and jackhammer esophagus can be associated with EGJ outflow obstruction, an association supported by experimental models. For instance, Mittal and colleagues[27] observed esophageal muscle hypertrophy and hyperexcitability by placing calibrated ligatures around the EGJ in cats. In humans, esophageal hypercontractility has been observed with mechanical EGJ obstruction induced by fundoplication or gastric lap band.[28] Gyawali and Kushnir[29] expanded on this observation, reporting that patients with EGJ outflow obstruction exhibited a motor pattern characterized by multipeaked contractions, high distal esophageal amplitude, and prolonged contraction duration. Finally, as previously defined, impaired EGJ relaxation in association with premature contractions constitutes spastic achalasia.[12]

Given the relationship between EGJ outflow obstruction and hypercontractility, some investigators have speculated that esophageal spastic disorders can progress to achalasia. Supporting this contention, among a series of 35 patients diagnosed with DES on conventional manometry, 5 (14%) progressed to achalasia, 4 (12%) reverted to normal manometry, and 26 (74%) had persistent DES at a mean follow-up of 2.1 years.[30] Progression from nutcracker esophagus to achalasia also was observed.[31,32] The number of patients reported to undergo such progression, however, is extremely limited (only case reports of nutcracker esophagus), leaving open the possibility that the type of spastic disorder might have been misdiagnosed with either the initial or the follow-up conventional manometry study. EGJ pseudorelaxation secondary to esophageal shortening commonly leads to an erroneous diagnosis of DES instead of spastic achalasia.[4]

Association with Other Conditions: Gastroesophageal Reflux Disease and Eosinophilic Esophagitis

Manometric findings consistent with primary spastic motility disorders can also occur in conjunction with, or as a consequence of, other conditions, notably gastroesophageal reflux disease (GERD). In a series of 108 patients with DES, GERD was documented by either pH-metry or endoscopy in 38%.[33] Furthermore, in some instances, esophageal acid perfusion can induce spasm.[34] In a series of 45 patients with nutcracker esophagus (conventional manometry), 47% had abnormal acid exposure time on pH-metry, 4% had endoscopic esophagitis, and 16% positive symptom index.[35] Finally, reflux esophagitis has also been observed in patients with jackhammer esophagus and the hypercontractile pattern can resolve with of proton pump inhibitor (PPI) therapy.[15]

Similar overlap exists between spastic disorders and eosinophilic esophagitis. In a retrospective study of patients who underwent Heller myotomy for achalasia, mucosal eosinophilia was reported in 8%.[36] A case of achalasia with eosinophilic infiltrate responding to steroid therapy has been reported.[37] Jackhammer esophagus was also associated with eosinophilic esophagitis in 3 of 41 patients (7%) who underwent endoscopy with mucosal biopsies.[15]

DIAGNOSIS OF ESOPHAGEAL SPASTIC DISORDERS

Dysphagia, chest pain, regurgitation, and heartburn are all symptoms potentially associated with esophageal spastic disorders. All of these are nonspecific, however, and esophageal spastic disorders are rare.[15,38] Hence, the clinical evaluation needs to prioritize identifying more morbid conditions and more prevalent conditions before pursuing these rare, nonfatal conditions. When chest pain is among the presenting symptoms, the evaluation should first prioritize excluding cardiovascular disease owing to its potentially life-threatening nature. Even within the realm of esophageal chest pain, reflux is a more common cause than spastic disorders. Using the liberal definitions put forth by Richter and Castell, DES accounted for fewer than 5% of patients referred for dysphagia or chest pain in a motility laboratory.[39] With the more refined criteria of the Chicago classification, the combined prevalence of DES, spastic achalasia, and jackhammer is even lower, approximately 2%.[12,14,15,40] Consequently, evaluation of suspected esophageal spastic disorders requires a thorough evaluation to first identify or exclude other potential causes of esophageal chest pain.

One potential consequence of spastic contractions is an impairment of esophageal bolus transit that may explain the perception of dysphagia. As evident by the fluoroscopic appearance of DES as a corkscrew or rosary bead esophagus, long segments of simultaneous contractions might occur. In such instances, the bolus becomes trapped in the spastic segment because the distal portion contracts prematurely with insufficient time to allow for bolus transit.[17] Paradoxically, Tutuian and Castell[41] reported that 55% of patients with DES defined with conventional manometry and 97% of patients with nutcracker esophagus exhibited complete bolus transit when tested with multichannel intraluminal impedance. Although their findings with respect to nutcracker are consistent with understanding of its physiology, the observation regarding DES are not and speak to the overdiagnosis of the condition using conventional manometry and diagnostic criteria. DES patients with dysphagia exhibited more frequently abnormal bolus transit than DES patients with chest pain.[42]

The mechanism by which spastic disorders induce chest pain is not well understood. The amplitude of contractions might be relevant. Tutuian and colleagues[42] demonstrated that DES patients with chest pain had greater amplitude esophageal contractions than DES patients with dysphagia or GERD. Hypersensitivity might also play a role. Using stepwise balloon distension, Mujica and colleagues[43] observed a lower chest pain threshold in patients with nutcracker esophagus compared with controls. Hypersensitivity might also explain the perception of heartburn in patients without demonstrable evidence of reflux.

Finally, epiphrenic diverticula might occur as a consequence of spastic disorders. The majority of patients with epiphrenic diverticula are found to have an esophageal motility disorder. In a surgical series of 21 patients with epiphrenic diverticula, 24% were diagnosed as DES before surgery, 24% as nutcracker esophagus, and 9% as achalasia.[44] The presence of a diverticulum might also explain the symptoms of dysphagia or regurgitation.

Upper Endoscopy

Upper endoscopy should be performed as initial evaluation of esophageal symptoms consistent with spastic disorders. It allows exclusion of mechanical obstruction, esophageal stenosis, or esophagitis. Systematic esophageal biopsies should be obtained to rule out eosinophilic esophagitis, especially when dysphagia is a prominent symptom. Usually no specific endoscopic abnormality is revealed, but disordered esophageal contractions might be observed by the endoscopist. In some cases of achalasia, increased resistance at the EGJ might be perceived.

Esophageal Manometry

The diagnosis of spastic disorders is established by esophageal manometry and recent developments suggest that HRM with EPT is superior to conventional manometry for several reasons. First, the diagnosis of EGJ relaxation is more reliable with HRM compared with conventional manometry, which is essential in distinguishing DES from spastic achalasia.[4,45] A major factor leading to the failure to detect impaired EGJ relaxation with conventional manometry is esophageal shortening that occurs during peristalsis that may be accentuated with spasm. Correct evaluation of EGJ relaxation is of cardinal importance because spastic contractions with normal EGJ relaxation constitute DES but spastic contractions with impaired EGJ relaxation diagnose spastic achalasia, and treatment then focuses on alleviating EGJ obstruction. Moreover, the use of the integrated relaxation pressure (IRP),[5] DL,[14] and DCI[8] measurements in HRM (see **Table 2**) more accurately diagnose spastic disorders than the metrics used in conventional manometry. The EPT definitions of spastic disorders are summarized in **Table 1**.

DES was initially defined using conventional manometry by the presence of at least 20% simultaneous contractions with minimum amplitude of 30 mm Hg.[11] A simultaneous contraction was defined by a propagation velocity greater than 8 cm/s measured between 3 cm and 8 cm above the EGJ. Associated, but not essential, criteria for DES were spontaneous, repetitive, or multipeaked contractions and intermittent normal peristalsis. With HRM and EPT, DES is defined as at least 20% premature contractions in the context of normal EGJ relaxation.[16] Premature contractions exhibit a reduced (<4.5 s) DL defined as the interval between upper esophageal sphincter (UES) relaxation and onset of the contraction at the contractile deceleration point (CDP) (**Fig. 1**). Recently, Pandolfino and colleagues[14] demonstrated that DL was much more specific than the contractile front velocity (CFV) for detecting spastic disorders. Among 1070 patients, 91 exhibited rapid contractions (defined as CFV >9 cm/s). In 24 of them, these contractions were also premature. All of the patients with premature contractions were ultimately managed as either DES or spastic achalasia. In contrast, the 67 patients with rapid contractions but normal DL were more likely to have nonspastic disorders, in particular, weak peristalsis. Finally, in the Chicago classification, there is no requirement of any normal contractions in the diagnosis of DES.

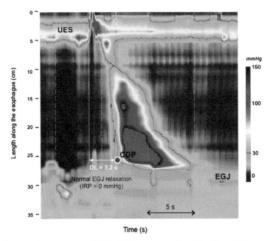

Fig. 1. Distal esophageal spasm in EPT. EGJ assessed with the IRP is normal. Premature contractions are observed for at least 20% of swallows. A reduced DL (<4.5 s), measured from UES relaxation to CDP (pink dot), defines premature contraction. The CDP corresponds to an abrupt slowing of the contraction wavefront representing the transition from esophageal clearance to the formation of the phrenic ampulla. (*Data from* Pandolfino JE, Leslie E, Luger D, et al. The contractile deceleration point: an important physiologic landmark on esophageal pressure topography. Neurogastroenterol Motil 2010;22(4):395–400.)

The only differentiating feature between DES and spastic achalasia (also named type III in the Chicago classification) is the adequacy of EGJ relaxation. Using conventional manometry, spastic achalasia was included in the concept of vigorous achalasia. No distinction was made, however, between bolus pressurization from simultaneous contractions, leading to the likely inclusion of many type II achalasia patients in the vigorous group. Using HRM and EPT, it is easy to differentiate panesophageal pressurization from simultaneous contractions by comparing their respective spatial pressure variation plots, which illustrate the instantaneous longitudinal pressure profile within the esophagus. The spatial pressure variation plot between UES and EGJ is flat in instances of panesophageal pressurization whereas it exhibits peaks and valleys in instances of simultaneous contractions (**Fig. 2**). Thus, using EPT, spastic achalasia is defined as impaired EGJ relaxation (IRP ≥15 mm Hg) associated with at least 20% premature contractions.

Jackhammer esophagus is an extreme pattern of hypercontractility. Using conventional manometry, nutcracker esophagus was defined as a mean distal esophageal peristaltic amplitude (measured 3 cm and 8 cm above the EGJ) greater than 180 mm Hg in the context of normal LES relaxation.[11] Subsequently, some investigators proposed increasing the threshold to 260 mm Hg, a value suggested as having greater clinical relevance.[46] Similarly, seeking a more clinically relevant definition of hypercontractility, the diagnosis of jackhammer esophagus was proposed in EPT, defined as at least 1 swallow with a DCI (the metric of contractile vigor) greater than 8000 mm Hg · s · cm (**Fig. 3**).[15] Distinguishing jackhammer from hypertensive peristalsis or nutcracker esophagus, this pattern was never observed in control subjects. Jackhammer may be associated with EGJ outflow obstruction or obstruction. Multipeaked contractions are frequent in patients with jackhammer esophagus but are not mandatory to diagnose this disorder.

Because symptoms of spastic disorders are intermittent, ambulatory 24-hour manometry has been proposed as a way to increase the diagnostic yield. In 1 such

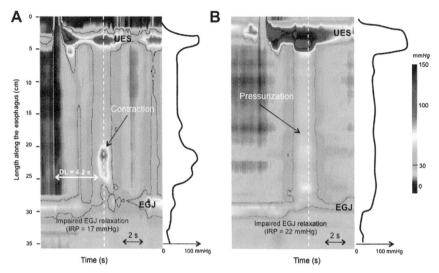

Fig. 2. Spastic (type III) achalasia is characterized as impaired EGJ relaxation associated with at least 20% of premature contractions (A). The premature contraction exhibits a reduced DL (<4.5 s). EGJ relaxation is assesses using the IRP. Simultaneous (premature) contractions might be differentiated from pressurization (B) using the spatial pressure variation plot represented on the right of each EPT plots. Each spatial pressure variation pressure plot was obtained at the time, identified by the white dashed line. In the instance of an esophageal contraction (A), pressure variations are obvious along the esophageal body. In instances of pressurization (B), intraesophageal pressure did not vary between UES and the EGJ. (B) This corresponds to type II achalasia (achalasia with compression).

series of 390 patients referred with esophageal motility disorders, 16 (4%) were diagnosed with DES on 24-hour manometry, 14 of whom were missed by laboratory manometry.[47] Likely because of the scarcity of suitable recording devices, however, 24-hour manometry is rarely done and the implications of such an examination on patient management have yet to be defined.

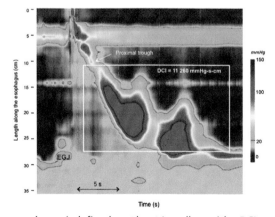

Fig. 3. Jackhammer esophagus is defined as at least 1 swallow with a DCI greater than 8000 mm Hg · s · cm. DCI is the EPT metric summarizing contractile vigor and is calculated as the product of the amplitude (>20 mm Hg) times the duration times the length of the contraction between the proximal pressure trough (also known as the transition zone) and the EGJ (*white box*).

Barium Swallow

The classic appearance of esophageal spasm is the corkscrew or rosary bead esophagus (**Fig. 4**). In a series of 14 patients with DES on barium swallow, Prabhakar and colleagues[48] observed a classical radiologic pattern of corkscrew esophagus in only 2 patients; the others exhibited nonperistaltic contractions that were not lumen obliterating. Lower esophageal sphincter dysfunction was suspected in 9 patients on barium swallow. Alternatively, using conventional manometry, these 14 patients were classified as DES with normal LES function in 2 cases, DES with LES dysfunction in 4 cases, and spastic achalasia in 8 cases. In total, 13 of the 14 patients had LES dysfunction evident either on barium swallow or manometry, suggesting that the 2 techniques were complementary in differentiating DES from spastic achalasia. Consequently, when spastic disorders are suspected on manometry, a barium swallow might be performed to appreciate the consequences of motility disorders on esophageal bolus transit, such as barium stasis or retrograde barium movement in the esophagus. It may also detect an epiphrenic diverticulum to support the diagnosis of spastic disorders.

Other Examinations

CT scan and endoscopic ultrasonography

Esophageal muscle thickening can be observed in patients with spastic disorders. This thickening is sometimes profound (as much as 1 cm) and identifiable on CT scan.[49] CT scan is not routinely indicated in patients with spastic disorders, however, unless there is a suspicion of extrinsic esophageal compression. Alternatively, endoscopic ultrasonography can quantify esophageal thickening and also reveal mediastinal or intramural abnormalities making it useful in atypical cases. The clinical

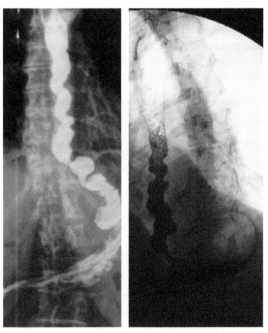

Fig. 4. Barium swallow of 2 patients with distal esophageal spasm. Note the typical pattern of rosary beads or corkscrew esophagus.

detection of esophageal thickening favors the diagnosis of spastic disorders. Endoscopic ultrasound also allows for the exclusion of intramural esophageal tumor that might potentially induce abnormal contractility.

24-Hour pH monitoring
Because of the potential overlap between DES and GERD, 24-hour pH monitoring should be considered in patients having chest pain, regurgitation, or heartburn to exclude pathologic reflux. The yield of pH impedance in this indication is not known. Wireless pH monitoring has been evaluated in patients with noncardiac chest pain.[50] As pH recording was extended to 48 hours with the wireless pH capsule; a diagnostic gain of 9.7% was observed in detecting pathologic esophageal acid exposure compared with 24-hour recording. Two-thirds of patients, however, reported severe chest pain during wireless pH monitoring in this indication. Consequently, wireless pH monitoring should be used with caution in patients with noncardiac chest pain.

Impedance manometry
Impedance manometry allows for a direct concurrent assessment of bolus transit and motility.[41] Compared with barium swallow, impedance monitoring has the advantage of avoiding radiation exposure. Recently, it has been suggested that impedance might be as accurate as barium swallow to evaluate bolus transit in patients with dysphagia.[51] The concordance was high for severe barium stasis and incomplete bolus transit on impedance (97%) and for normal barium transit and complete bolus transit (96%). Instances of complete bolus transit on impedance and mild barium stasis on fluoroscopy, however, were observed in patients who had been treated for DES or achalasia, making the claim of equivalency between the examinations questionable.

TREATMENT OF ESOPHAGEAL SPASTIC DISORDERS

The first treatment strategy of spastic disorders depends on whether or not there is an accompanying EGJ outflow obstruction (**Table 3**). If EGJ relaxation is impaired, the initial treatment should be directed at alleviating EGJ obstruction. Otherwise, the goal of treatment is to reduce the vigor of the abnormal esophageal contractions.

Pharmacologic Treatment

Smooth muscle relaxants, such as nitrates, NO donors, and calcium channel blockers, have been proposed for treating esophageal spastic disorders. These drugs both

Table 3		
Therapeutic options for spastic disorders		
Therapeutic option	Impaired EGJ relaxation (spastic [type III] achalasia)	Normal EGJ relaxation (distal esophageal spasm, jackhammer esophagus)
Pharmacologic	Phosphodiesterase-5 inhibitors?	Nitrates Phosphodiesterase-5 inhibitors Calcium channel blockers Peppermint oil Low-dose antidepressants PPIs
Endoscopic	Pneumatic dilation Toxin botulinum at the EGJ level POEM	Botulinum toxin in the esophageal body Extended POEM?
Surgical	Myotomy	Extended myotomy?

reduce LES pressure and esophageal contraction amplitude. Placebo-controlled crossover trials report only minimal benefit in achalasia, however.[52] In DES, nitrates may improve manometric findings and chest discomfort.[53,54] They also prolong the DL and decrease the distal contraction amplitude in patients with DES.[55] Nitrates have not been tested in controlled trials, however, in DES or in nutcracker esophagus.

Phosphodiesterase-5 inhibitors (eg sildenafil) represent a new therapeutic option. Phosphodiesterase-5 inhibitors block the degradation of NO, enhancing its effect and resulting in more prolonged smooth muscle relaxation. Sildenafil reduces both contractile amplitude and propagation velocity in controls and in patients with motility disorders. Preliminary data also suggest it is effective in relieving esophageal symptoms and improving manometric findings in patients with spastic motility disorders.[56,57] Practical limitations of this treatment, however, are side effects (dizziness and headache) and cost. Because its main approved indication, erectile dysfunction in men, is viewed as recreational, most insurers do not cover the cost for patients.

Another smooth muscle relaxant, peppermint oil, has also been reported by one group of investigators[58] to eliminate simultaneous contractions. No other study, however, has yet confirmed these data.

Low-dose antidepressants can improve patients' reaction to pain without objectively improving motility function.[59] A controlled trial showing efficacy for this strategy was with the anxiolytic, trazadone (serotonin uptake inhibitor), suggesting that reassurance and control of anxiety are important therapeutic goals.[59] Also consistent with that conclusion, success has been reported using behavioral modification and biofeedback.[60]

Finally, due to the potential overlap between GERD and spastic disorders, a trial of PPIs may be beneficial, especially in the setting of esophagitis or abnormal pH-metry.

Endoscopic Treatment

Pneumatic dilation has been proposed for treating spastic disorders and some success has been reported.[61] A caveat to this success is that it is unclear whether or not the patients benefited by pneumatic dilation would not be more properly categorized as having spastic achalasia or achalasia with esophageal compression, emphasizing the need for accurate manometric classification. Pandolfino and colleagues[12] observed that pneumatic dilation was associated with a lower treatment response in patients with spastic achalasia compared with patients with achalasia with esophageal compression.

Botulinum toxin injection is a pathophysiologically attractive approach to treating patients with spastic disorders, and therapeutic trials suggest it can reduce chest pain.[62] The technique has not been standardized in this application with some reports injection of botulinum toxin only at the level of the EJG and others also injecting the distal esophagus.[62] Some efficacy is noted in a majority of achalasia patients with injection in the EGJ. Achalasia subtypes, however, were not defined in these trials and effects were temporary with a fall-off in success rates from 80% to 90% after 1 month to 53% to 54% after 1 year.[63] In a sham-controlled trial of 22 patients with DES or nutcracker esophagus, thus far reported only in abstract form, injection of toxin botulinum in the distal esophagus was superior to placebo in improving dysphagia.[64]

Recently, peroral endoscopic myotomy (POEM) has been introduced to treat achalasia[65] and a case of DES successfully treated by extended POEM has been reported.[66] Short-term results with this technique are promising but larger and longer-term studies are required to determine its place in the management of patients with spastic disorders.

Surgical Treatment

Heller myotomy is an established treatment of achalasia. As with pneumatic dilation, however, a lower response rate has been observed in patients with spastic achalasia.[12] This might be explained by the disease involving not only the LES but also the esophageal body. Long myotomy extending from the LES proximally onto the esophageal body has been used to treat patients with spastic disorders. The extent of the myotomy may be guided by manometric findings.[67,68] In a series of 20 patients with extended myotomy (14 cm on the esophagus and 2 cm below the EGJ) and anterior fundoplication for DES, dysphagia and chest pain were significantly improved after a median follow-up of 50 months.[69] Functional results seemed to be stable with time in that series. An uncontrolled study suggested that surgical treatment might be more effective than the medical treatment of DES.[68] Choice of treatment, however, was based on physician preference, patient choice, and access to a referral center for treatment. Controlled trials are required to determine if surgical management is more effective than endoscopic or medical treatment.

SUMMARY

Largely as a consequence of refined classification made possible with HRM and EPT, the current concept of esophageal spastic disorders has evolved to encompass spastic achalasia, DES, and jackhammer esophagus. These are conceptually distinct in that spastic achalasia and DES are characterized by a loss of neural inhibition, whereas jackhammer esophagus is associated with hypercontractility, presumably by activation of the cholinergic pathway. Esophageal spastic disorders can present with dysphagia, chest pain, regurgitations, and/or heartburn. Because the defining endoscopic features may also occur in the setting of EGJ obstruction, endoscopic examination is required when esophageal spastic disorders are suspected to evaluate for mechanical obstruction. Esophageal biopsies should also be performed because of the possible association with eosinophilic esophagitis. The key examination, however, is high-resolution esophageal manometry, which facilitates a specific definition of each spastic disorder. HRM with EPT is preferred to conventional manometry because these disorders have not been reliably distinguished from one another with the older technology. Finally, other examinations, such as barium swallow and esophageal pH-metry, might be useful to assess bolus transit and esophageal acid exposure, respectively. Therapeutic management depends on the presence of EGJ outflow obstruction. Alleviating EGJ outflow obstruction is achieved with either pneumatic dilation, endoscopic botulinum injection, or myotomy. Pharmacologic treatment (nitrates and phosphodiesterase-5 inhibitors) may reduce esophageal contractions as effectively as botulinum toxin injection. Extensive myotomy using the POEM technique might have a role in cases of treatment failure.

REFERENCES

1. Richter JE, Castell DO. Diffuse esophageal spasm: a reappraisal. Ann Intern Med 1984;100(2):242–5.
2. Clouse RE, Staiano A. Topography of the esophageal peristaltic pressure wave. Am J Physiol 1991;261(4 Pt 1):G677–84.
3. Clouse RE, Staiano A, Alrakawi A. Development of a topographic analysis system for manometric studies in the gastrointestinal tract. Gastrointest Endosc 1998; 48(4):395–401.

4. Clouse RE, Staiano A, Alrakawi A, et al. Application of topographical methods to clinical esophageal manometry. Am J Gastroenterol 2000;95(10):2720–30.
5. Ghosh SK, Pandolfino JE, Rice J, et al. Impaired deglutitive EGJ relaxation in clinical esophageal manometry: a quantitative analysis of 400 patients and 75 controls. Am J Physiol Gastrointest Liver Physiol 2007;293(4):G878–85.
6. Pandolfino JE, Leslie E, Luger D, et al. The contractile deceleration point: an important physiologic landmark on oesophageal pressure topography. Neurogastroenterol Motil 2010;22(4):395–400.
7. Roman S, Lin Z, Pandolfino JE, et al. Distal contraction latency: a measure of propagation velocity optimized for esophageal pressure topography studies. Am J Gastroenterol 2011;106(3):443–51.
8. Ghosh SK, Pandolfino JE, Zhang Q, et al. Quantifying esophageal peristalsis with high-resolution manometry: a study of 75 asymptomatic volunteers. Am J Physiol Gastrointest Liver Physiol 2006;290(5):G988–97.
9. Grubel C, Borovicka J, Schwizer W, et al. Diffuse esophageal spasm. Am J Gastroenterol 2008;103(2):450–7.
10. Soudagar AS, Sayuk GS, Gyawali CP. Learners favour high resolution oesophageal manometry with better diagnostic accuracy over conventional line tracings. Gut 2012;61(6):798–803.
11. Spechler SJ, Castell DO. Classification of oesophageal motility abnormalities. Gut 2001;49(1):145–51.
12. Pandolfino JE, Kwiatek MA, Nealis T, et al. Achalasia: a new clinically relevant classification by high-resolution manometry. Gastroenterology 2008;135(5): 1526–33.
13. Roman S, Lin Z, Kwiatek MA, et al. Weak peristalsis in esophageal pressure topography: classification and association with dysphagia. Am J Gastroenterol 2011;106(2):349–56.
14. Pandolfino JE, Roman S, Carlson D, et al. Distal esophageal spasm in high-resolution esophageal pressure topography: defining clinical phenotypes. Gastroenterology 2011;141(2):469–75.
15. Roman S, Pandolfino JE, Chen J, et al. Phenotypes and clinical context of hypercontractility in high resolution pressure topography (EPT). Am J Gastroenterol 2012;107(1):37–45.
16. Bredenoord AJ, Fox M, Kahrilas PJ, et al. Chicago classification criteria of esophageal motility disorders defined in high resolution esophageal esophageal pressure topography (EPT). Neurogastroenterol Motil 2012;24(Suppl 1):57–65.
17. Behar J, Biancani P. Pathogenesis of simultaneous esophageal contractions in patients with motility disorders. Gastroenterology 1993;105(1):111–8.
18. Goyal RK, Chaudhury A. Physiology of normal esophageal motility. J Clin Gastroenterol 2008;42(5):610–9.
19. Murray JA, Ledlow A, Launspach J, et al. The effects of recombinant human hemoglobin on esophageal motor functions in humans. Gastroenterology 1995; 109(4):1241–8.
20. Pehlivanov N, Liu J, Kassab GS, et al. Relationship between esophageal muscle thickness and intraluminal pressure in patients with esophageal spasm. Am J Physiol Gastrointest Liver Physiol 2002;282(6):G1016–23.
21. Mashimo H, Kjellin A, Goyal RK. Gastric stasis in neuronal nitric oxide synthase-deficient knockout mice. Gastroenterology 2000;119(3):766–73.
22. Benjamin SB, Gerhardt DC, Castell DO. High amplitude, peristaltic esophageal contractions associated with chest pain and/or dysphagia. Gastroenterology 1979;77(3):478–83.

23. Jung HY, Puckett JL, Bhalla V, et al. Asynchrony between the circular and the longitudinal muscle contraction in patients with nutcracker esophagus. Gastroenterology 2005;128(5):1179–86.
24. Korsapati H, Bhargava V, Mittal RK. Reversal of asynchrony between circular and longitudinal muscle contraction in nutcracker esophagus by atropine. Gastroenterology 2008;135(3):796–802.
25. Loo FD, Dodds WJ, Soergel KH, et al. Multipeaked esophageal peristaltic pressure waves in patients with diabetic neuropathy. Gastroenterology 1985;88(2):485–91.
26. Dogan I, Puckett JL, Padda BS, et al. Prevalence of increased esophageal muscle thickness in patients with esophageal symptoms. Am J Gastroenterol 2007;102(1):137–45.
27. Mittal RK, Ren J, McCallum RW, et al. Modulation of feline esophageal contractions by bolus volume and outflow obstruction. Am J Physiol 1990;258(2 Pt 1):G208–15.
28. Burton PR, Brown W, Laurie C, et al. The effect of laparoscopic adjustable gastric bands on esophageal motility and the gastroesophageal junction: analysis using high-resolution video manometry. Obes Surg 2009;19(7):905–14.
29. Gyawali CP, Kushnir VM. High-resolution manometric characteristics help differentiate types of distal esophageal obstruction in patients with peristalsis. Neurogastroenterol Motil 2011;23(6):502-e197.
30. Fontes LH, Herbella FA, Rodriguez TN, et al. Progression of diffuse esophageal spasm to achalasia: incidence and predictive factors. Dis Esophagus 2012. [Epub ahead of print].
31. Anggiansah A, Bright NF, McCullagh M, et al. Transition from nutcracker esophagus to achalasia. Dig Dis Sci 1990;35(9):1162–6.
32. Paterson WG, Beck IT, Da Costa LR. Transition from nutcracker esophagus to achalasia. A case report. J Clin Gastroenterol 1991;13(5):554–8.
33. Almansa C, Heckman MG, DeVault KR, et al. Esophageal spasm: demographic, clinical, radiographic, and manometric features in 108 patients. Dis Esophagus 2012;25(3):214–21.
34. Crozier RE, Glick ME, Gibb SP, et al. Acid-provoked esophageal spasm as a cause of noncardiac chest pain. Am J Gastroenterol 1991;86(11):1576–80.
35. Borjesson M, Pilhall M, Rolny P, et al. Gastroesophageal acid reflux in patients with nutcracker esophagus. Scand J Gastroenterol 2001;36(9):916–20.
36. Cools-Lartigue J, Chang SY, McKendy K, et al. Pattern of esophageal eosinophilic infiltration in patients with achalasia and response to Heller myotomy and Dor fundoplication. Dis Esophagus 2012. [Epub ahead of print].
37. Savarino E, Gemignani L, Zentilin P, et al. A case of achalasia with dense eosinophilic infiltrate responding to steroidal treatment. Clin Gastroenterol Hepatol 2011;9(12):1104–6.
38. Patti MG, Gorodner MV, Galvani C, et al. Spectrum of esophageal motility disorders: implications for diagnosis and treatment. Arch Surg 2005;140(5):442–8 [discussion: 448–9].
39. Dalton CB, Castell DO, Hewson EG, et al. Diffuse esophageal spasm. A rare motility disorder not characterized by high-amplitude contractions. Dig Dis Sci 1991;36(8):1025–8.
40. Pandolfino JE, Ghosh SK, Rice J, et al. Classifying esophageal motility by pressure topography characteristics: a study of 400 patients and 75 controls. Am J Gastroenterol 2008;103(1):27–37.

41. Tutuian R, Castell DO. Combined multichannel intraluminal impedance and manometry clarifies esophageal function abnormalities: study in 350 patients. Am J Gastroenterol 2004;99(6):1011–9.
42. Tutuian R, Mainie I, Agrawal A, et al. Symptom and function heterogenicity among patients with distal esophageal spasm: studies using combined impedance-manometry. Am J Gastroenterol 2006;101(3):464–9.
43. Mujica VR, Mudipalli RS, Rao SS. Pathophysiology of chest pain in patients with nutcracker esophagus. Am J Gastroenterol 2001;96(5):1371–7.
44. Tedesco P, Fisichella PM, Way LW, et al. Cause and treatment of epiphrenic diverticula. Am J Surg 2005;190(6):891–4.
45. Fox M, Hebbard G, Janiak P, et al. High-resolution manometry predicts the success of oesophageal bolus transport and identifies clinically important abnormalities not detected by conventional manometry. Neurogastroenterol Motil 2004; 16(5):533–42.
46. Agrawal A, Hila A, Tutuian R, et al. Clinical relevance of the nutcracker esophagus: suggested revision of criteria for diagnosis. J Clin Gastroenterol 2006; 40(6):504–9.
47. Barham CP, Gotley DC, Fowler A, et al. Diffuse oesophageal spasm: diagnosis by ambulatory 24 hour manometry. Gut 1997;41(2):151–5.
48. Prabhakar A, Levine MS, Rubesin S, et al. Relationship between diffuse esophageal spasm and lower esophageal sphincter dysfunction on barium studies and manometry in 14 patients. AJR Am J Roentgenol 2004;183(2):409–13.
49. Goldberg MF, Levine MS, Torigian DA. Diffuse esophageal spasm: CT findings in seven patients. AJR Am J Roentgenol 2008;191(3):758–63.
50. Prakash C, Clouse RE. Wireless pH monitoring in patients with non-cardiac chest pain. Am J Gastroenterol 2006;101(3):446–52.
51. Cho YK, Choi MG, Oh SN, et al. Comparison of bolus transit patterns identified by esophageal impedance to barium esophagram in patients with dysphagia. Dis Esophagus 2012;25(1):17–25.
52. Traube M, Hongo M, Magyar L, et al. Effects of nifedipine in achalasia and in patients with high-amplitude peristaltic esophageal contractions. JAMA 1984; 252(13):1733–6.
53. Orlando RC, Bozymski EM. Clinical and manometric effects of nitroglycerin in diffuse esophageal spasm. N Engl J Med 1973;289(1):23–5.
54. Swamy N. Esophageal spasm: clinical and manometric response to nitroglycerine and long acting nitrites. Gastroenterology 1977;72(1):23–7.
55. Konturek JW, Gillessen A, Domschke W. Diffuse esophageal spasm: a malfunction that involves nitric oxide? Scand J Gastroenterol 1995;30(11):1041–5.
56. Eherer AJ, Schwetz I, Hammer HF, et al. Effect of sildenafil on oesophageal motor function in healthy subjects and patients with oesophageal motor disorders. Gut 2002;50(6):758–64.
57. Bortolotti M, Mari C, Lopilato C, et al. Effects of sildenafil on esophageal motility of patients with idiopathic achalasia. Gastroenterology 2000;118(2):253–7.
58. Pimentel M, Bonorris GG, Chow EJ, et al. Peppermint oil improves the manometric findings in diffuse esophageal spasm. J Clin Gastroenterol 2001;33(1): 27–31.
59. Clouse RE, Lustman PJ, Eckert TC, et al. Low-dose trazodone for symptomatic patients with esophageal contraction abnormalities. A double-blind, placebo-controlled trial. Gastroenterology 1987;92(4):1027–36.
60. Latimer PR. Biofeedback and self-regulation in the treatment of diffuse esophageal spasm: a single-case study. Biofeedback Self Regul 1981;6(2):181–9.

61. Irving JD, Owen WJ, Linsell J, et al. Management of diffuse esophageal spasm with balloon dilatation. Gastrointest Radiol 1992;17(3):189–92.
62. Storr M, Allescher HD, Rosch T, et al. Treatment of symptomatic diffuse esophageal spasm by endoscopic injections of botulinum toxin: a prospective study with long-term follow-up. Gastrointest Endosc 2001;54(6):754–9.
63. Boeckxstaens GE. Achalasia. Best Pract Res Clin Gastroenterol 2007;21(4): 595–608.
64. Vanuytsel T, Bisschops R, Holvoet L, et al. A sham-control study of injection of botulinum toxin in non achalasia esophageal hypermotility disorder. Gastroenterology 2009;136(5 Suppl 1):A-152.
65. Inoue H, Minami H, Kobayashi Y, et al. Peroral endoscopic myotomy (POEM) for esophageal achalasia. Endoscopy 2010;42(4):265–71.
66. Shiwaku H, Inoue H, Beppu R, et al. Successful treatment of diffuse esophageal spasm by peroral endoscopic myotomy. Gastrointest Endosc 2012. [Epub ahead of print].
67. Ellis FH Jr. Esophagomyotomy for noncardiac chest pain resulting from diffuse esophageal spasm and related disorders. Am J Med 1992;92(5A):129S–31S.
68. Patti MG, Pellegrini CA, Arcerito M, et al. Comparison of medical and minimally invasive surgical therapy for primary esophageal motility disorders. Arch Surg 1995;130(6):609–15 [discussion: 615–6].
69. Leconte M, Douard R, Gaudric M, et al. Functional results after extended myotomy for diffuse oesophageal spasm. Br J Surg 2007;94(9):1113–8.

Management of Achalasia

An J. Moonen, MD, Guy E. Boeckxstaens, MD, PhD*

KEYWORDS

- Achalasia • Laparoscopic Heller myotomy • Pneumatic dilation
- Peroral endoscopic myotomy • Botilinum toxin

KEY POINTS

- Achalasia is a motor disorder of the esophagus with dysphagia, regurgitation, and weight loss as the main symptoms.
- Manometry is the "gold standard" for diagnosing achalasia.
- Pneumatic dilation and laparoscopic Heller myotomy are the most commonly used treatment modalities and have comparable rates of success.
- Peroral endoscopic myotomy is an interesting new treatment with high short-term rates of success.
- Patients with achalasia should be monitored on a regular basis to prevent possible complications, such as sigmoidlike esophagus and esophageal carcinoma.

INTRODUCTION

Achalasia is a rare chronic motility disorder of the esophagus with an estimated annual incidence of 1 per 100,000 persons. It is characterized by the absence of peristalsis and defective relaxation of the lower esophageal sphincter (LES). These motor abnormalities result in impaired bolus propulsion and stasis of food in the esophagus, with dysphagia, retrosternal pain, and regurgitation of undigested food as the main symptoms.[1] Since the first description of achalasia by Sir Thomas Willis in 1974, several theories on pathophysiology have been reported. To date, it is widely accepted that the lack of relaxation in achalasia is due to a loss of inhibitory innervation of the LES. Nevertheless, the exact mechanism causing this loss of inhibitory neurons is far from elucidated and treatment is still confined to mechanical disruption of the LES. Treatment modalities available for this purpose include pneumatic dilation, laparoscopic Heller myotomy (LHM), and, recently, peroral endoscopic myotomy (POEM). In this review, the current management and treatment options of achalasia are discussed.

Funding Sources: GEB is supported by a grant (Odysseus program, G.0905.07) from the Flemish 'Fonds Wetenschappelijk Onderzoek' (FWO).
Conflict of Interest: There are no conflicts of interest.
Department of Gastroenterology, Translational Research Center for Gastrointestinal Disorders (TARGID), University Hospital of Leuven, Catholic University of Leuven, Herestraat 49, Leuven 3000, Belgium
* Corresponding author.
E-mail address: guy.boeckxstaens@med.kuleuven.be

Gastroenterol Clin N Am 42 (2013) 45–55
http://dx.doi.org/10.1016/j.gtc.2012.11.009
0889-8553/13/$ – see front matter © 2013 Elsevier Inc. All rights reserved.

gastro.theclinics.com

DIAGNOSIS

The diagnosis of achalasia is suspected in patients with dysphagia (94% of the patients), regurgitation (76%), heartburn (52%), and weight loss (35%).[2] The first diagnostic step is to rule out anatomic lesions and pseudoachalasia using endoscopy and barium swallow. Pseudoachalasia is a syndrome that may lead to a similar clinical picture as achalasia. Approximately 2% to 4% of patients suspected of achalasia suffer from pseudoachalasia. The most common cause of pseudoachalasia is malignancy infiltrating the gastroesophageal junction. In general, patients with pseudoachalasia are older and have a shorter history of symptoms, and weight loss is more prominent.[3] When pseudoachalasia is suspected, endoscopy, endoscopic ultrasound, or computed tomographic scanning of the chest can exclude an infiltrating malignancy.

In the early stages of idiopathic achalasia, both barium swallow and endoscopy can be normal. In more advanced cases, endoscopy may show a dilated esophagus with retained food and some resistance at the gastroesophageal junction. Barium swallow typically reveals a "bird-beak" image at the junction, with a dilated esophageal body and an air-fluid level in absence of an intragastric air bubble (**Fig. 1**). Barium swallow is of key importance in defining the morphology of the esophagus (diameter and axis) and associated conditions, such as epiphrenic diverticulae. Endoscopy is diagnostic in one-third of the patients; barium swallow is diagnostic in in two-thirds of the patients. Diagnostic certainty is provided by manometry in 90% of the patients and requires 2 pathognomonic abnormalities: aperistalsis of the esophageal body and an incomplete relaxation of the LES after deglutition.[4] However, despite the absence of peristalsis, there can still be substantial pressurization within the esophagus. Pandolfino and colleagues[5,6] proposed classification into 3 different subtypes: type I, classic achalasia with no evidence of pressurization; type II, panesophageal pressurization; and type III, vigorous achalasia or 2 or more spastic contractions of the distal esophageal segment (**Fig. 2**). Interestingly, the therapeutic response differs between the manometric subtypes: panesophageal pressurization is found to be a predictor

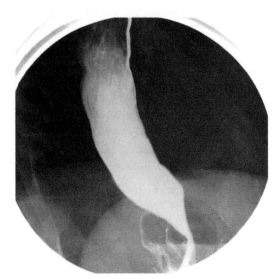

Fig. 1. Barium swallow showing a narrowing at the esophagogastric junction (bird-beak appearance) and an air-fluid level in the distal esophagus.

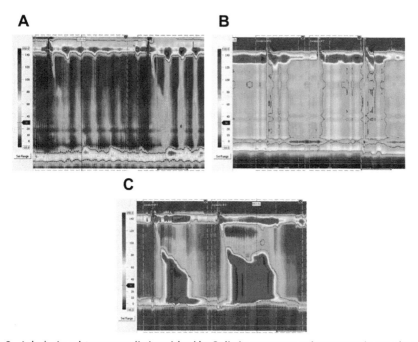

Fig. 2. Achalasia subtypes are distinguished by 3 distinct manometric patterns in esophageal body contractility. In type I (A) there is no evidence of pressurization and no esophagogastric junction relaxation. Type II (B) shows a panesophageal pressurization and type III or vigorous achalasia (C) is characterized by 2 or more spastic contractions of the distal esophageal segment. (*Modified from* Boeckxstaens G, Zaninotto G. Achalasia and esophagogastric junction outflow obstruction: focus on the subtypes. Neurogastroenterol Motil 2012;24(Suppl 1):27–31; with permission.)

of a positive treatment response, whereas spastic achalasia is associated with a negative treatment response. Adopting this classification will be useful in predicting outcomes in future prospective studies.

TREATMENT

As the pathophysiology of achalasia remains poorly understood, treatment is still confined to mechanical disruption of the LES. Treatment modalities available for this purpose include pharmacotherapy, pneumatic dilation, LHM, and, recently, POEM.

Pharmacologic Treatment

Reduction of the LES pressure can be achieved by smooth muscle relaxants. Nitrates or nitric oxide—related molecules increase the nitric oxide concentration in smooth muscle cells, which subsequently increases cyclic guanosine monophosphate levels, resulting in smooth muscle relaxation. Calcium channels blockers ensure smooth muscle relaxation by reducing the intracellular calcium, required for esophageal muscle contraction. Both nitrates and calcium channel blockers decrease LES pressure in a dose-dependent manner and thereby improve esophageal emptying. The results published are rather scarce and show only variable results with initial improvement ranging between 50% and 90%.[7] The effect, however, is transient due to tolerance, and side effects, such as hypotension, headache, and peripheral edema, are common. As a result, there is infrequently a place for these drugs in the clinical management of achalasia.

Endoscopic Injection of Botuline Toxine

As Botulinum toxin (Botox) is a potent inhibitor of acetylcholine release from nerve endings, it counteracts the unopposed LES contraction mediated by cholinergic nerves, thereby lowering LES pressure. In general, a total dose of 100 IU is endoscopically injected in the LES using a sclerotherapy needle, in 4 gifts, one in each quadrant. LES pressure decreases on average by 50% and esophageal emptying improves.[8] Increasing the dose to 200 IU does not improve rate of success, whereas repeating a 100 IU injection after 1 month may improve its efficacy.[9] Unfortunately, these effects are short lasting and decline in time: rates of success drop from 80% to 90% after 1 month to 60% to 70% after 6 months, and to only 53% to 54% after 1 year.[8,10,11] As a consequence, therapy has to be repeated, but the response decreases with further injections, probably from antibody production to the foreign protein.[12] Predictors of good clinical response are older age (>50) and vigorous achalasia. When compared with pneumatic dilation, its long-term efficacy is inferior and costs are higher.[12–14] Botox should be preferentially reserved for patients with significant comorbidity, excluding conventional treatment with laparoscopic myotomy or pneumatic dilation, or for patients on a waiting list for surgery.

Pneumatic Dilation

Pneumatic dilation aims at disrupting the LES by forceful inflation of an air-filled balloon. To date, the most commonly used balloon is the Rigiflex balloon (Boston Scientific Corp, Natick, MA, USA), which is commercially available in 3 diameters (3.0, 3.5, 4.0 cm). Briefly, this noncompliant polyethylene balloon is inserted over an endoscopically placed guidewire and positioned across the LES. After confirmation of the correct position, by either fluoroscopy or endoscopy, the balloon is inflated until the waist, caused by the impression of the esophagogastric junction, is completely flattened. The pressure required is usually 7 to 15 psi of air, held for 15 to 60 seconds. Although this technique has been introduced many years ago and is currently widely accepted, there is no real consensus on the distension protocol. Some investigators only perform 1 dilation,[15] but most use a graded dilation protocol with increasing balloon sizes starting with a 3.0-cm balloon, followed by a 3.5-cm balloon, and then a 4.0-cm balloon in subsequent sessions.[16–18] Graded dilation is more effective than single dilation with a 3.0-cm balloon. The 3-year rate of success for a single dilation with a 3.0-cm balloon is 37% in comparison to 86% for the graded dilation protocol.[19] Irrespective of the protocol used, a large portion of patients will relapse, mainly during the first year after treatment.[16,17] Risk factors for relapse are mainly young age, male sex, single dilation with a 3.0-cm balloon, posttreatment LES pressure greater than 10 to 15 mm Hg, and poor esophageal emptying on a timed barium swallow.[15,16,20–23] Long-term remission can be achieved in most of the patients with repeated pneumatic dilation.[18] However, selecting these patients remains a challenge because symptoms do not correlate with functional data (LES pressure measurements, stasis on barium swallow).

Pneumatic dilation can be safely performed after LHM, although larger diameter balloons are often required.[24] Rate of response is lower (50%) with no increased risk of complications.

Perforation is the most important and serious complication of pneumodilation with an overall rate of 1.9%.[25,26] Early diagnosis is crucial, either by assessment of pain evoked by ingestion of water 1 to 2 hours after the procedure or by routinely performing a postdilation radiograph of the esophagus using water-soluble contrast. In a recent retrospective study, Vanuytsel and colleagues[26] identified age (>60 years) as the most important risk factor for esophageal perforation (hazard ratio 3.4 compared with <60 years). In a large recent European trial, the risk for perforation was also significantly higher when the first dilation was performed with a 3.5-cm balloon compared with a 3.0-cm balloon.[27] Small perforations and deep painful tears can be managed conservatively with antibiotics and by ingesting nothing by mouth. However, surgical repair through thoracotomy is best for large, symptomatic perforations with extensive soiling of the mediastinum.

Other minor complications of pneumodilation are gastroesophageal reflux disease in 15% to 35% of the patients, and responding to proton pump inhibitors, chest pain, aspiration pneumonia, transient fever, and bleeding, usually without a decrease in hemoglobin.[23]

Laparoscopic Heller Myotomy

During LHM, an anterior myotomy of both muscular layers of the LES is performed extending 2 to 3 cm onto the proximal stomach, thereby decreasing the LES pressure and improving dysphagia. The LES pressure is more consistently lowered than with pneumatic dilation. Depending on the distal extent of the myotomy to the cardia, LES pressure is lowered by 55% to 75% with remaining LES pressure usually less than 10 mm Hg.[28] To reduce postoperative gastroesophageal reflux disease, a partial fundoplication (anterior Dor or posterior Toupet) is performed. In a study comparing Dor and Nissen (360°) fundoplication, the efficacy in preventing abnormal reflux was similar, but dysphagia was more frequently observed after Nissen fundoplication (2.8 vs 15%, $P<.001$).[29] Rates of success for LHM are high. A recent meta-analysis including 3086 patients reported rates of success of 89% after a mean follow-up of 35 months.[30] Younger patients, especially men and patients with higher LES pressure, may benefit most from primary surgery. However, similar to pneumatic dilation treatment, rates of success decline over time to 60% after 6 to 10 years.[16,31,32] In patients with recurrent symptoms after LHM, both pneumodilation and redo myotomy lead to good rates of success, ranging from 50% to 67% for pneumodilation and 58% to 87% for redo myotomy.[16,24,33]

Pneumatic Dilation Versus Laparoscopic Heller Myotomy

Before the introduction of laparoscopic surgery, repeated endoscopic pneumodilation had been the treatment of choice. This choice was mainly because open Heller myotomy is accompanied by a significant postoperative morbidity and requires several days of hospitalization. However, the situation has changed enormously in favor of surgery because most procedures are performed via the laparoscopic approach. Comparison between these 2 techniques is rather difficult because different groups of investigators often use different outcome measures, and randomized controlled data, comparing pneumodilation and LHM, were lacking until recently. A large retrospective longitudinal study of 1461 patents with a follow-up period of 10 years stated that patients who underwent peumodilation needed re-treatment more often than those who had LHM (64% vs 38%).[34] However, in this study, repeated pneumodilation was seen as an adverse outcome. Because "on-demand" pneumodilation is nowadays the accepted approach in achalasia treatment, this cannot be viewed as a failure of therapy. Another cross-sectional follow-up study of 179 patients (106 pneumodilation vs 73 LHM) showed similar rates of success for pneumodilation and LHM.[16] Recently, Boeckxstaens and colleagues[27] reported the results of a prospective, multicenter trial in which 201 patients were randomized to either graded pneumodilation (n = 95) or LHM (n = 106). In this study patients were allowed to be re-treated to a maximum of 3 series of pneumatic dilation. Both treatments had comparable rates of success at 2 years: 86% for pneumatic dilation and 90% for myotomy. Although in this study age was not a predictive factor of clinical success for either treatment, patients younger than the age of 40 treated with pneumodilation presented more often with recurrent symptoms requiring redilation. This finding seems to support the proposal to preferentially treat younger patients, especially men, with LHM.[35] Although longer follow-up is required, the data from the European achalasia trial indicate that both treatments are equally effective.

Peroral Endoscopic Myotomy

Recently a new endoscopic technique (POEM) was developed to treat achalasia. The endoscopist creates a submucosal tunnel to reach the LES and to dissect the circular muscle fibers over a length of 7 to 10 cm in the esophagus and 2 cm in the stomach. Inoue and colleagues[36] reported a rate of success of 100% and a significant reduction in LES pressure in 17 patients after a follow-up of 5 months. A recent European study reporting on their experience in 16 patients confirmed the high rate of success (94%).[37] Hungness and colleagues[38] reported results from a prospective nonrandomized trial comparing POEM versus laparoscopic Heller myotomy. Operation time was shorter in POEM, but therapeutic success (Eckard <3) after 6 months did not differ significantly between the 2 procedures (89%). It should be emphasized though that follow-up in these studies is still short and that prospective randomized trials comparing POEM to pneumodilation or LHM are needed to determine the place of POEM in the treatment of achalasia.

FOLLOW-UP

The current guidelines do not provide guidance on follow-up of patients with achalasia.[39,40] However, regular follow-up is important to ensure symptom control and to prevent evolution to end-stage achalasia with a dilated and decompensated esophagus.[41,42] Several studies have proposed that regular follow-up should be performed to decide on re-treatment, preferably based on the results of functional tests such as a timed barium swallow.[18,43] Furthermore, patients with longstanding achalasia are at risk of developing dysplasia and squamous cell carcinoma.[44,45] To date, regular endoscopic follow-up is not recommended because it does not seem cost-efficient.[46] However, with new endoscopic techniques, rates of detection can dramatically rise and thereby be cost-effective.

Re-Treatment

Treatment success gradually decreases in patients with longstanding achalasia (>10 years) to 40% to 60%.[17,22,34,47] This success implies that most of the patients will require additional treatment, fortunately with satisfactory results and rates of success of 60% to 80% after both pneumodilation and LHM.[22,24,42,48] Selecting patients in need of re-treatment is a clinical challenge because symptoms and functional data (LES pressure measurements, stasis on barium swallow) do not correlate. However, identifying patients in need of re-treatment is particularly important to avoid chronic stasis of food within the esophagus, even in the absence of symptoms, in view of the risk for dysplasia/neoplasia and the development of mega-esophagus, known to be associated with higher morbidity and refractory symptoms. Multiple studies have assessed risk factors for re-treatment after initial therapy. Vaezi and colleagues[23] have demonstrated that 90% of patients with esophageal stasis need additional treatment within a year, even if they have few or no symptoms shortly after initial treatment. The data from the European achalasia trial confirm that monitoring esophageal emptying after treatment is a helpful tool for predicting recurrence.[27] Recently Rohof and colleagues[49] showed that esophagogastric junction distensibility, measured with a new technique called EndoFLIP, a functional luminal imaging probe, is correlated with esophageal emptying and symptoms. Further studies are needed to determine the best parameter for re-treatment.

Management of End-Stage Achalasia

As stated before, rates of success decrease over time and eventually 10% to 15% of the patients will evolve to progressive deterioration of their esophageal function.[50,51] Five percent of these patients will end up with an "end-stage" achalasia, which is a massive dilated and sigmoidlike esophagus, despite appropriate initial treatment (**Fig. 3**).[48] Incomplete esophageal emptying with mucosal damage from reflux disease, unresponsive to treatment, is also part of the "end-stage" definition.[52] Despite a consensus on the need for esophagectomy in end-stage achalasia, most surgeons emphasize that a modified Heller myotomy should be attempted initially, even in patients with a dilated and sigmoid-shaped esophagus, reserving esophagectomy for failures.[25] After esophagectomy, reconstruction can be performed in different manners: with gastric, colon, or jejunal interposition. At present, from the published literature, gastric interposition is the first choice, but vascular supply to the stomach and significant reflux to the esophageal remnant affect its success as an ideal transplant.[52]

Screening for Carcinoma

A potential long-term complication of achalasia is the development of esophageal cancer. Several studies have shown an increased relative risk of developing esophageal carcinoma.[44,45,53] It is thought that food stasis, as seen in achalasia, leads to chronic

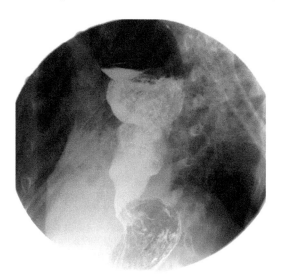

Fig. 3. Barium swallow of end-stage achalasia with a dilated, sigmoid-shaped esophagus.

inflammation of the esophageal mucosa, which potentially increases the risk of development of hyperplasia, dysplasia, and esophageal squamous cell carcinoma.[54–56] Also the incidence of adenocarcinomas is increased. A possible mechanism is that therapy, lowering the LES pressure, can aggravate acid gastroesophageal reflux, leading to Barrett's metaplasia and adenocarcinoma.[57,58] Recently, Leeuwenburgh and colleagues[45] reported results of a long-term prospective trial demonstrating a hazard ratio of 28 for esophageal carcinoma in patients with achalasia compared with matched controls. However, despite regular surveillance, most cancers were diagnosed in an advanced state. Symptoms of esophageal carcinoma in achalasia patients are often misinterpreted as merely symptoms of achalasia, and conventional white light endoscopy of the esophagus is not sensitive for the detection of dysplasia, leading to a diagnosis in an advanced stage of the carcinoma and a poor prognosis.[45] In a retrospective study, a rate of mortality as high as 19% because of esophageal carcinoma in patients with longstanding achalasia was reported.[53] The introduction of new endoscopic techniques, such as chromoendoscopy, high-resolution endoscopy, narrow band imaging, and virtual chromoendoscopy, has greatly improved detection of early lesions in both the esophagus and the large intestine.[59,60] The reported sensitivity of Lugol for the detection of dysplastic lesions in squamous epithelium varies in the literature between 80% and 96%.[61,62] Therefore, it would be a useful tool for endoscopic carcinoma surveillance. It can be argued that with these new tools, dysplastic lesions can be found in an early and curable stage, leading to better survival of patients. These data suggest that regular endoscopic carcinoma surveillance, especially in patients with longstanding achalasia (>15 years) and in patients with esophageal stasis, should be performed. However, further studies are needed to determine the benefit of such screening.

SUMMARY

As the pathophysiology of achalasia remains poorly understood, treatment is still confined to mechanical disruption of the LES. Patients with achalasia and an acceptable operative risk should be given the option of graded pneumodilation or LHM as both treatments have similar rates of success, which was recently demonstrated in a prospective, randomized trial.[27] Botox injection is a safe procedure but it is less effective than pneumodilation and LHM. Following treatment, patients should be followed up to guarantee symptom control and to prevent evolution to end-stage achalasia and/or esophageal carcinoma. Prognosis of the latter is generally poor because diagnosis is mostly made in an advanced stage. Hopefully, new endoscopic techniques, such as chromoendoscopy, can improve the detection of early dysplastic lesions and thereby the prognosis of achalasia patients.

REFERENCES

1. Boeckxstaens GE. The lower oesophageal sphincter. Neurogastroenterol Motil 2005;17(Suppl 1):13–21.
2. Fisichella PM, Raz D, Palazzo F, et al. Clinical, radiological, and manometric profile in 145 patients with untreated achalasia. World J Surg 2008;32(9):1974–9.
3. Gockel I, Eckardt VF, Schmitt T, et al. Pseudoachalasia: a case series and analysis of the literature. Scand J Gastroenterol 2005;40(4):378–85.
4. Howard PJ, Maher L, Pryde A, et al. Five year prospective study of the incidence, clinical features, and diagnosis of achalasia in Edinburgh. Gut 1992;33(8):1011–5.

5. Boeckxstaens G, Zaninotto G. Achalasia and esophago-gastric junction outflow obstruction: focus on the subtypes. Neurogastroenterol Motil 2012;24(Suppl 1): 27–31.

6. Pandolfino JE, Kwiatek MA, Nealis T, et al. Achalasia: a new clinically relevant classification by high-resolution manometry. Gastroenterology 2008;135(5): 1526–33.

7. Lake JM, Wong RK. Review article: the management of achalasia - a comparison of different treatment modalities. Aliment Pharmacol Ther 2006;24(6):909–18.

8. Hoogerwerf WA, Pasricha PJ. Pharmacologic therapy in treating achalasia. Gastrointest Endosc Clin N Am 2001;11(2):311–24, vii.

9. Annese V, Bassotti G, Coccia G, et al. A multicentre randomised study of intra-sphincteric botulinum toxin in patients with oesophageal achalasia. GISMAD Achalasia Study Group. Gut 2000;46(5):597–600.

10. Friedenberg F, Gollamudi S, Parkman HP. The use of botulinum toxin for the treatment of gastrointestinal motility disorders. Dig Dis Sci 2004;49(2):165–75.

11. Vittal H, Pasricha PF. Botulinum toxin for gastrointestinal disorders: therapy and mechanisms. Neurotox Res 2006;9(2–3):149–59.

12. Fishman VM, Parkman HP, Schiano TD, et al. Symptomatic improvement in achalasia after botulinum toxin injection of the lower esophageal sphincter. Am J Gastroenterol 1996;91(9):1724–30.

13. Mikaeli J, Fazel A, Montazeri G, et al. Randomized controlled trial comparing botulinum toxin injection to pneumatic dilatation for the treatment of achalasia. Aliment Pharmacol Ther 2001;15(9):1389–96.

14. Vaezi MF, Richter JE, Wilcox CM, et al. Botulinum toxin versus pneumatic dilatation in the treatment of achalasia: a randomised trial. Gut 1999;44(2): 231–9.

15. Eckardt VF, Gockel I, Bernhard G. Pneumatic dilation for achalasia: late results of a prospective follow up investigation. Gut 2004;53(5):629–33.

16. Vela MF, Richter JE, Khandwala F, et al. The long-term efficacy of pneumatic dilatation and Heller myotomy for the treatment of achalasia. Clin Gastroenterol Hepatol 2006;4(5):580–7.

17. West RL, Hirsch DP, Bartelsman JF, et al. Long term results of pneumatic dilation in achalasia followed for more than 5 years. Am J Gastroenterol 2002;97(6): 1346–51.

18. Zerbib F, Thetiot V, Richy F, et al. Repeated pneumatic dilations as long-term maintenance therapy for esophageal achalasia. Am J Gastroenterol 2006; 101(4):692–7.

19. Farhoomand K, Connor JT, Richter JE, et al. Predictors of outcome of pneumatic dilation in achalasia. Clin Gastroenterol Hepatol 2004;2(5):389–94.

20. Eckardt VF, Kanzler G, Westermeier T. Complications and their impact after pneumatic dilation for achalasia: prospective long-term follow-up study. Gastrointest Endosc 1997;45(5):349–53.

21. Ghoshal UC, Kumar S, Saraswat VA, et al. Long-term follow-up after pneumatic dilation for achalasia cardia: factors associated with treatment failure and recurrence. Am J Gastroenterol 2004;99(12):2304–10.

22. Hulselmans M, Vanuytsel T, Degreef T, et al. Long-term outcome of pneumatic dilation in the treatment of achalasia. Clin Gastroenterol Hepatol 2010;8(1): 30–5.

23. Vaezi MF, Baker ME, Achkar E, et al. Timed barium oesophagram: better predictor of long term success after pneumatic dilation in achalasia than symptom assessment. Gut 2002;50(6):765–70.

24. Guardino JM, Vela MF, Connor JT, et al. Pneumatic dilation for the treatment of achalasia in untreated patients and patients with failed Heller myotomy. J Clin Gastroenterol 2004;38(10):855–60.
25. Richter JE. Update on the management of achalasia: balloons, surgery and drugs. Expert Rev Gastroenterol Hepatol 2008;2(3):435–45.
26. Vanuytsel T, Lerut T, Coosemans W, et al. Conservative management of esophageal perforations during pneumatic dilation for idiopathic esophageal achalasia. Clin Gastroenterol Hepatol 2012;10(2):142–9.
27. Boeckxstaens GE, Annese V, des Varannes SB, et al. Pneumatic dilation versus laparoscopic Heller's myotomy for idiopathic achalasia. N Engl J Med 2011; 364(19):1807–16.
28. Oelschlager BK, Chang L, Pellegrini CA. Improved outcome after extended gastric myotomy for achalasia. Arch Surg 2003;138(5):490–5.
29. Rebecchi F, Giaccone C, Farinella E, et al. Randomized controlled trial of laparoscopic Heller myotomy plus Dor fundoplication versus Nissen fundoplication for achalasia: long-term results. Ann Surg 2008;248(6):1023–30.
30. Campos GM, Vittinghoff E, Rabl C, et al. Endoscopic and surgical treatments for achalasia: a systematic review and meta-analysis. Ann Surg 2009;249(1): 45–57.
31. Chen Z, Bessell JR, Chew A, et al. Laparoscopic cardiomyotomy for achalasia: clinical outcomes beyond 5 years. J Gastrointest Surg 2010;14(4):594–600.
32. Snyder CW, Burton RC, Brown LE, et al. Multiple preoperative endoscopic interventions are associated with worse outcomes after laparoscopic Heller myotomy for achalasia. J Gastrointest Surg 2009;13(12):2095–103.
33. Pallati PK, Mittal SK. Operative interventions for failed heller myotomy: a single institution experience. Am Surg 2011;77(3):330–6.
34. Lopushinsky SR, Urbach DR. Pneumatic dilatation and surgical myotomy for achalasia. JAMA 2006;296(18):2227–33.
35. Richter JE. A young man with a new diagnosis of achalasia. Clin Gastroenterol Hepatol 2008;6(8):859–63.
36. Inoue H, Minami H, Kobayashi Y, et al. Peroral endoscopic myotomy (POEM) for esophageal achalasia. Endoscopy 2010;42(4):265–71.
37. von RD, Inoue H, Minami H, et al. Peroral endoscopic myotomy for the treatment of achalasia: a prospective single center study. Am J Gastroenterol 2012;107(3): 411–7.
38. Hungness ES, Teitelbaum EN, Santos BF, et al. Comparison of Perioperative Outcomes Between Peroral Esophageal Myotomy (POEM) and Laparoscopic Heller Myotomy. J Gastrointest Surg 2012. [Epub ahead of print].
39. Spechler SJ. AGA technical review on treatment of patients with dysphagia caused by benign disorders of the distal esophagus. Gastroenterology 1999; 117(1):233–54.
40. Vaezi MF, Richter JE. Diagnosis and management of achalasia. American College of Gastroenterology Practice Parameter Committee. Am J Gastroenterol 1999; 94(12):3406–12.
41. Richter JE, Boeckxstaens GE. Management of achalasia: surgery or pneumatic dilation. Gut 2011;60(6):869–76.
42. Zaninotto G, Costantini M, Rizzetto C, et al. Four hundred laparoscopic myotomies for esophageal achalasia: a single centre experience. Ann Surg 2008; 248(6):986–93.
43. Gerson LB. Pneumatic dilation or myotomy for achalasia? Gastroenterology 2007; 132(2):811–3.

44. Eckardt AJ, Eckardt VF. Editorial: Cancer surveillance in achalasia: better late than never? Am J Gastroenterol 2010;105(10):2150–2.
45. Leeuwenburgh I, Scholten P, Alderliesten J, et al. Long-term esophageal cancer risk in patients with primary achalasia: a prospective study. Am J Gastroenterol 2010;105(10):2144–9.
46. Hirota WK, Zuckerman MJ, Adler DG, et al. ASGE guideline: the role of endoscopy in the surveillance of premalignant conditions of the upper GI tract. Gastrointest Endosc 2006;63(4):570–80.
47. Eckardt VF, Aignherr C, Bernhard G. Predictors of outcome in patients with achalasia treated by pneumatic dilation. Gastroenterology 1992;103(6):1732–8.
48. Vela MF, Richter JE, Wachsberger D, et al. Complexities of managing achalasia at a tertiary referral center: use of pneumatic dilatation, Heller myotomy, and botulinum toxin injection. Am J Gastroenterol 2004;99(6):1029–36.
49. Rohof WO, Hirsch DP, Kessing BF, et al. Efficacy of treatment for patients with achalasia depends on the distensibility of the esophagogastric junction. Gastroenterology 2012;143(2):328–35.
50. Ellis FH Jr, Watkins E Jr, Gibb SP, et al. Ten to 20-year clinical results after short esophagomyotomy without an antireflux procedure (modified Heller operation) for esophageal achalasia. Eur J Cardiothorac Surg 1992;6(2):86–9.
51. Okike N, Payne WS, Neufeld DM, et al. Esophagomyotomy versus forceful dilation for achalasia of the esophagus: results in 899 patients. Ann Thorac Surg 1979;28(2):119–25.
52. Duranceau A, Liberman M, Martin J, et al. End-stage achalasia. Dis Esophagus 2012;25(4):319–30.
53. Zaninotto G, Rizzetto C, Zambon P, et al. Long-term outcome and risk of oesophageal cancer after surgery for achalasia. Br J Surg 2008;95(12):1488–94.
54. Just-Viera JO, Morris JD, Haight C. Achalasia and esophageal carcinoma. Ann Thorac Surg 1967;3(6):526–38.
55. Porschen R, Molsberger G, Kuhn A, et al. Achalasia-associated squamous cell carcinoma of the esophagus: flow-cytometric and histological evaluation. Gastroenterology 1995;108(2):545–9.
56. Streitz JM Jr, Ellis FH Jr, Gibb SP, et al. Achalasia and squamous cell carcinoma of the esophagus: analysis of 241 patients. Ann Thorac Surg 1995;59(6):1604–9.
57. Ellis FH Jr, Gibb SP, Balogh K, et al. Esophageal achalasia and adenocarcinoma in Barrett's esophagus: a report of two cases and a review of the literature. Dis Esophagus 1997;10(1):55–60.
58. Feczko PJ, Ma CK, Halpert RD, et al. Barrett's metaplasia and dysplasia in post-myotomy achalasia patients. Am J Gastroenterol 1983;78(5):265–8.
59. Kawahara Y, Uedo N, Fujishiro M, et al. The usefulness of NBI magnification on diagnosis of superficial esophageal squamous cell carcinoma. Dig Endosc 2011;23(Suppl 1):79–82.
60. Uedo N, Fujishiro M, Goda K, et al. Role of narrow band imaging for diagnosis of early-stage esophagogastric cancer: current consensus of experienced endoscopists in Asia-Pacific region. Dig Endosc 2011;23(Suppl 1):58–71.
61. Dawsey SM, Fleischer DE, Wang GQ, et al. Mucosal iodine staining improves endoscopic visualization of squamous dysplasia and squamous cell carcinoma of the esophagus in Linxian, China. Cancer 1998;83(2):220–31.
62. Freitag CP, Barros SG, Kruel CD, et al. Esophageal dysplasias are detected by endoscopy with Lugol in patients at risk for squamous cell carcinoma in southern Brazil. Dis Esophagus 1999;12(3):191–5.

Gastroesophageal Reflux Disease and Sleep

Yasuhiro Fujiwara, MD[a], Tetsuo Arakawa, MD[a],
Ronnie Fass, MD[b],*

KEYWORDS

- Gastroesophageal reflux disease • Sleep disturbances • Heartburn
- Proton-pump inhibitor • Obstructive sleep apnea • pH monitoring • Actigraphy

KEY POINTS

- Nighttime gastroesophageal reflux (GER) events in the recumbent position can occur before falling asleep, after falling asleep as a result of a brief amnestic arousal, during conscious awakening from sleep, and immediately after waking up in the morning.
- GER events occur because of transient lower esophageal sphincter relaxation (TLESR), free reflux, hiatal hernia, or other causes, although the detailed mechanisms are likely complex and multi-factorial.
- Some of the GER events during sleep are symptomatic but most are asymptomatic.
- Aggressive acid-suppressive therapy or surgical intervention is required to control patients' symptoms during sleep time.
- The role of hypnotic drugs, TLESR reducers (γ-aminobutyric acid$_B$ agonists), or combinations of PPI and such drugs are currently under investigation.
- Future studies using a randomized placebo-controlled design are needed.

INTRODUCTION

Gastroesophageal reflux disease (GERD) is a chronic disorder characterized by typical bothersome symptoms such as heartburn and acid regurgitation.[1] A population-based study estimated that 20% of adults in the United States experience GERD symptoms at least weekly.[2] A recent report demonstrated that GERD is the most

Disclosures: Tetsuo Arakawa received a research grant and served as a consultant to Otsuka Pharmaceutical and Eisai. Ronnie Fass received research support from Reckitt Benckiser and Ephesus, speaker honorarium from Takeda, GSK, Astrazeneca, Eisai and Given Imaging, and served as a consultant to Given Imaging, Takeda, Perrigo, and Ironwood.
[a] Department of Gastroenterology, Osaka City University Graduate School of Medicine, 1-4-3 Asahi-machi, Abeno-ku, Osaka 545-8585, Japan; [b] Division of Gastroenterology and Hepatology, Esophageal and Swallowing center, MetroHealth Medical Center, Case Western Reserve University, 2500 MetroHealth Drive, Cleveland, OH 44109-1998, USA
* Corresponding author.
E-mail address: Ronnie.fass@gmail.com

common gastrointestinal (GI) diagnosis, accounting for approximately 9 million patient visits in the United States in 2009.[3] Heartburn occurs at any time throughout the day, whereas heartburn during sleep occurs only during conscious awakenings. Nighttime GERD is associated with more severe disease than daytime GERD, including worsened quality of life, impairment of work productivity, extraesophageal symptoms (hoarseness, wheezing, and coughing), daytime sleepiness, sleep disturbances, and esophageal complications (stricture, Barrett's esophagus, and esophageal adenocarcinoma).[4]

Recent studies have further explored the epidemiology, pathophysiology, diagnostic modalities, and therapy in GERD-related sleep disturbances. This review attempts to provide a summary of the current knowledge about GERD and sleep.

EPIDEMIOLOGY

A national survey demonstrated that 74% of the individuals who experienced GERD symptoms at least once a week also reported nighttime GERD symptoms. These symptoms occurred when patients lay down to sleep at night (69%), awoke from sleep at night (54%), woke up in the morning (40%), and awoke at night because of coughing or choking due to fluid, an acidic or bitter taste, or food in the throat (29%).[5] Another nationwide survey by the Gallup Organization demonstrated that 79% of the 1000 adults who experienced heartburn at least once a week had nighttime heartburn. Among these individuals, 75% reported that these symptoms affected their sleep, 63% believed that heartburn negatively affected their ability to sleep well, 40% believed that sleep difficulties caused by nighttime heartburn impaired their ability to function the following day, 42% stated that they accepted they could not sleep through the night, 39% reported that they took naps whenever possible, 34% reported sleeping in a chair or in a seated position, and 27% reported that their heartburn-induced sleep disturbances kept their spouses from having a good night's sleep.[6] In a large cohort evaluated by the Sleep Heart Health Study, 3806 of 15,314 subjects (25%) reported having heartburn that caused them to awaken from sleep 2 or more times per month. Heartburn that occurred during sleep was strongly associated with increased body mass index (BMI), consumption of carbonated soft drinks, snoring and daytime sleepiness, insomnia, hypertension, asthma, and benzodiazepine usage. College education was associated with a reduced risk for reporting heartburn during sleep.[7] A patient-reported survey conducted in 2006 among the general United States population revealed that 89% of participants experienced nighttime symptoms, 68% experienced sleep difficulties, 49% had difficulty falling asleep, and 58% reported difficulty in maintaining sleep.[8] These epidemiologic studies strongly indicate that nighttime GERD is very common and that most United States adults with GERD suffer from several types of GERD-related sleep abnormalities.

Sleep problems are also common in the general population. The 2008 National Sleep Foundation Sleep in America Poll demonstrated that approximately half of the participants reported nonrefreshing sleep a few nights per week or more, with 42% reporting frequent awakenings at night and 26% reporting difficulty in falling asleep.[9] Wallander and colleagues[10] performed a longitudinal, population-based cohort study of adults living in the United Kingdom. The investigators found that the diagnosis rate of a new sleep disorder was 12.5 per 1000 person-years, and prior GERD was identified as one of the risk factors for the development of sleep disturbances (odds ratio: 1.4; 95% confidence interval: 1.2–1.7). The latter study suggests that GERD precedes the development of sleep disturbances.

PATHOPHYSIOLOGY OF NIGHTTIME GERD AND ITS RELATED SLEEP DISTURBANCES

There are several differences in GI functions associated with GERD between wakeful and asleep periods. Basal gastric acid secretion is high during the late evening,[11] although no differences in gastric acid secretion have been observed among the different sleep stages.[12] Nocturnal acid breakthrough (NAB), defined as an intragastric pH less than 4.0 lasting for more than 1 hour during the night in patients taking a twice-daily proton-pump inhibitor (PPI),[13] might play a role in the pathogenesis of nighttime GERD, particularly in PPI-refractory cases.[14]

Several physiologic changes have been observed during sleep in comparison with the awake period, including delayed gastric emptying,[15] decrease in frequency of transient lower esophageal sphincter relaxation (TLESR),[16] decrease in basal upper esophageal sphincter pressure,[17] primary and secondary esophageal peristalsis.[18] Changes that occur during sleep with an impact on GERD, apart from those that affect the GI tract, include decreased saliva secretion[19] and swallowing responses.[20] It should be noted that TLESR, which plays a pivotal role in the pathogenesis of GERD, occurs only during arousals from sleep.[16] These physiologic changes that occur during sleep increase the likelihood of nighttime reflux in patients with GERD.

Several pathophysiological mechanisms might explain the bidirectional relationship between GERD and sleep disturbances. Awakening from sleep because of nighttime heartburn commonly results in the initiation of swallowing and a consequent increase in esophageal clearance.[21] Such response is necessary to prevent aspiration of reflux contents into the trachea. However, arousal from sleep is associated with impairment in sleep quality.[21] Recently, several new findings regarding the mechanisms underlying the relationship between GERD and sleep were reported using combined pH monitoring and actigraphy (an actigraph is a wristwatch-like device that has been shown to be highly comparable with a polysomnogram in determining durations of sleep and awakening). Poh and colleagues[22] found that the mean number of conscious awakenings detected by actigraphy was significantly higher in GERD patients than in controls. Of the conscious awakenings, 52% were associated with an acid reflux event in GERD patients, although they were seldom symptomatic. This finding confirmed that the presence of nighttime heartburn during sleep could not explain the full extent of the association between GERD and sleep disturbances.

Allen and colleagues[23] demonstrated that increased acid reflux during recumbency occurred primarily during the recumbent-awake and not the recumbent-asleep period, suggesting that nighttime reflux is associated with difficulty in falling asleep. Therefore, presentation of gastroesophageal reflux (GER) during the recumbent period in bed is different during recumbent-awake compared with the recumbent-asleep period.[24] Poh and colleagues[25] examined the differences in the characteristics of reflux episodes before (up to 1 hour) and immediately after (10 and 20 minutes) awakening from sleep in the morning. The investigators found an increase in the frequency of reflux events in the early morning, termed "riser's reflux," in approximately 50% of the GERD patients. These findings might be associated with early awakening in the morning. Dickman and colleagues[26] identified reflux events that are associated with short, amnestic arousals. This type of arousal is likely the precursor of prolonged acid reflux events during sleep. In addition, these types of acid reflux events during sleep might be associated with severe erosive esophagitis because lack of a conscious awakening response results in prolonged acid contact time with the esophageal mucosa. Short, amnestic arousals might also be associated with poorer quality of sleep due to sleep fragmentation. The aforementioned studies revealed that GERD could disturb sleep by causing difficulty in falling asleep, sleep fragmentation caused by multiple short amnestic arousals, or/and conscious awakenings and awakening in the early morning.

Poor sleep quality appears to affect GERD-related symptoms. Schey and colleagues[27] examined the role of sleep deprivation on esophageal mucosal acid sensitivity of 10 healthy controls and 10 GERD patients. A crossover study was performed in which the participants were randomized to either sleep deprivation (1 night with ≤3 hours of sleep) or sufficient sleep (3 consecutive days with ≥7 hours sleep per night) as confirmed by actigraphy. Subsequently, the subjects underwent intraesophageal acid infusion in the morning after sufficient sleep or sleep deprivation. The investigators found that sleep deprivation significantly shortened the lag time to symptom generation and enhanced the intensity rating of symptoms in comparison with sufficient sleep in the GERD group but not in the healthy controls.[27] This study suggests that sleep deprivation per se leads to or enhances esophageal sensitivity to acid, and was the first to suggest that poor sleep can exacerbate GERD. Thus, poor sleep can affect GERD and GERD can affect sleep.[28] **Fig. 1** summarizes the proposed mechanisms underlying the associations between GERD and sleep disturbances.[29]

OBSTRUCTIVE SLEEP APNEA

The *International Classification of Sleep Disorders* published by the American Academy of Sleep Medicine suggested that sleep disorders are divided into insomnias, sleep-related breathing disorders, hypersomnia of central origin, circadian rhythm sleep disorders, parasomnias, sleep-related movement disorders, and others.[30] Whereas the relationship between GERD and insomnia has been well substantiated, the association between GERD and other types of sleep disorders is either controversial or has not been fully elucidated.

Obstructive sleep apnea (OSA) is a sleep-related breathing disorder characterized by episodes of partial or complete obstruction of the upper airway, thus interrupting or reducing the flow of air. This process leads to transient awakening from sleep during the night. In the United States, the prevalence of OSA is estimated to be 3% to 7% in men and 2% to 5% in women.[31] Untreated OSA is currently recognized as an independent risk factor for the development of certain comorbid conditions such as hypertension, stroke, diabetes mellitus, and perioperative complications.[32]

Epidemiologic studies demonstrated that the prevalence of GERD, GER episodes, and heartburn in patients with OSA is higher than in normal, healthy controls.[28,33,34] However, the exact underlying mechanism of the relationship between OSA and GERD remains to be elucidated. Because negative intrathoracic pressure is generated against the closed airway during an apneic event, increases in the transdiaphragmatic pressure gradient could be responsible for GER in patients with OSA. However, a recent study using a combination of high-resolution manometry, pH-impedance monitoring, and polysomnography showed that esophageal body pressure decreased through apneic events, whereas end-inspiratory upper esophageal sphincter (UES) and gastroesophageal junction (GEJ) pressures progressively increased in patients with OSA.[35] Such compensatory changes in UES and GEJ pressures prevent reflux from occurring. Kuribayashi and colleagues[36] demonstrated that GER events were mainly induced by TLESR that occurred during arousals from sleep in OSA patients with and without reflux esophagitis. Therefore, apneic events in patients with OSA were not directly associated with most GER events. An increase in the transdiaphragmatic pressure gradient during apneic events might play a role in GER of some patients with OSA, especially those with hiatal hernia.[37]

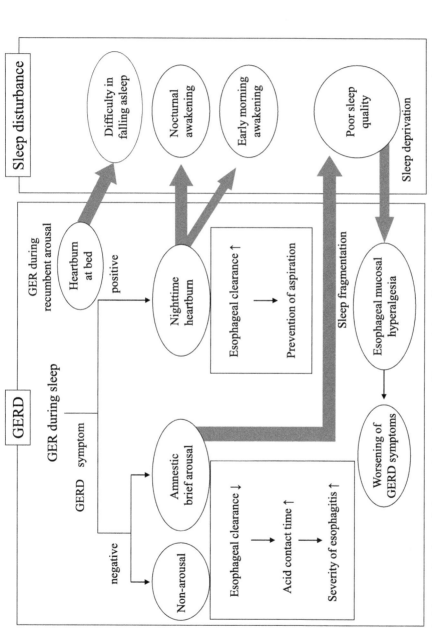

Fig. 1. The underlying mechanisms of the association between GERD and sleep disturbances. (*Adapted from* Fujiwara Y, Arakawa T, Fass R. Gastro-esophageal reflux disease and sleep disturbances. J Gastroenterol 2012;47:760–9; with permission.)

Only a few small studies have evaluated the effect of nasal continuous positive airway pressure therapy (nCPAP) on GER in patients with OSA. Kerr and colleagues[38] demonstrated that nCPAP reduced the percentage of total recording time that esophageal pH was less than 4.0 from 6.3% to 0.1%. Tawk and colleagues[39] showed that nCPAP normalized the esophageal acid exposure in 81% of patients with OSA and GERD. However, Ing and colleagues[33] demonstrated that nCPAP reduced the GER parameters in patients with OSA and those without OSA, suggesting that the effect of nCPAP was likely nonspecific. Morse and colleagues[40] demonstrated that GERD symptoms were unrelated to sleep apnea, and OSA was not influenced by the severity of GERD; they also identified old age (>65 years), male gender, and high BMI (>30 kg/m^2) as risk factors for sleep apnea.[40]

Because obesity is strongly associated with GERD and OSA, the relationship between OSA and GERD might be simply due to common risk factors. Thus at present there is insufficient evidence of a causal relationship between OSA and GERD, and the disorders are likely associated with each other through similar risk factors.

DIAGNOSIS OF NIGHTTIME GERD

If patients report having nighttime heartburn, the diagnosis of nighttime GERD is easily established. Nighttime breakthrough symptoms were the most common complaint reported by patients who failed PPI treatment. The challenge is to diagnose nighttime GERD in subjects who do not report GERD-related symptoms during the night. Nighttime GERD may solely present with sleep disturbances without typical GERD-related symptoms. Thus, in GERD patients reporting nighttime sleep abnormalities, GER should be excluded as the possible underlying cause.

In patients whose chief complaint is sleep problems, the presence of nighttime heartburn or other GERD-related symptoms should be determined. Orr and colleagues[41] reported that patients with sleep disturbances without heartburn have a significantly greater percentage of esophageal acid exposure in comparison with control individuals. Therefore, the presence of "silent GERD" should be considered in cases of unexplained sleep disturbances following a standard assessment of sleep disorders. In such cases, an upper endoscopy followed by impedance-pH testing should be considered. Alternatively, an empiric trial with a PPI may be attempted. A diagnostic algorithm for nighttime GERD is shown in **Fig. 2**.

TREATMENT OF NIGHTTIME GERD
Lifestyle Modification

A systematic review revealed that only elevation of the head of the bed and weight loss had sufficient evidence to support their value as lifestyle modifications in GERD patients.[42] Elevation of the head of the bed significantly decreased esophageal acid exposure, increased acid clearance time, and improved severity of erosive esophagitis.[43] Shaker and colleagues[6] reported that GERD patients with nighttime heartburn selected several lifestyle modifications such as avoiding food before bed, drinking or eating something, and elevating the head of the bed, but the efficacy of each of these measures was limited and unsatisfactory. However, avoiding late night meals and snacks might improve nighttime GERD, because it reduces the chances of experiencing gastroesophageal reflux during sleep time. This recommendation is supported by data showing that a shorter dinner-to-bed time (<3 hours) was significantly more commonly associated with GERD related symptoms compared with longer dinner-to-bed time (≥3 hours),[44] and that a significant

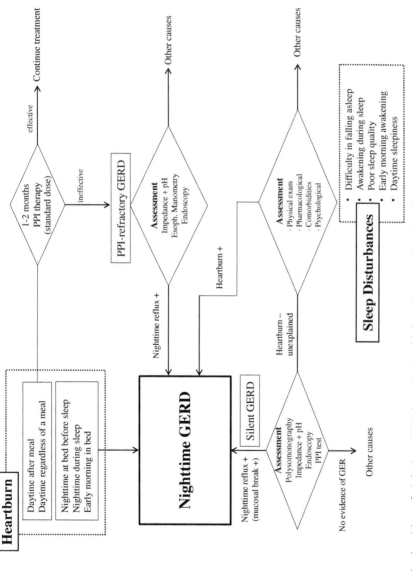

Fig. 2. Diagnostic algorithm of nighttime GERD in patients with heartburn or sleep disturbances.

increase in GER in the recumbent position was more commonly associated with late meal consumption.[45]

Thus, avoidance of a late-night meal and elevation of the head of the bed are important therapeutic strategies for nighttime GERD and its related sleep disturbances. In addition, any pharmacologic intervention for nighttime GERD should also incorporate the aforementioned lifestyle modifications.

Acid-Suppressive Agents

Sufficient control of gastric acid secretion at night and, possibly, the prevention of NAB are important pharmacologic therapeutic strategies for nighttime GERD and its related sleep disturbances. Numerous clinical trials have evaluated the effects of different doses and administration timing of acid-suppressive drugs such as PPIs on nighttime gastric acid secretion and the occurrence of NAB using 24-hour intragastric and esophageal pH monitoring. However, only a few clinical trials included improvement of sleep disturbances as a clinical end point.

There have been 3 high-quality, large, placebo-controlled, randomized trials that assessed the value of PPIs in improving nighttime GERD and sleep.[46–48] Johnson and colleagues[46] compared the efficacy of esomeprazole, 40 mg or 20 mg, versus placebo given once daily in 650 patients with GERD-related sleep disturbances and moderate to severe nighttime heartburn. Both doses of esomeprazole significantly relieved nighttime heartburn and GERD-related sleep disturbances, and this improved sleep quality in comparison with placebo. However, a dose-response effect was not documented in this study. Johnson and colleagues[47] confirmed these previous results in a follow-up study using a similar design in patients with moderate to severe nighttime heartburn and GERD-related sleep disturbances. Esomeprazole, 20 mg given once daily, significantly relieved nighttime heartburn compared with placebo (34% vs 10%). In addition, esomeprazole, 20 mg was significantly better in reducing the number of days with GERD-related sleep disturbances. Esomeprazole also significantly improved sleep quality, work productivity, and regular daily activities. Fass[48] compared the efficacy of dexlansoprazole modified release (MR), 30 mg, with placebo in relieving nighttime heartburn and GERD-related sleep disturbances among 305 GERD patients. The study found that dexlansoprazole MR, 30 mg in the morning, significantly improved the median percentage of nights without heartburn (73% vs 36%, respectively), and GERD-related sleep disturbances. In addition, increase in sleep quality resulted in improved morning activities and work productivity. Although these 3 large clinical trials and others[49] demonstrated that PPIs significantly improved subjective sleep disturbances in GERD patients, 2 studies have failed to demonstrate significant improvement in objective sleep parameters using polysomnographic techniques in GERD patients treated with PPIs versus placebo.[21,50] Orr and colleagues[21] found that rabeprazole, 20 mg twice a day, improved nighttime GERD-related symptoms and sleep quality but did not alter objective sleep parameters such as latency of sleep onset, sleep efficiency, arousals per hour, and the proportion of deeper sleep stages. Another study demonstrated that esomeprazole, 40 mg twice daily, significantly improved nighttime GER events but did not affect sleep parameters such as total sleep time, sleep efficiency, and latency of sleep onset.[50] The lack of a PPI effect on polysomnographic parameters might be related to the small sample size. Alternatively, it is highly likely that polysomnography parameters are not sensitive enough to detect the effect of PPIs on patients' sleep experience. Overall, these studies clearly suggest that PPI treatment improves nighttime GERD symptoms as well as subjective reports of sleep quality. However, the full effect of PPI treatment on objective sleep parameters remains unclear.

Antireflux Surgery

A few studies assessed the effect of antireflux surgery on GERD-related sleep disturbances. Cohen and colleagues,[51] using a case-controlled study, showed that antireflux surgery improved subjective parameters such as difficulty in falling asleep, but not objective sleep parameters, in 11 GERD patients. Johannessen and colleagues[52] reported sleep difficulties in operated GERD patients when compared with matched nonoperated GERD patients during 3 to 10 years of follow-up. The investigators found a tendency toward less sleeplessness in operated patients than in nonoperated patients, although the difference did not reach statistical significance. Further prospective studies are needed to assess the efficacy of surgical interventions in improving GERD-related sleep disturbances. In particular, whether surgical fundoplication improves subjective as well as objective sleep parameters in operated GERD patients.

Hypnotics

The role of hypnotics in improving GERD has been raised because of the bidirectional relationship between GERD and sleep quality. If poor sleep worsen GERD-related symptoms than potentially by improving sleep, GERD may improve as well. However, benzodiazepines decrease the lower esophageal sphincter (LES) basal pressure[53] and increase the risk of nighttime GERD symptoms, as has been shown in an epidemiologic cohort study.[7] Therefore, benzodiazepines should not be used for the treatment of sleep disturbances in GERD patients. Gagliardi and colleagues[54] examined the effect of zolpidem, a nonbenzodiazepine drug (γ-aminobutyric acid [GABA]$_A$ receptor agonist), on arousals from sleep in response to nighttime reflux using polysomnography and pH monitoring. Zolpidem treatment was found to significantly reduce the number of arousal episodes in response to nighttime acid reflux but to increase the duration of each esophageal acid reflux event during sleep in both controls and GERD patients. These results suggest that zolpidem might prolong reflux because of the lack of an arousal from sleep in response to acid reflux. Melatonin (MT), a hormone released from the pineal gland, is increased at night and decreased during the day. This hormone plays a role in the regulation of the circadian rhythm. Recently, Jha and colleagues[55] examined the effects of ramelteon (an MT1/MT2 agonist) on nighttime GERD symptoms and sleep quality. In comparison with placebo, ramelteon reduced nighttime symptom score and insomnia severity index, and improved objective sleep parameters such as sleep efficiency and sleep latency. This study suggests that ramelteon might be a useful treatment for GERD-related sleep disturbances. Whether, in addition to PPI treatment, hypnotic drugs such as GABA$_A$ agonists and ramelteon can improve GERD and its related sleep disturbances remains to be elucidated.

GABA$_B$ Agonists

Baclofen, a GABA$_B$ agonist, has been reported to reduce postprandial reflux events and acid exposure time in GERD patients by reducing TLESR rate.[56] Orr and colleagues[57] examined the effects of baclofen on nighttime heartburn and sleep in 21 individuals with GERD symptoms using pH monitoring and polysomnography. Compared with placebo, 40 mg baclofen before bedtime significantly reduced the number of reflux events and improved several variables of sleep parameters such as total sleep time and sleep efficiency, awakening after sleep onset, and subjective sleep quality. The investigators speculated that baclofen may confer its effect by reducing TLESR rate and improving sleep quality. The latter can improve GERD by also reducing the TLESR rate as well as esophageal perception of acidic stimuli.[14]

Table 1
Summary of the associations between nighttime reflux and sleep

Position	Night	Recumbent		Morning
		Asleep ———→ Arousal		
Consciousness status	Awake	Asleep		Awake
Consciousness status at GER event	Awake	Brief amnestic arousal	Arousal	Awake
Pathogenesis of GER	TLESR	TLESR	TLESR / Free reflux	TLESR
Duration of GER	Short	Short/long	Short	Short
Sleep-related symptoms	Difficulty in falling asleep	Sleep fragmentation = poor sleep quality	Awakening from sleep	Awakening in the morning
GERD symptoms	May be present	Absent	May be present	May be present
Proposed treatment	PPI before dinner; Avoid late meal	High doses of PPI	PPI in combination with GABA$_B$ agonist, ramelteon, or nonbenzodiazepine	PPI before dinner

Abbreviations: GABA, γ-aminobutyric acid; PPI, proton-pump inhibitor; TLESR, transient lower esophageal sphincter relaxation.

SUMMARY

Table 1 summarizes the possible associations between GERD and sleep, and includes the proposed therapies. Nighttime GER events in the recumbent position can occur before falling asleep, after falling asleep as a result of a brief amnestic arousal, during conscious awakening from sleep, and immediately after waking up in the morning. These GER events occur because of TLESR, free reflux, hiatal hernia, or other triggers, although the detailed mechanisms are likely complex and multifactorial. Some of the GER events are symptomatic but most are asymptomatic. GER events that are associated with short amnestic arousals may result in prolonged esophageal acid exposure, and thus are more likely to be associated with esophageal inflammation. Consequently, aggressive acid-suppressive therapy or surgical intervention (in carefully selected individuals) is required to control patients' symptoms. In other patterns of GER, a PPI should be used as the first-line of treatment, but timing of administration and dosing of PPI should be individualized. Additional options such as hypnotic drugs, TLESR reducers (GABA$_B$ agonists), or combinations of PPI and such drugs are currently under investigation. Future studies using a randomized, placebo-controlled design are urgently needed.

REFERENCES

1. Vakil N, van Zanten SV, Kahrilas P, et al. The Montreal definition and classification of gastroesophageal reflux disease: a global evidence-based consensus. Am J Gastroenterol 2006;101:1900–20.
2. Locke GR 3rd, Talley NJ, Fett SL, et al. Prevalence and clinical spectrum of gastroesophageal reflux: a population-based study in Olmsted County, Minnesota. Gastroenterology 1997;112:1448–56.
3. Peery AF, Dellon ES, Lund J, et al. Burden of gastrointestinal disease in the United States: 2012 update. Gastroenterology 2012;143:1179–87.
4. Orr WC. Sleep-related gastro-oesophageal reflux as a distinct clinical entity. Aliment Pharmacol Ther 2010;31:47–56.
5. Farup C, Kleinman L, Sloan S, et al. The impact of nocturnal symptoms associated with gastroesophageal reflux disease on health-related quality of life. Arch Intern Med 2001;161:45–52.
6. Shaker R, Castell DO, Schoenfeld PS, et al. Nighttime heartburn is an underappreciated clinical problem that impacts sleep and daytime function: the results of a Gallup survey conducted on behalf of the American Gastroenterological Association. Am J Gastroenterol 2003;98:1487–93.
7. Fass R, Quan SF, O'Connor GT, et al. Predictors of heartburn during sleep in a large prospective cohort study. Chest 2005;127:1658–66.
8. Mody R, Bolge SC, Kannan H, et al. Effects of gastroesophageal reflux disease on sleep and outcomes. Clin Gastroenterol Hepatol 2009;7:953–9.
9. Swanson LM, Arnedt JT, Rosekind MR, et al. Sleep disorders and work performance: findings from the 2008 National Sleep Foundation Sleep in America poll. J Sleep Res 2011;20:487–94.
10. Wallander MA, Johansson S, Ruigómez A, et al. Morbidity associated with sleep disorders in primary care: a longitudinal cohort study. Prim Care Companion J Clin Psychiatry 2007;9:338–45.
11. Moore JG. Circadian dynamics of gastric acid secretion and pharmacodynamics of H2 receptor blockade. Ann N Y Acad Sci 1991;618:150–8.
12. Stacher G, Presslich B, Stärker H. Gastric acid secretion and sleep stages during natural night sleep. Gastroenterology 1975;68:1449–55.

13. Peghini PL, Katz PO, Castell DO. Ranitidine controls nocturnal gastric acid break-through on omeprazole: a controlled study in normal subjects. Gastroenterology 1998;115:1335–9.
14. Fass R. Proton pump inhibitor failure—what are the therapeutic options? Am J Gastroenterol 2009;104(Suppl 2):S33–8.
15. Goo RH, Moore JG, Greenberg E, et al. Circadian variation in gastric emptying of meals in humans. Gastroenterology 1987;93:515–8.
16. Dent J, Dodds WJ, Friedman RH, et al. Mechanism of gastroesophageal reflux in recumbent asymptomatic human subjects. J Clin Invest 1980;65:256–67.
17. Kahrilas PJ, Dodds WJ, Dent J, et al. Effect of sleep, spontaneous gastroesophageal reflux, and a meal on upper esophageal sphincter pressure in normal human volunteers. Gastroenterology 1987;92:466–71.
18. Pasricha PJ. Effect of sleep on gastroesophageal physiology and airway protective mechanisms. Am J Med 2003;115(Suppl 3A):114S–8S.
19. Schneyer LH, Pigman W, Hanahan L, et al. Rate of flow of human parotid, sublingual, and submaxillary secretions during sleep. J Dent Res 1956;35:109–14.
20. Lear CS, Flanagan JB Jr, Moorrees CF. The frequency of deglutition in man. Arch Oral Biol 1965;10:83–100.
21. Orr WC, Goodrich S, Robert J. The effect of acid suppression on sleep patterns and sleep-related gastro-oesophageal reflux. Aliment Pharmacol Ther 2005;21:103–8.
22. Poh CH, Allen L, Gasiorowska A, et al. Conscious awakenings are commonly associated with acid reflux events in patients with gastroesophageal reflux disease. Clin Gastroenterol Hepatol 2010;8:851–7.
23. Allen L, Poh CH, Gasiorowska A, et al. Increased oesophageal acid exposure at the beginning of the recumbent period is primarily a recumbent-awake phenomenon. Aliment Pharmacol Ther 2010;32:787–94.
24. Poh CH, Gasiorowska A, Allen L, et al. Reassessment of the principal characteristics of gastroesophageal reflux during the recumbent period using integrated actigraphy-acquired information. Am J Gastroenterol 2010;105:1024–31.
25. Poh CH, Allen L, Malagon I, et al. Riser's reflux—an eye-opening experience. Neurogastroenterol Motil 2010;22:387–94.
26. Dickman R, Parthasarathy S, Malagon IB, et al. Comparisons of the distribution of oesophageal acid exposure throughout the sleep period among the different gastro-oesophageal reflux disease groups. Aliment Pharmacol Ther 2007;26:41–8.
27. Schey R, Dickman R, Parthasarathy S, et al. Sleep deprivation is hyperalgesic in patients with gastroesophageal reflux disease. Gastroenterology 2007;133:1787–95.
28. Fass R. Effect of gastroesophageal reflux disease on sleep. J Gastroenterol Hepatol 2010;25(Suppl 1):S41–4.
29. Fujiwara Y, Arakawa T, Fass R. Gastroesophageal reflux disease and sleep disturbances. J Gastroenterol 2012;47:760–9.
30. American Academy of Sleep Medicine. International classification of sleep disorders. 2nd edition. Chicago: Diagnostic and Coding Manuals; 2005.
31. Punjabi NM. The epidemiology of adult obstructive sleep apnea. Proc Am Thorac Soc 2008;5:136–43.
32. Park JG, Ramar K, Olson EJ. Updates on definition, consequences, and management of obstructive sleep apnea. Mayo Clin Proc 2011;86:549–54.
33. Ing AJ, Ngu MC, Breslin AB. Obstructive sleep apnea and gastroesophageal reflux. Am J Med 2000;108(Suppl 4a):120S–5S.

34. Fujiwara Y, Arakawa T. Epidemiology and clinical characteristics of GERD in the Japanese population. J Gastroenterol 2009;44:518–34.
35. Kuribayashi S, Massey BT, Hafeezullah M, et al. Upper esophageal sphincter and gastroesophageal junction pressure changes act to prevent gastroesophageal and esophagopharyngeal reflux during apneic episodes in patients with obstructive sleep apnea. Chest 2010;137:769–76.
36. Kuribayashi S, Kusano M, Kawamura O, et al. Mechanism of gastroesophageal reflux in patients with obstructive sleep apnea syndrome. Neurogastroenterol Motil 2010;22:611-e172.
37. Kahrilas PJ. Obstructive sleep apnea and reflux disease: bedfellows at best. Chest 2010;137:747–8.
38. Kerr P, Shoenut JP, Millar T, et al. Nasal CPAP reduces gastroesophageal reflux in obstructive sleep apnea syndrome. Chest 1992;101:1539–44.
39. Tawk M, Goodrich S, Kinasewitz G, et al. The effect of 1 week of continuous positive airway pressure treatment in obstructive sleep apnea patients with concomitant gastroesophageal reflux. Chest 2006;130:1003–8.
40. Morse CA, Quan SF, Mays MZ, et al. Is there a relationship between obstructive sleep apnea and gastroesophageal reflux disease? Clin Gastroenterol Hepatol 2004;2:761–8.
41. Orr WC, Goodrich S, Fernström P, et al. Occurrence of nighttime gastroesophageal reflux in disturbed and normal sleepers. Clin Gastroenterol Hepatol 2008;6:1099–104.
42. Kaltenbach T, Crockett S, Gerson LB. Are lifestyle measures effective in patients with gastroesophageal reflux disease? An evidence-based approach. Arch Intern Med 2006;166:965–71.
43. Gerson LB, Fass R. A systematic review of the definitions, prevalence, and response to treatment of nocturnal gastroesophageal reflux disease. Clin Gastroenterol Hepatol 2009;7:372–8.
44. Fujiwara Y, Machida A, Watanabe Y, et al. Association between dinner-to-bed time and gastro-esophageal reflux disease. Am J Gastroenterol 2005;100:2633–6.
45. Piesman M, Hwang I, Maydonovitch C, et al. Nocturnal reflux episodes following the administration of a standardized meal. Does timing matter? Am J Gastroenterol 2007;102:2128–34.
46. Johnson DA, Orr WC, Crawley JA, et al. Effect of esomeprazole on nighttime heartburn and sleep quality in patients with GERD: a randomized, placebo-controlled trial. Am J Gastroenterol 2005;100:1914–22.
47. Johnson D, Crawley JA, Hwang C, et al. Clinical trial: esomeprazole for moderate-to-severe nighttime heartburn and gastro-oesophageal reflux disease-related sleep disturbances. Aliment Pharmacol Ther 2010;32:182–90.
48. Fass R, Johnson DA, Orr Wc, et al. The effect of dexlansoprazole MR on nocturnal heartborn and GERD-related sleep disturbances in patients with symptomatic GERD. Am J Gastroenterol 2011;106:421–31.
49. Regenbogen E, Helkin A, Georgopoulos R, et al. Esophageal reflux disease proton pump inhibitor therapy impact on sleep disturbance: a systematic review. Otolaryngol Head Neck Surg 2012;146:524–32.
50. Orr WC, Craddock A, Goodrich S. Acidic and non-acidic reflux during sleep under conditions of powerful acid suppression. Chest 2007;131:460–5.
51. Cohen JA, Arain A, Harris PA, et al. Surgical trial investigating nocturnal gastroesophageal reflux and sleep (STINGERS). Surg Endosc 2003;17:394–400.

52. Johannessen R, Petersen H, Olberg P, et al. Airway symptoms and sleeping diffi-culties in operated and non-operated patients with gastroesophageal reflux disease. Scand J Gastroenterol 2012;47:762–9.

53. Rushnak MJ, Leevy CM. Effect of diazepam on the lower esophageal sphincter. A double-blind controlled study. Am J Gastroenterol 1980;73:127–30.

54. Gagliardi GS, Shah AP, Goldstein M, et al. Effect of zolpidem on the sleep arousal response to nocturnal esophageal acid exposure. Clin Gastroenterol Hepatol 2009;7:948–52.

55. Jha LK, Gadam R, Grewal YS, et al. Rozerem improves reports of symptoms in GERD patients with chronic insomnia. Gastroenterology 2012;142(Suppl 1): S592 (abstarct).

56. Lidums I, Lehmann A, Checklin H, et al. Control of transient lower esophageal sphincter relaxations and reflux by the GABAB agonist baclofen in normal subjects. Gastroenterology 2000;118:7–13.

57. Orr WC, Goodrich S, Wright S, et al. The effect of baclofen on nocturnal gastro-esophageal reflux and measures of sleep quality: a randomized, cross-over trial. Neurogastroenterol Motil 2012;24:553–9.

Extraesophageal Manifestations of Gastroesophageal Reflux Disease

Christopher Hom, MD, Michael F. Vaezi, MD, PhD, MSc (Epi)*

KEYWORDS

- Extraesophageal reflux syndrome • Laryngopharyngeal reflux • Chronic laryngitis
- Asthma • Chronic cough

KEY POINTS

- The pulmonary and ear/nose/throat manifestations of gastroesophageal reflux disease (GERD) are important commonly encountered extraesophageal syndromes.
- Upper gastrointestinal endoscopy and pH monitoring are poorly sensitive markers for diagnosing reflux in this group of patients.
- Instead, it is recommended that in those without warning symptoms, an empiric trial of proton-pump inhibitors be the initial approach to the diagnosis and treatment of the potential underlying cause of these extraesophageal symptoms.
- Diagnostic testing, including pH and/or impedance monitoring, may be important in further evaluating those with poor response, to essentially exclude GERD as the cause of persistent symptoms.

INTRODUCTION

Gastroesophageal reflux disease (GERD) is an acid-based disorder that presents with a wide spectrum of symptoms. In 2006, the modified Delphi process was used to define GERD as "a condition which develops when the reflux of stomach contents causes troublesome symptoms and/or complications."[1] Historically, GERD is defined as primary complaints of heartburn and regurgitation[1–4]; however, it is now recognized that a range of extraesophageal symptoms may be its sole or accompanying manifestation. For example, chronic cough, asthma, posterior laryngitis, and dental erosion are but a few extraesophageal manifestations of GERD (**Fig. 1**).[1,5] Extraesophageal reflux (EER) symptoms can occur concomitantly with or without typical GERD

Division of Gastroenterology, Hepatology and Nutrition, Center for Swallowing and Esophageal Disorders, Vanderbilt University Medical Center, 1301 Medical Center Drive, Nashville, TN 37232, USA
* Corresponding author. Division of Gastroenterology and Hepatology, Center for Swallowing and Esophageal Disorders, Vanderbilt University Medical Center, 1301 Medical Center Drive, C2104-MCN, Nashville, TN 37232.
E-mail address: Michael.vaezi@vanderbilt.edu

Gastroenterol Clin N Am 42 (2013) 71–91
http://dx.doi.org/10.1016/j.gtc.2012.11.004
0889-8553/13/$ – see front matter © 2013 Elsevier Inc. All rights reserved.

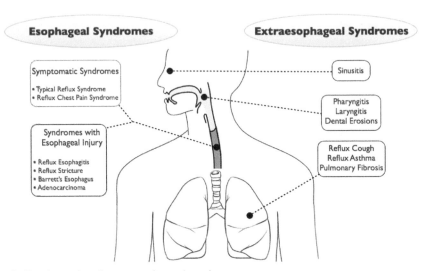

Fig. 1. Esophageal and extraesophageal syndromes.

symptoms, which in the latter may delay the diagnosis of reflux as a potential etiologic factor. The prevalence of reflux disease is increasing around the world, with Western Europe, North America, and South America having the highest prevalence rates of approximately 20% to 40%.[6–8] GERD has become an important public health issue owing to the considerable health care resources used to treat it. The annual direct cost of GERD management is cited at $971 per patient in the United States,[9] with national expenditures ranging from $9.3 billion[10] to $12.1 billion.[11] More concerning are the recent data showing that the cost of caring for patients with EER is 5 times that of GERD, at nearly $50 billion (Fig. 2).

The pathophysiologic consequence of reflux in patients with EER symptoms affects both upper and lower respiratory systems, including asthma, chronic cough, hoarseness, otitis media, atypical loss of dental enamel, idiopathic pulmonary fibrosis, recurrent pneumonia, chronic bronchitis, and even sudden infant death syndrome.[12–16] Two responsible mechanisms comprise direct (aspiration) and indirect (vagally mediated) (Fig. 3).[1,17–21]

The direct mechanism involves aspirate that directly stimulates the pharynx or larynx, causing a tracheal or bronchial cough reflex. The presence of an intact lower esophageal sphincter (LES) and upper esophageal sphincter (UES) barrier usually

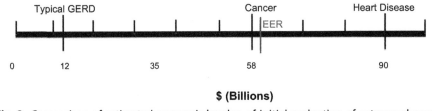

$ (Billions)

Fig. 2. Comparison of estimated economic burden of initial evaluation of extraesophageal reflux (EER) with that of typical GERD, cancer, and heart disease.

Pathophysiology of Extraesophageal Manifestations

Reflux Theory

- Reflux through esophageal sphincters causing pulmonary, larygneal, pharyngeal, or extraesophageal symptoms

- Direct contact of gastric refluxate with bronchial and laryngeal areas

Reflex Theory

- Reflux into distal esophagus stimulates vagally-mediated reflex

- Common embryonic origins between esophagus and bronchial tree

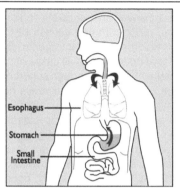 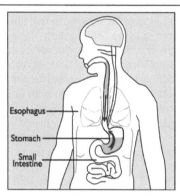

Fig. 3. Reflux and reflex pathophysiologic mechanisms in extraesophageal manifestations of GERD.

prevents gastroesophagopharyngeal reflux. Although the LES is frequently breached by gastric contents in both physiologic and pathophysiologic states, the high basal pressure of the UES usually prevents pharyngeal and laryngeal contact with refluxate.[22] Furthermore, the UES pressure is augmented when distal reflux results in increased intraesophageal pressure. The pharynx and upper airway are further protected by the esophagoglottic closure reflex, which protects the airway from contact with proximal refluxate.[23] In addition, swallowing or cough functions to clear refluxate that does breach the UES. These and other physiologic protective mechanisms usually prevent refluxate from violating the pharyngeal and laryngeal space and thereby causing symptoms and tissue damage. Perturbation of any of these, or other less or currently unknown protective mechanisms, could possibly account for the production of pulmonary, laryngeal, pharyngeal, or other extraesophageal symptoms of reflux disease.[24]

The second mechanism involves distal esophageal reflux that produces a cough response by a vagally mediated process (see **Fig. 3**).[25] Given that the esophagus and bronchial tree share a common embryonic origin, it is not surprising that they also share a common neural innervation. Acidification of the distal esophagus can stimulate acid-sensitive receptors that may result in cardiac-type chest pain or interact with pulmonary bronchi and other upper airway structures via a vagally mediated arc.[21,26] Further, reflux-related chronic cough has been linked to changes in the chronic pressure gradient between the abdominal and thoracic cavities during the act of coughing, leading to a positive feedback cycle between reflux and coughing symptoms.[26,27] It is currently unknown if gastric acid, duodenal contents, microbial contamination, or some combination of the 3 cause the worsening symptoms in those with extraesophageal manifestations of GERD.[28,29] Aspiration of gastric acid or duodenal contents has been shown to cause damage to the larynx, pharynx, and lung, and certainly microbial contamination of aspirated contents can cause pulmonary symptoms.[30] Patients receiving immunosuppressive regimens may be particularly susceptible to such damage.[31]

This review discusses the current state of knowledge regarding the relationship between GERD and pulmonary and ear/nose/throat (ENT) manifestations of reflux, and outlines recent developments in the diagnostic and treatment strategies for this difficult group of patients.

REFLUX COUGH SYNDROME

In nonsmoking patients with normal chest radiographs who are not taking angiotensin-converting enzyme (ACE) inhibitors, some of the most common causes of chronic cough are postnasal drip syndrome, asthma, chronic bronchitis, and gastroesophageal reflux (**Fig. 4**). These 4 conditions may represent up to 90% of all cases of chronic cough, defined as cough lasting longer than 8 weeks.[32,33] Reflux cough syndrome has a well-established association with GERD. Large population-based surveys demonstrate an increased risk of chronic cough among patients with reflux symptoms or esophagitis.[34–36] Chronic cough and bronchitis are documented symptoms in 30% to 50% of patients suffering from GERD.[37] Similarly, other studies have shown a high prevalence of objective signs of GERD in patients with chronic cough. In a retrospective analysis of pH-monitoring results, pathologic esophageal acid exposure was demonstrated in 52% of patients with chronic cough.[38] Poe and Kallay[26] concluded that GERD alone accounted for cough in 13% of their study population while in 56% of patients it was a contributing factor to chronic cough.

Reflux cough syndrome may essentially be considered a diagnosis of exclusion. As such, the 2 other common causes of chronic cough, asthma and postnasal drip syndrome (PDS), must be initially ruled out. According to Irwin,[27] the evaluation of chronic cough begins with patients with normal chest radiographs and who are not taking ACE inhibitors so as to avoid their confounding influence. It is surprisingly common to find patients with chronic cough who are referred to gastroenterology for evaluation of GERD who continue to be on ACE inhibitors. Thus, this important cause of chronic cough must be explored in every patient presenting with the

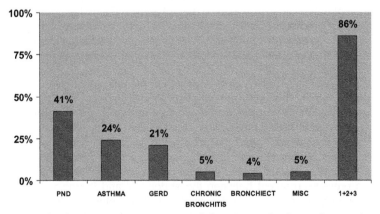

Fig. 4. GERD is the third most common cause of chronic cough after asthma and postnasal drainage (PND). These 3 causes can account for 86% of all etiology for chronic cough, and often multiple causes exist in a given patient. BRONCHIECT, bronchiectasis; MISC, miscellaneous.

condition. In addition, the authors strongly recommend identification and treatment of all potential contributing factors because reflux therapy alone may not be adequate in achieving symptom resolution in this group of patients.

One complexity in attributing reflux as a contributing etiologic factor in chronic cough is that many patients do not exhibit the classic symptoms of GERD. In fact, Ing and colleagues[18] reported that up to 75% of patients with reflux cough syndrome may not exhibit regurgitation or heartburn. Similarly, Poe and Kallay[26] found that 43% of their sample population exhibited no GERD symptoms at all. Another study by Everett and Morice[39] found that nearly 40% of patients presenting with chronic cough did not report typical symptoms of reflux. Therefore, lack of concomitant typical reflux symptoms cannot be used to exclude GERD as a potential cause in patients with chronic cough.

Further complicating the diagnosis of reflux cough syndrome is the low sensitivity of common diagnostic tests for GERD, including esophagogastroduodenoscopy (EGD) and pH monitoring.[40] Typically, EGD is used to evaluate for the presence of esophagitis and other mucosal irregularities associated with GERD, including Barrett's esophagus. However, esophagitis is a diagnosis of low prevalence in this group of patients and its presence is not causally linked to chronic cough, thus making EGD a poor diagnostic tool for reflux cough syndrome. For example, in the study by Baldi and colleagues[33] of 45 patients with chronic cough evaluated using EGD, 55% of the study group complained of classic reflux symptoms, whereas only 15% had EGD-proven esophagitis.

Ambulatory 24-hour esophageal pH monitoring was previously considered to be the gold standard for diagnosing GERD.[40] However, in patients with chronic cough its specificity is as low as 66%.[21,27] pH monitoring in such patients has also been used to correlate reflux episodes with coughing fits. Using this technique, Baldi and colleagues[33] found that in their population of patients with chronic cough, 53% had pathologic reflux correlating with cough fits. However, compared with less invasive tests such as empiric proton-pump inhibitor (PPI) therapy, esophageal pH monitoring is found to have low diagnostic gain.[32,33] For example, Ours and colleagues[32] found that pH monitoring was not a reliable predictor of acid reflux–induced chronic cough because only 35% of patients in their study population with abnormal pH monitoring responded to PPI therapy. One important advantage of pH monitoring in chronic cough may be the ability to correlate esophageal reflux episodes with cough symptoms by using the 2 most commonly used indices, symptom index (SI) or symptom association probability (SAP). However, a recent study by Slaughter and colleagues[41] concluded that both SI and SAP indices can be overinterpreted and are prone to misinterpretation. The investigators suggested that unless patients with GERD refractory to PPI therapy have high rates of esophageal acid exposure, both SI and SAP accuracy are essentially chance occurrences at best. Furthermore, using ambulatory acoustic monitoring it was recently reported that up to 71% to 91% of patients do not accurately report their cough events (**Fig. 5**), which further reduces the enthusiasm regarding the use of symptom indices in pH monitoring.[42] Another study using an acoustic cough monitoring device showed that cough temporally associates with reflux irrespective of proposed diagnoses and that it may be self-perpetuating in some patients, likely because of central processes and not just reflux.[43] Thus, given the low predictive value of pH testing, lack of reliability of symptom-association probability, and temporal association, which may not be causal, pH testing in patients with chronic cough may be problematic.

In patients with chronic cough suspected to be GERD related, most experts recommend empiric PPI therapy, often with twice-daily dosing. This recommendation is

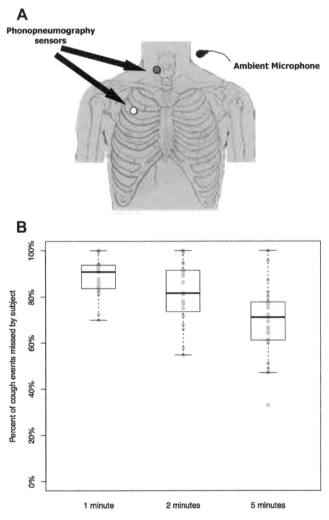

Fig. 5. (*A*) Positioning of the acoustic cough sensors in the chest wall and neck. Cough events were detected via phonopneumography sensors positioned at 2 sites: to the right of the trachea at the midpoint between the Adam's apple and the substernal notch, and at the midclavicular line in the second intercostal space. An ambient microphone was af- fixed to the patient's shirt collar. (*B*) Box-plot illustration of the median (interquartile range) percentage of cough events missed by the individual subjects compared with the audio recording by 1-, 2-, and 5-minute time windows. Patients did not report 91%, 82%, and 71% of cough events detected by audio recording within 1, 2, and 5 minutes of those de- tected by audio recording, respectively.

based solely on open-label trials, and placebo-controlled studies do not support a benefit to PPI therapy in this group. For example, Poe and Kallay[26] diagnosed 79% of patients with cough secondary to GERD, with resolution of symptoms after an empiric trial of PPI therapy. A recent study by Baldi and colleagues[33] sug- gested that once-daily PPI therapy may be similar to twice-daily therapy. However, a meta-analysis of 5 placebo-controlled studies in adult patients with chronic cough found insufficient evidence in favor of PPI therapy.[29] In agreement with the conclusions of this meta-analysis, most recently 2 additional randomized controlled studies[44,45] did not find any benefit to PPI therapy in comparison with placebo in adult subjects with chronic cough. Taken together, these studies suggest the uncertainty of association between chronic cough and GERD, most likely attributable to poor diagnostic tests leading to inappropriate patient selection in the controlled studies. Nevertheless, a short course of PPI therapy is a reasonable initial approach. A positive response to initial empiric PPI therapy is the best indicator for eventual resolution.[33] However, it is important that the patient response is assessed shortly after initiation of PPI therapy to avoid prolonged use of such therapies. A recent cost analysis of subjects with chronic cough found that the most costly aspect of evaluation and treatment of this group of patients is the prolonged, often unnecessary, use of PPI therapy at high doses.[46] With respect to the role of surgical fundoplication, the authors recently showed that the response to surgical intervention of patients with chronic cough may be dependent on the concomitant presence at baseline of typical symptoms of GERD (heartburn and regurgitation).[47]

In recent years, the term sensory neuropathic cough has been used to describe patients with recalcitrant cough after excluding other causes including GERD. This condition seems to result from a lowered response threshold to stimuli, just as in post-herpetic neuralgic pain, and does not respond to the usual therapies including PPIs.[48] It is sudden and comes in attacks, and can be triggered by a factor such as eating, talking, or deep breathing. It can result in oculorrhea and rhinorrhea, vomiting, laryngospasm, and syncope or near-syncope.[48] It is estimated that up to 31% of patients with chronic cough may have sensory neuropathic cough.[49] Recent study suggested symptomatic improvement of this type of cough with gabapentin.[50–52] Thus, in patients with chronic cough in whom other causes are excluded, there may be some benefit in off-label use of neuromodulator medications such as amitriptyline (10 mg/d), gabapentin (100–900 mg/d), and pregabalin (150 mg, twice a day maximum). Amitriptyline is a tricyclic antidepressant. Pregabalin and gabapentin are very similar in structure, and are analogues of γ-aminobutyric acid (GABA). These agents do not bind to $GABA_A$ or $GABA_B$; instead they bind to the subunits on presynaptic calcium channels, and decrease the release of the neurotransmitters glutamate, noradrenaline, and substance P.[53]

In conclusion, a systematic approach with an anatomy-based protocol should be followed in diagnosing the cause of chronic cough. Common causes including medication (ACE inhibitors), postnasal drip, and asthma must be excluded. In those with concomitant heartburn and/or regurgitation or those with high degree of suspicion for GERD, an empiric trial of PPI therapy for 1 to 2 months is a reasonable approach. EGD and 24-hour esophageal pH and/or impedance monitoring should be reserved for patients in whom GERD is still suspected and for whom treatment does not eliminate the cough. In this group, complete lack of response to PPI therapy may be an indicator that causes other than GERD should be sought. Such causes include other lung-related diseases as well as sensory neuropathic cough.

REFLUX ASTHMA SYNDROME

Based on pH probe monitoring,[54,55] gastroesophageal reflux disease is present in up to 80% of asthmatic patients and often occurs without gastrointestinal symptoms.[56,57] The triggers that incite an inflammatory response can also exacerbate asthma, which is made possible because the esophagus and lung share embryonic origins that may permit complex interactions. For instance, acid-induced bronchoconstriction can be provoked by a vagally mediated reflex, neural enhanced bronchial reactivity, or micro-aspiration. Neurogenic inflammation in the lung may occur with either vagally mediated mechanisms or with microaspiration. These findings lend biological plausibility to the theory that GERD may induce asthma symptoms either by direct effects on airway hyperresponsiveness or via aspiration-induced inflammation.[58] Conversely, bronchoconstriction seen in asthma may induce acid reflux. Lung hyperinflation in asthmatic patients increases the pressure gradient between the abdomen and chest and may cause the LES to herniate into the chest, where its barrier function is impaired.[59,60]

A significant portion of patients with asthma also exhibit typical symptoms of GER, such as heartburn and regurgitation (**Fig. 6**). However, as in those with chronic cough, lack of the classic symptoms does not rule out physiologic acid reflux. Havemann and colleagues[61] found that the average prevalence of GERD in asthma was 59.2%, a potential underestimation because many patients may not exhibit typical symptoms of reflux. Another study by Kiljander and colleagues[62] found that 35% of asthma patients in their study did not have typical reflux symptoms, but were instead found to have reflux by 24-hour esophageal pH monitoring.

Ambulatory pH monitoring has been used to assess reflux and its association with asthma. Meier and colleagues[63] concluded that 50% of their patients with asthma had abnormal esophageal pH parameters. Similarly, Kiljander and colleagues[62] found 53% of patients with asthma had pathologic GER diagnosed by ambulatory pH monitoring. Furthermore, 35% of these patients did not have typical reflux symptoms of heartburn and regurgitation. In 2005, Leggett and colleagues[64] evaluated GER in patients with difficult-to-control asthma by dual 24-hour ambulatory pH probes configured with both distal and proximal probes. The prevalence of reflux at the distal and proximal probes was 55% and 35%, respectively. In 2007, Havemann and colleagues[61] reviewed the association between GER and asthma and estimated the prevalence of abnormal acid exposure diagnosed by pH monitoring to be 51%. However, given the less than optimal sensitivity of pH monitoring, its use is often confined to those who continue to be symptomatic despite therapy.

As is the case for most EER conditions, there is controversy regarding the benefit of PPI use in patients suspected of having reflux-induced asthma. Studies have used different end points regarding efficacy of acid-suppressive therapy in this group. Some use objective measurements such as improvement in forced expiratory volume in 1 second (FEV_1), whereas others rely on patient-reported questionnaires or decreasing need for asthma medications. Early trials reported improvements in

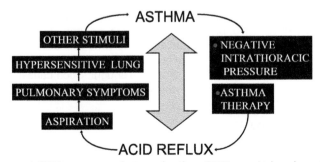

Fig. 6. Asthma and GERD may exacerbate each other. GERD may induce bronchospasm and asthma may induce GERD. Breaking the cycle by aggressively treating both is the key to improvement of patients' symptoms.

pulmonary symptoms and pulmonary function in patients treated with acid-suppressive therapy.[65] In 1994, Meier and colleagues[63] conducted a double-blind, placebo-controlled crossover study, which evaluated pulmonary function of asthma patients treated with 20 mg of omeprazole twice a day for 6 weeks. This study found that 27% (4 of 15) patients with reflux had a 20% or greater increase in FEV_1.

In another study, Sontag and colleagues[65] evaluated 62 patients with both GERD and asthma, and divided the group into 3 treatment arms: control, treatment of reflux with ranitidine 150 mg 3 times a day, or surgical treatment with Nissen fundoplication. After a 2-year follow-up, 75% of surgical patients had improvement in nocturnal asthma exacerbations, compared with 9.1% and 4.2% of patients on medical therapy and controls, respectively. In addition, there was a statistically significant improvement in mean asthma symptom score, but no improvement in pulmonary function or reduction in the need for medication between the groups. Littner and colleagues[66] followed 207 patients with symptomatic reflux who were treated with either placebo or a PPI twice a day for 24 weeks. The primary outcome of the study was daily asthma symptoms by patient diary, and secondary outcomes included the need for rescue albuterol inhaler use, pulmonary function, asthma quality of life, investigator-assessed asthma symptoms, and asthma exacerbations. The study showed that medical treatment of reflux did not reduce daily asthma symptoms or albuterol use and did not improve pulmonary function in this group of asthmatic patients. Similarly, a study conducted by the American Lung Association Asthma Clinical Research Center[67] randomized 412 patients with poor asthma control to either esomeprazole 40 mg twice daily or placebo. After 24 weeks of follow-up, no treatment benefit was shown by PPI therapy in asthma control. Most recently, a randomized controlled trial in children with asthma without overt GERD did not show a benefit of lansoprazole in improvement of symptoms or lung function.[68] A Cochrane review of therapy for GERD patients with asthma found only minimal improvement of asthma symptoms with reflux therapy.[69] Encouragingly, a recent controlled trial in asthmatics suggested a therapeutic benefit of PPIs in the subgroup of asthmatics with both nocturnal respiratory and GERD symptoms.[70] Thus, the issue of asthma control by treating reflux in patients who have asthma is not yet clear.

Therefore, the current recommendation in patients with asthma (with or without concomitant heartburn or regurgitation) is similar to that for patients with chronic cough and laryngitis, suggesting the initial empiric trial of once- or twice-daily PPIs for 2 to 3 months. In those responsive to therapy for both heartburn and/or asthma symptoms, PPIs should be tapered to the minimal dose necessary to control symptoms. In unresponsive patients, testing for reflux, by pH testing and/or impedance/pH monitoring, may be needed to measure for continued reflux of acid or nonacid material, or, more commonly, to exclude reflux as the cause of patients' continued symptoms.

REFLUX LARYNGITIS SYNDROME

The pathophysiology of the laryngeal manifestations of GERD is thought to be related to direct acid-peptic injury to the larynx via esophagopharyngeal reflux or acidification of the distal esophagus through vagally mediated reflexes. This process results in chronic throat clearing and coughing, which eventually lead to the evolution of laryngeal mucosal signs and symptoms.[71,72]

Patients with unexplained vocal and throat changes may have reflux of gastroduodenal contents as a contributing or exacerbating factor.[73] GERD is implicated as an important cause of laryngeal inflammation.[74] Symptoms and signs that have been suggested as GERD related, also termed laryngopharyngeal reflux (LPR) by ENT physicians, include vocal-cord nodules, posterior laryngitis, laryngospasms, hoarseness, dysphonia, subglottic stenosis, laryngeal cancer, and globus pharyngeus (**Boxes 1 and 2**).[75] These signs and symptoms are nonspecific, and can also be seen in patients with postnasal drip and environmental exposure to allergens or other irritants such as smoke.[76] Heartburn and regurgitation occur in some, but not all, patients.

Earlier studies suggested that pepsin may be the main cause for LPR symptoms[77–79]; however, later studies suggested the coimportance of acid, pepsin, and bile acids.[19] There is now a resurgence of publications on the role of pepsin in LPR. Some suggest that reflux of pepsin into the larynx, with subsequent pepsin transfer into the cytoplasm of the laryngeal cells and later activation in the cell organelles with lower pH ranges than the lumen, may be an important contributor to LPR.[80] Dilation of intercellular spaces (DIS) is reported to be an early morphologic marker in GERD, reflecting the alteration of esophageal mucosal integrity. However, recent studies assessing DIS in patients suspected of LPR and GERD did not show a difference in epithelial-space separation between patients and a group of controls,[81] thus questioning the uniform reflux-related epithelial presence of DIS.

Currently available tests for reflux detection in patients suspected with LPR have significant limitations because of their optimal sensitivity and/or specificity, and often they do not predict response to therapy (**Table 1**). For example, Laryngoscopy is considered an important tool for the diagnosis of reflux-associated laryngeal symptoms; however, the commonly used laryngoscopic findings of LPR (see **Box 2**) are often highly subjective, and when present in many normal subjects without GERD are not specific.[82–85] For example, Milstein and colleagues,[84] who evaluated 52 nonsmoker volunteers with no history of ENT abnormalities or GERD, highlighted the nonspecific nature of laryngeal evaluation. This cohort underwent both rigid and flexible videolaryngoscopy. The investigators found that in this asymptomatic normal population there was at least 1 sign of tissue irritation in 93% of flexible and 83% of rigid laryngoscopic evaluation. In addition, the findings were dependent on the technique. Laryngeal signs were more commonly reported on flexible transnasal laryngoscopy than on rigid transoral examination. The high prevalence of laryngeal irritation in normal volunteers combined with the variability of the diagnosis based on methods used highlights the uncertainty associated with laryngeal signs in LPR.

Box 1
Symptoms associated with gastroesophageal reflux laryngitis

- Hoarseness
- Dysphonia
- Sore or burning throat
- Excessive throat clearing
- Chronic cough
- Globus
- Apnea
- Laryngospasm
- Dysphagia
- Postnasal drip
- Neoplasm

Box 2
Potential laryngopharyngeal signs associated with gastroesophageal reflux laryngitis

- Edema and hyperemia of larynx
- Hyperemia and lymphoid hyperplasia of posterior pharynx (cobblestoning)
- Contact ulcers
- Laryngeal polyps
- Granuloma
- Interarytenoid changes
- Subglottic stenosis
- Posterior glottic stenosis
- Reinke edema
- Tumors

A test commonly used to diagnose reflux in those with laryngitis is ambulatory pH monitoring. The role of pH monitoring in establishing a relationship between GERD and LPR is not clear, and its application in the diagnosis of reflux esophagitis may not be as useful as was once thought.[74,86] It was initially thought that patients with

Table 1
Advantages and disadvantages of methods for detecting esophageal reflux

Method	Advantages	Disadvantages
Endoscopy	Easy visualization of mucosal damage/erosions	Poor sensitivity/specificity/PPV Requires sedation High cost
Laryngoscopy	No sedation required Direct visualization of the larynx and laryngeal abnormality	No specific laryngeal signs for reflux Overdiagnoses GERD
pH monitoring	Easy to perform Relatively noninvasive Prolonged monitoring Ambulatory	Many are catheter based May have up to 30% false-negative rate No pH predictors of treatment response in LPR
Impedance monitoring	Easy to perform Relatively noninvasive Prolonged monitoring Ambulatory Measures acidic and nonacidic gas and liquid reflux (combined with pH)	Catheter based False negative rate unknown but most likely similar to catheter-based pH monitoring Unknown clinical relevance when abnormal on PPI therapy Unknown importance in LPR
ResTech Dx-pH	Faster detection rate and faster time to equilibrium pH than traditional pH catheters	Unknown if clinically useful in patients with LPR
Lateral flow device for pepsin	Fast and easy detection of salivary pepsin Acceptable sensitivity and specificity	Limited outcome studies

Abbreviations: LPR, laryngopharyngeal reflux; PPI, proton-pump inhibitor; PPV, positive predictive value; ResTech Dx-pH, Dx-pH measurement system (Respiratory Technology Corp, San Diego, CA).

symptoms of reflux-related laryngitis would have more reflux events in the upper esophageal and hypopharyngeal regions. However, Joniau and colleagues[87] demonstrated that up to 43% of normal subjects without LPR symptoms may have abnormal hypopharyngeal pH monitoring. Furthermore, they found no statistical difference in the prevalence of pharyngeal reflux events in symptomatic patients in comparison with normal volunteers. Another study has shown that only 54% of patients with suspected LPR have abnormal esophageal acid exposure.[88,89]

In patients who remain symptomatic despite aggressive acid-suppressive therapy, recent studies suggest that nonacid reflux may play a role in their symptoms measured by pH and/or impedance monitoring.[90,91] Unlike traditional dual-channel pH probe testing that only reports acidic changes in the esophagus, impedance monitoring can determine the presence of any remaining physiologic reflux regardless of pH. Furthermore, unlike other probe modalities, this device can detect the frequency, location, and direction of any gas or liquid refluxate along the esophagus as well as in the hypopharynx.[92] Unfortunately, outcome studies with impedance monitoring are lacking, and their clinical significance with regard to medically recalcitrant LPR patients still remains unclear.[93–96]

Studies assessing patients with heartburn and regurgitation in addition to patients with extraesophageal symptoms suggest that 10% to 40% of patients on twice-daily PPI therapy may have persistent nonacid reflux.[96,97] However, causation between these nonacid reflux events and persistent symptoms is difficult to establish.[98] A recent study found that abnormal impedance in patients on therapy predicts acid reflux in patients off therapy.[99] The study also concluded that in patients with refractory reflux, combined impedance/pH monitoring might provide the single best strategy for evaluating reflux symptoms. However, the clinical significance of abnormal impedance findings in this group of patients awaits further study. The most recent uncontrolled surgical study in patients suspected of having LPR found that on or off therapy, impedance monitoring does not predict LPR symptom response to fundoplication, but presence of hiatal hernia, significant acid reflux at baseline, and presence of regurgitation concomitantly with LPR symptoms were important predictors of symptom response.[100]

The Dx-pH measurement system (Respiratory Technology Corp, San Diego, CA) is a sensitive and minimally invasive device for detection of acid reflux in the posterior oropharynx, which is increasingly being used in patients with LPR.[101] It uses a nasopharyngeal catheter (the Restech pH catheter) to measure pH in either liquid or aerosolized droplets (**Fig. 7**). A comparison of this device with the traditional pH catheters has shown a faster detection rate and faster time to equilibrium pH. A recent prospective observational study[102] in healthy volunteers developed normative data for this device at pH cutoff of 4, 5, and 6 for the distal esophagus and oropharynx. The initial studies with this device in patients with LPR are encouraging.[101] Moreover, the most recent study suggested a significantly higher number of reflux events detected by Restech pH in LPR patients than in patients with GERD and healthy volunteers, concluding that the device may hold promise in the evaluation of those with suspected GERD-related LPR.[103] However, controlled outcome–driven studies are needed to assess the future role of this new device in this group of patients who are difficult to diagnose and manage.

Detection of salivary pepsin has been advocated as an objective method of diagnosing reflux in recent years.[104] Pepsin is a proteolytic enzyme secreted from the chief cells in the gastric fundus as pepsinogen, and activated in the acidic environment.[105] Using an enzymatic method, Potluri and colleagues[104] compared salivary pepsin activity with proximal and distal esophageal pH results in 16 reflux patients, and found

A

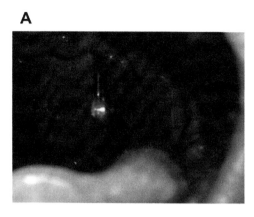

B

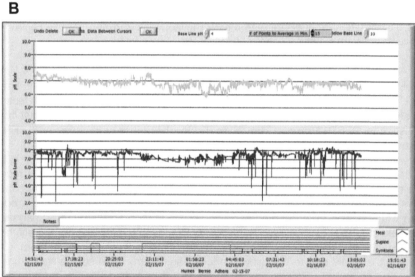

Fig. 7. (*A*) Dx-pH probe and light-emitting diode positioned in the oropharynx. (*B*) Typical tracing of distal esophageal (*lower trace*) and oropharyngeal (*upper trace*) pH monitoring in a healthy volunteer.

that the mean proximal and distal pH values correlated with findings of salivary pepsin assay. The investigators concluded that salivary pepsin assay might be a noninvasive method to assess for proximal reflux. Whereas Ozmen and colleagues[106] found 100% sensitivity and 92.3% specificity for pepsin assay in nasal lavage fluid in chronic rhino-sinusitis patients, Printza and colleagues[107] did not demonstrate any peptic activity in saliva samples from 93 LPR patients. Using a Western blot technique for sputum and salivary pepsin samples in patients with EER, Kim and colleagues[108] reported sensitivity and specificity of 89% and 68%, respectively, based on the pH-monitoring results. Recently a novel pepsin rapid test (Peptest-Biomed) is also being used as a convenient, office-based, noninvasive, quick, and inexpensive technique in LPR diagnosis. This lateral flow device (LFD) uses 2 monoclonal antibodies to human pepsin (**Fig. 8**). The results can be read in 5 to 15 minutes.[109] The authors recently conducted a prospective, blinded study of salivary pepsin assay in 59 patients with objective GERD (esophagitis or abnormal pH testing) in a comparison with 51 control

Sample well

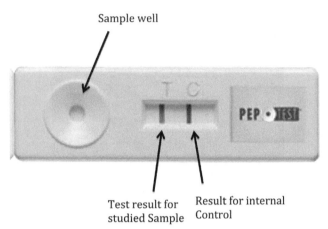

Test result for   Result for internal
studied Sample   Control

Fig. 8. Pepsin lateral flow device with a gastric-juice sample showing positive pepsin test relative to the control band. C, control band; T, test-sample band.

subjects, and found positive and negative predictive values of 87% and 78%, respectively.[110] The sensitivity and specificity of the assay was 87% by in vitro bench testing. This study thus suggests that rapid LFD for salivary pepsin has acceptable test characteristics in GERD. However, the clinical role of this assay in those with LPR is unknown and is the subject of ongoing studies.

As with some other extraesophageal manifestations of GERD, PPI therapy is the standard of care if reflux is suspected as the underlying cause. However, a recent large-scale multicenter study of 145 patients suspected of having LPR did not show a benefit in those treated for 4 months with esomeprazole, 40 mg twice a day, compared with placebo for a duration of 16 weeks.[111] In fact, a recent meta-analysis of controlled studies in LPR showed no benefit of PPI therapy, although admittedly there was evidence that perhaps a subgroup of patients may benefit from such therapy.[112] This result is partly due to the dilution effect resulting from the subjective nature of diagnosing reflux laryngitis; many patients may not have had the disease for which they were being randomized. A recent surgical trial suggested that LPR patients with moderate to severe reflux measured by pH monitoring off PPI therapy and those with moderate-sized hernia (>4 cm) and presence of concomitant typical symptoms may be more likely to respond to surgical fundoplication.[47] Otolaryngologists usually suspect GER-related laryngitis based on nonspecific symptoms such as throat clearing, cough, globus, and signs of laryngeal edema and erythema. Patients unresponsive to PPI therapy have either non–reflux-related causes or may have a functional component to their symptoms. The placebo response rate of around 40% in LPR studies seems similar to those reported in functional gastrointestinal disorders such as irritable bowel syndrome.[113]

Overall, suspected patients with LPR or other extraesophageal symptoms who do not have warning symptoms or signs should initially be treated with empiric PPI therapy for a duration of 1 to 2 months (**Fig. 9**). If symptoms improve, the therapy may need to be prolonged for additional 2 to 3 months to allow healing of laryngeal tissue, after which the dose should be tapered to minimize acid suppression, resulting in continued response. It is important to remember that the use of PPIs in the empiric manner is only intended to be of short duration, and prolonged use is not encouraged. In unresponsive patients, testing with pH and/or impedance monitoring may be the

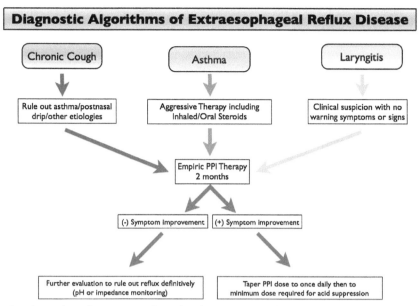

Fig. 9. Diagnosis and treatment algorithm for patients with extraesophageal symptoms of cough, asthma, and laryngitis with suspected GERD as the cause. PPI, proton-pump inhibitor.

best alternative to rule out reflux as the cause, and to move forward with considering other causes for patients' continued symptoms. Moreover, until a specific diagnostic tool to differentiate reflux laryngitis from other causes of chronic laryngitis is developed, empiric therapy with PPIs is still the best means of identifying patients in whom GERD is the cause of laryngeal signs and symptoms.

SUMMARY

The pulmonary and ENT manifestations of GERD are important commonly encountered extraesophageal syndromes. Upper gastrointestinal endoscopy and pH monitoring are poorly sensitive markers for diagnosing reflux in this group of patients. Instead it is recommended that in those without warning symptoms, an empiric trial of PPIs should be the initial approach to diagnose and treat the potential underlying cause of these extraesophageal symptoms. Diagnostic testing, including pH and/or impedance monitoring, may be important in further evaluating those with poor response to essentially exclude GERD as the cause of persistent symptoms.

REFERENCES

1. Vakil N, van Zanten SV, Kahrilas P, et al. The Montreal definition and classification of gastroesophageal reflux disease: a global evidence-based consensus. Am J Gastroenterol 2006;101:1900–20 [quiz: 1943].
2. Berstad T. Gastro-oesophageal reflux and chronic respiratory disease in infants and children: surgical treatment. Scand J Gastroenterol Suppl 1995;211: 26–8.
3. Cicala M, Emerenziani S, Caviglia R, et al. Intra-oesophageal distribution and perception of acid reflux in patients with non-erosive gastro-oesophageal reflux disease. Aliment Pharmacol Ther 2003;18:605–13.

4. Napierkowski J, Wong RK. Extraesophageal manifestations of GERD. Am J Med Sci 2003;326:285–99.
5. Shaw GY. Application of ambulatory 24-hour multiprobe pH monitoring in the presence of extraesophageal manifestations of gastroesophageal reflux. Ann Otol Rhinol Laryngol Suppl 2000;184:15–7.
6. Stanghellini V. Relationship between upper gastrointestinal symptoms and lifestyle, psychosocial factors and comorbidity in the general population: results from the Domestic/International Gastroenterology Surveillance Study (DIGEST). Scand J Gastroenterol Suppl 1999;231:29–37.
7. Dent J, El-Serag HB, Wallander MA, et al. Epidemiology of gastro-oesophageal reflux disease: a systematic review. Gut 2005;54:710–7.
8. Bor S, Mandiracioglu A, Kitapcioglu G, et al. Gastroesophageal reflux disease in a low-income region in Turkey. Am J Gastroenterol 2005;100:759–65.
9. Fenter TC, Naslund MJ, Shah MB, et al. The cost of treating the 10 most prevalent diseases in men 50 years of age or older. Am J Manag Care 2006;12: S90–8.
10. Sandler RS, Everhart JE, Donowitz M, et al. The burden of selected digestive diseases in the United States. Gastroenterology 2002;122:1500–11.
11. Everhart JE, Ruhl CE. Burden of digestive diseases in the United States part I: overall and upper gastrointestinal diseases. Gastroenterology 2009; 136:376–86.
12. Jaspersen D. Extra-esophageal disorders in gastroesophageal reflux disease. Dig Dis 2004;22:115–9.
13. Malagelada JR. Review article: supra-oesophageal manifestations of gastro-oesophageal reflux disease. Aliment Pharmacol Ther 2004;19(Suppl 1):43–8.
14. DeVault KR. Extraesophageal symptoms of GERD. Cleve Clin J Med 2003; 70(Suppl 5):S20–32.
15. Paterson WG. Extraesophageal complications of gastroesophageal reflux disease. Can J Gastroenterol 1997;11(Suppl B):45B–50B.
16. Paterson WG. Extraesophageal manifestations of reflux disease: myths and reality. Chest Surg Clin N Am 2001;11:523–38.
17. Field SK, Evans JA, Price LM. The effects of acid perfusion of the esophagus on ventilation and respiratory sensation. Am J Respir Crit Care Med 1998;157: 1058–62.
18. Ing AJ, Ngu MC, Breslin AB. Pathogenesis of chronic persistent cough associated with gastroesophageal reflux. Am J Respir Crit Care Med 1994;149:160–7.
19. Adhami T, Goldblum JR, Richter JE, et al. The role of gastric and duodenal agents in laryngeal injury: an experimental canine model. Am J Gastroenterol 2004;99:2098–106.
20. Tuchman DN, Boyle JT, Pack AI, et al. Comparison of airway responses following tracheal or esophageal acidification in the cat. Gastroenterology 1984;87: 872–81.
21. Tokayer AZ. Gastroesophageal reflux disease and chronic cough. Lung 2008; 186(Suppl 1):S29–34.
22. Shaker R. Protective mechanisms against supraesophageal GERD. J Clin Gastroenterol 2000;30:S3–8.
23. Jadcherla SR, Gupta A, Coley BD, et al. Esophago-glottal closure reflex in human infants: a novel reflex elicited with concurrent manometry and ultrasonography. Am J Gastroenterol 2007;102:2286–93.
24. Vakil NB, Kahrilas PJ, Dodds WJ, et al. Absence of an upper esophageal sphincter response to acid reflux. Am J Gastroenterol 1989;84:606–10.

25. Wright RA, Miller SA, Corsello BF. Acid-induced esophagobronchial-cardiac reflexes in humans. Gastroenterology 1990;99:71–3.

26. Poe RH, Kallay MC. Chronic cough and gastroesophageal reflux disease: experience with specific therapy for diagnosis and treatment. Chest 2003;123: 679–84.

27. Irwin RS. Chronic cough due to gastroesophageal reflux disease: ACCP evidence-based clinical practice guidelines. Chest 2006;129:80S–94S.

28. Kahrilas PJ, Lee TJ. Pathophysiology of gastroesophageal reflux disease. Thorac Surg Clin 2005;15:323–33.

29. Chang AB, Lasserson TJ, Gaffney J, et al. Gastro-oesophageal reflux treatment for prolonged non-specific cough in children and adults. Cochrane Database Syst Rev 2005;(2):CD004823.

30. Sontag SJ. The spectrum of pulmonary symptoms due to gastroesophageal reflux. Thorac Surg Clin 2005;15:353–68.

31. Hadjiliadis D, Duane Davis R, Steele MP, et al. Gastroesophageal reflux disease in lung transplant recipients. Clin Transplant 2003;17:363–8.

32. Ours TM, Kavuru MS, Schilz RJ, et al. A prospective evaluation of esophageal testing and a double-blind, randomized study of omeprazole in a diagnostic and therapeutic algorithm for chronic cough. Am J Gastroenterol 1999;94: 3131–8.

33. Baldi F, Cappiello R, Cavoli C, et al. Proton pump inhibitor treatment of patients with gastroesophageal reflux-related chronic cough: a comparison between two different daily doses of lansoprazole. World J Gastroenterol 2006;12:82–8.

34. Gislason T, Janson C, Vermeire P, et al. Respiratory symptoms and nocturnal gastroesophageal reflux: a population-based study of young adults in three European countries. Chest 2002;121:158–63.

35. el-Serag HB, Sonnenberg A. Comorbid occurrence of laryngeal or pulmonary disease with esophagitis in United States military veterans. Gastroenterology 1997;113:755–60.

36. Poelmans J, Tack J. Extraoesophageal manifestations of gastro-oesophageal reflux. Gut 2005;54:1492–9.

37. Ludviksdottir D, Bjornsson E, Janson C, et al. Habitual coughing and its associations with asthma, anxiety, and gastroesophageal reflux. Chest 1996;109: 1262–8.

38. Alhabib KF, Vedal S, Champion P, et al. The utility of ambulatory pH monitoring in patients presenting with chronic cough and asthma. Can J Gastroenterol 2007; 21:159–63.

39. Everett CF, Morice AH. Clinical history in gastroesophageal cough. Respir Med 2007;101:345–8.

40. Laukka MA, Cameron AJ, Schei AJ. Gastroesophageal reflux and chronic cough: which comes first? J Clin Gastroenterol 1994;19:100–4.

41. Slaughter JC, Goutte M, Rymer JA, et al. Caution about overinterpretation of symptom indexes in reflux monitoring for refractory gastroesophageal reflux disease. Clin Gastroenterol Hepatol 2011;9:868–74.

42. Kavitt RT, Higginbotham T, Slaughter JC, et al. Symptom reports are not reliable during ambulatory reflux monitoring. Am J Gastroenterol 2012;107:1826–32.

43. Smith JA, Decalmer S, Kelsall A, et al. Acoustic cough-reflux associations in chronic cough: potential triggers and mechanisms. Gastroenterology 2010; 139:754–62.

44. Faruqi S, Molyneux ID, Fathi H, et al. Chronic cough and esomeprazole: a double-blind placebo-controlled parallel study. Respirology 2011;16:1150–6.

45. Shaheen NJ, Crockett SD, Bright SD, et al. Randomised clinical trial: high-dose acid suppression for chronic cough - a double-blind, placebo-controlled study. Aliment Pharmacol Ther 2011;33:225-34.
46. Francis DO, Slaughter JC, Choksi Y, et al. High economic burden of caring for patients with suspected extraesophageal reflux [in review]. Am J Gastroenterol 2012, in press.
47. Francis DO, Goutte M, Slaughter JC, et al. Traditional reflux parameters and not impedance monitoring predict outcome after fundoplication in extraesophageal reflux. Laryngoscope 2011;121:1902-9.
48. Bastian RW, Vaidya AM, Delsupehe KG. Sensory neuropathic cough: a common and treatable cause of chronic cough. Otolaryngol Head Neck Surg 2006;135: 17-21.
49. O'Connell F, Thomas VE, Pride NB, et al. Capsaicin cough sensitivity decreases with successful treatment of chronic cough. Am J Respir Crit Care Med 1994; 150:374-80.
50. Lee B, Woo P. Chronic cough as a sign of laryngeal sensory neuropathy: diagnosis and treatment. Ann Otol Rhinol Laryngol 2005;114:253-7.
51. Mintz S, Lee JK. Gabapentin in the treatment of intractable idiopathic chronic cough: case reports. Am J Med 2006;119:e13-5.
52. Ryan NM, Birring SS, Gibson PG. Gabapentin for refractory chronic cough: a randomised, double-blind, placebo-controlled trial. Lancet 2012;380: 1583-9.
53. Halum SL, Sycamore DL, McRae BR. A new treatment option for laryngeal sensory neuropathy. Laryngoscope 2009;119:1844-7.
54. Harding SM, Guzzo MR, Richter JE. 24-h esophageal pH testing in asthmatics: respiratory symptom correlation with esophageal acid events. Chest 1999;115: 654-9.
55. Sontag SJ, O'Connell S, Khandelwal S, et al. Most asthmatics have gastroesophageal reflux with or without bronchodilator therapy. Gastroenterology 1990;99:613-20.
56. Harding SM, Guzzo MR, Richter JE. The prevalence of gastroesophageal reflux in asthma patients without reflux symptoms. Am J Respir Crit Care Med 2000; 162:34-9.
57. Thomas JW. National Heart, Lung, and Blood Institute resources and programs for cell-based therapies. Circ Res 2007;101:1-6.
58. Parsons JP, Mastronarde JG. Gastroesophageal reflux disease and asthma. Curr Opin Pulm Med 2010;16:60-3.
59. Choy D, Leung R. Gastro-oesophageal reflux disease and asthma. Respirology 1997;2:163-8.
60. Zerbib F, Guisset O, Lamouliatte H, et al. Effects of bronchial obstruction on lower esophageal sphincter motility and gastroesophageal reflux in patients with asthma. Am J Respir Crit Care Med 2002;166:1206-11.
61. Havemann BD, Henderson CA, El-Serag HB. The association between gastro-oesophageal reflux disease and asthma: a systematic review. Gut 2007;56: 1654-64.
62. Kiljander TO, Salomaa ER, Hietanen EK, et al. Gastroesophageal reflux in asthmatics: a double-blind, placebo-controlled crossover study with omeprazole. Chest 1999;116:1257-64.
63. Meier JH, McNally PR, Punja M, et al. Does omeprazole (Prilosec) improve respiratory function in asthmatics with gastroesophageal reflux? A double-blind, placebo-controlled crossover study. Dig Dis Sci 1994;39:2127-33.

64. Leggett JJ, Johnston BT, Mills M, et al. Prevalence of gastroesophageal reflux in difficult asthma: relationship to asthma outcome. Chest 2005;127:1227–31.
65. Sontag SJ, O'Connell S, Khandelwal S, et al. Asthmatics with gastroesophageal reflux: long term results of a randomized trial of medical and surgical antireflux therapies. Am J Gastroenterol 2003;98:987–99.
66. Littner MR, Leung FW, Ballard ED 2nd, et al. Effects of 24 weeks of lansoprazole therapy on asthma symptoms, exacerbations, quality of life, and pulmonary function in adult asthmatic patients with acid reflux symptoms. Chest 2005; 128:1128–35.
67. Mastronarde JG, Anthonisen NR, Castro M, et al. Efficacy of esomeprazole for treatment of poorly controlled asthma. N Engl J Med 2009;360:1487–99.
68. Holbrook JT, Wise RA, Gold BD, et al. Lansoprazole for children with poorly controlled asthma a randomized controlled trial. JAMA 2012;307:373–81.
69. Gibson PG, Powell H, Coughlan J, et al. Limited (information only) patient education programs for adults with asthma. Cochrane Database Syst Rev 2002;(2):CD001005.
70. Kiljander TO, Harding SM, Field SK, et al. Effects of esomeprazole 40 mg twice daily on asthma: a randomized placebo-controlled trial. Am J Respir Crit Care Med 2006;173:1091–7.
71. Locke GR 3rd, Talley NJ, Fett SL, et al. Prevalence and clinical spectrum of gastroesophageal reflux: a population-based study in Olmsted County, Minnesota. Gastroenterology 1997;112:1448–56.
72. Agreus L, Svardsudd K, Talley NJ, et al. Natural history of gastroesophageal reflux disease and functional abdominal disorders: a population-based study. Am J Gastroenterol 2001;96:2905–14.
73. Wo JM, Grist WJ, Gussack G, et al. Empiric trial of high-dose omeprazole in patients with posterior laryngitis: a prospective study. Am J Gastroenterol 1997;92:2160–5.
74. Vaezi MF. Laryngitis and gastroesophageal reflux disease: increasing prevalence or poor diagnostic tests? Am J Gastroenterol 2004;99:786–8.
75. Metz DC, Childs ML, Ruiz C, et al. Pilot study of the oral omeprazole test for reflux laryngitis. Otolaryngol Head Neck Surg 1997;116:41–6.
76. Diamond L. Laryngopharyngeal reflux—it's not GERD. JAAPA 2005;18:50–3.
77. Samuels TL, Johnston N. Pepsin as a causal agent of inflammation during nonacidic reflux. Otolaryngol Head Neck Surg 2009;141:559–63.
78. Johnston N, Dettmar PW, Bishwokarma B, et al. Activity/stability of human pepsin: implications for reflux attributed laryngeal disease. Laryngoscope 2007;117:1036–9.
79. Wood JM, Hussey DJ, Woods CM, et al. Biomarkers and laryngopharyngeal reflux. J Laryngol Otol 2011;125:1218–24.
80. Johnston N, Wells CW, Blumin JH, et al. Receptor-mediated uptake of pepsin by laryngeal epithelial cells. Ann Otol Rhinol Laryngol 2007;116:934–8.
81. Vaezi MF, Slaughter JC, Smith BS, et al. Dilated intercellular space in chronic laryngitis and gastro-oesophageal reflux disease: at baseline and post-lansoprazole therapy. Aliment Pharmacol Ther 2010;32:916–24.
82. Kendall KA. Controversies in the diagnosis and management of laryngopharyngeal reflux disease. Curr Opin Otolaryngol Head Neck Surg 2006;14: 113–5.
83. Hicks DM, Ours TM, Abelson TI, et al. The prevalence of hypopharynx findings associated with gastroesophageal reflux in normal volunteers. J Voice 2002;16: 564–79.

84. Milstein CF, Charbel S, Hicks DM, et al. Prevalence of laryngeal irritation signs associated with reflux in asymptomatic volunteers: impact of endoscopic technique (rigid vs. flexible laryngoscope). Laryngoscope 2005;115:2256–61.
85. Vavricka SR, Storck CA, Wildi SM, et al. Limited diagnostic value of laryngopharyngeal lesions in patients with gastroesophageal reflux during routine upper gastrointestinal endoscopy. Am J Gastroenterol 2007;102:716–22.
86. Vaezi MF. Extraesophageal manifestations of gastroesophageal reflux disease. Clin Cornerstone 2003;5:32–8 [discussion:39–40].
87. Joniau S, Bradshaw A, Esterman A, et al. Reflux and laryngitis: a systematic review. Otolaryngol Head Neck Surg 2007;136:686–92.
88. Johnson DA. Medical therapy of reflux laryngitis. J Clin Gastroenterol 2008;42: 589–93.
89. Vaezi MF, Hicks DM, Abelson TI, et al. Laryngeal signs and symptoms and gastroesophageal reflux disease (GERD): a critical assessment of cause and effect association. Clin Gastroenterol Hepatol 2003;1:333–44.
90. Tutuian R, Castell DO. Use of multichannel intraluminal impedance to document proximal esophageal and pharyngeal nonacidic reflux episodes. Am J Med 2003;115(Suppl 3A):119S–23S.
91. Vaezi MF, Schroeder PL, Richter JE. Reproducibility of proximal probe pH parameters in 24-hour ambulatory esophageal pH monitoring. Am J Gastroenterol 1997;92:825–9.
92. Carroll TL, Fedore LW, Aldahlawi MM. pH Impedance and high-resolution manometry in laryngopharyngeal reflux disease high-dose proton pump inhibitor failures. Laryngoscope 2012;122:2473–81.
93. Becker V, Bajbouj M, Waller K, et al. Clinical trial: persistent gastro-oesophageal reflux symptoms despite standard therapy with proton pump inhibitors - a follow-up study of intraluminal-impedance guided therapy. Aliment Pharmacol Ther 2007;26:1355–60.
94. Iwakiri K, Kawami N, Sano H, et al. Acid and non-acid reflux in Japanese patients with non-erosive reflux disease with persistent reflux symptoms, despite taking a double-dose of proton pump inhibitor: a study using combined pH-impedance monitoring. J Gastroenterol 2009;44:708–12.
95. Mainie I, Tutuian R, Agrawal A, et al. Combined multichannel intraluminal impedance-pH monitoring to select patients with persistent gastro-oesophageal reflux for laparoscopic Nissen fundoplication. Br J Surg 2006;93:1483–7.
96. Mainie I, Tutuian R, Shay S, et al. Acid and non-acid reflux in patients with persistent symptoms despite acid suppressive therapy: a multicentre study using combined ambulatory impedance-pH monitoring. Gut 2006;55: 1398–402.
97. Vaezi MF, Hicks DM, Ours TM, et al. ENT manifestation of GERD: a large prospective study assessing treatment outcome and predictors of response. Gastroenterology 2001;120:A636.
98. Vaezi MF. Laryngitis: from the gastroenterologist's point of view. In: Vaezi MF, editor. Extraesophageal reflux. San Diego (CA): Plural Publishing, Inc.; 2009. p. 37–47.
99. Pritchett JM, Aslam M, Slaughter JC, et al. Efficacy of esophageal impedance/ pH monitoring in patients with refractory gastroesophageal reflux disease, on and off therapy. Clin Gastroenterol Hepatol 2009;7:743–8.
100. Fletcher KC, Slaughter JC, Garrett CG, et al. Significance and degree of reflux in patients with primary extraesophageal symptoms. Laryngoscope 2011;121: 2561–5.

101. Wiener GJ, Tsukashima R, Kelly C, et al. Oropharyngeal pH monitoring for the detection of liquid and aerosolized supraesophageal gastric reflux. J Voice 2009;23:498–504.
102. Sun G, Muddana S, Slaughter JC, et al. A new pH catheter for laryngopharyngeal reflux: normal values. Laryngoscope 2009;119:1639–43.
103. Yuksel ES, Slaughter JC, Mucktar N, et al. In vitro and in vivo studies with a novel oropharyngeal pH monitoring device implicates utility in chronic laryngitis [in review]. Clin Gastroenterol Hepatol 2012.
104. Potluri S, Friedenberg F, Parkman HP, et al. Comparison of a salivary/sputum pepsin assay with 24-hour esophageal pH monitoring for detection of gastric reflux into the proximal esophagus, oropharynx, and lung. Dig Dis Sci 2003;48: 1813–7.
105. Piper DW, Fenton BH. pH stability and activity curves of pepsin with special reference to their clinical importance. Gut 1965;6:506–8.
106. Ozmen S, Yucel OT, Sinici I, et al. Nasal pepsin assay and pH monitoring in chronic rhinosinusitis. Laryngoscope 2008;118:890–4.
107. Printza A, Speletas M, Triaridis S, et al. Is pepsin detected in the saliva of patients who experience pharyngeal reflux? Hippokratia 2007;11:145–9.
108. Kim TH, Lee KJ, Yeo M, et al. Pepsin detection in the sputum/saliva for the diagnosis of gastroesophageal reflux disease in patients with clinically suspected atypical gastroesophageal reflux disease symptoms. Digestion 2008;77:201–6.
109. Strugala VM, Watson MG, Morice AH, et al. Detection of pepsin using a non-invasive lateral flow test for the diagnosis of extra-esophageal reflux - results of a pilot study. Gut 2007;56:A212.
110. Yuksel ES, Strugala V, Slaughter JC, et al. Rapid salivary pepsin test: blinded assessment of test performance in GERD. Laryngoscope 2012;122:1312–6.
111. Vaezi MF, Richter JE, Stasney CR, et al. Treatment of chronic posterior laryngitis with esomeprazole. Laryngoscope 2006;116:254–60.
112. Qadeer MA, Phillips CO, Lopez AR, et al. Proton pump inhibitor therapy for suspected GERD-related chronic laryngitis: a meta-analysis of randomized controlled trials. Am J Gastroenterol 2006;101:2646–54.
113. Patel SM, Stason WB, Legedza A, et al. The placebo effect in irritable bowel syndrome trials: a meta-analysis. Neurogastroenterol Motil 2005;17:332–40.

Novel Pharmaceutical Approaches to Reflux Disease

Usha Dutta, MBBS, MD, DM, MSc. Clinical Epidemiology,
David Armstrong, MA, MB BChir, FRCP(UK), FRCPC*

KEYWORDS

- Gastroesophageal reflux • Pathophysiology • Proton pump inhibitors • TLESR
- Novel therapies

KEY POINTS

- Acid suppression remains the cornerstone of pharmacologic therapy for gastroesophageal reflux disease (GERD).
- Traditional proton pump inhibitors (PPIs) are limited by their pharmacologic properties with respect to symptom control, healing, and potential side effects with long-term use.
- Novel acid suppression agents promise to improve GERD therapy for patients with acid-mediated disease.
- Acid suppression does not address the pathogenetic mechanisms underlying GERD.
- The development of novel pharmacologic approaches to GERD therapy is hampered, inevitably, by the multifactorial cause of GERD and by the ubiquity and redundancy of neurohumoral signaling mechanisms that control upper gastrointestinal sensation and motility.
- Advances in the pharmacologic therapy for GERD will require a personalized approach to therapy based on appropriate investigations to identify relevant therapeutic targets.

BACKGROUND

GERD develops when the reflux of gastric contents into the esophagus results in troublesome symptoms and/or complications.[1,2] Symptoms are considered to be troublesome if they occur at least twice a week or if they reduce quality of life or affect daily functioning. The refluxate contains varying amounts of acid, pepsin, bile salts, and trypsin, and the injury caused by these noxious agents may manifest as a wide range of symptoms at esophageal and extraesophageal sites. The long-term complications of GERD include Barrett's esophagus, peptic stricture, and esophageal

Division of Gastroenterology, Department of Medicine, McMaster University, 1280 Main Street West, Hamilton, Ontario L8S 4K1, Canada
* Corresponding author. Division of Gastroenterology, McMaster University Medical Centre, 1280 Main Street West, HSC-4W8F, Hamilton, Ontario L8S 4K1, Canada.
E-mail address: armstro@mcmaster.ca

Gastroenterol Clin N Am 42 (2013) 93–117
http://dx.doi.org/10.1016/j.gtc.2012.12.001
0889-8553/13/$ – see front matter © 2013 Elsevier Inc. All rights reserved.

adenocarcinoma. The classical symptoms of GERD are heartburn and regurgitation. The disease spectrum is wide and depends on the nature, site, and severity of the injury. The choice of therapy depends on the symptom profile, the pathogenesis of the injury, the affordability of the therapy, and individual preferences.

PREVALENCE AND IMPACT OF GERD

GERD is one of the most common medical conditions with an estimated prevalence of 10% to 20% in the Western world.[2–4] It is the most frequent outpatient diagnosis in the United States, the most common indication for upper endoscopy, and the most common principal gastroenterology-related diagnosis in primary care.[3] On an annual basis, GERD accounts for 9 million hospital visits and $10 billion expenditure toward direct as well as indirect costs for management.[3] GERD is associated with reduced quality of life and reduced work productivity and places a huge financial burden on society related not only to the typical reflux syndrome but also to other extraesophageal syndromes such as asthma, reflux laryngitis, and dental erosions.[1] GERD is, also, the leading risk factor for esophageal adenocarcinoma, leading to further significant mortality, morbidity, and health care costs. The prevalence, costs of treatment, and costs of adverse outcomes underline the need for appropriate management strategies targeted at the causes and consequences of reflux disease.

CURRENT THERAPEUTIC STRATEGIES AND THEIR LIMITATIONS

At present, acid suppression using traditional delayed-release PPIs, is the mainstay of GERD therapy. PPIs are effective in healing esophagitis, improving symptoms, and preventing complications and are generally well-tolerated with a convenient dosing schedule. PPIs produce higher healing and symptom relief rates than histamine receptor antagonists (H$_2$RAs) and antacids, and they have become the primary agents in the management of GERD. Antacids and H$_2$RAs, available over the counter in most countries, still have a role in the management of episodic and mild symptoms because they can provide rapid symptom relief, particularly for infrequent symptoms. Antireflux surgery remains an option for patients who are intolerant of PPIs or who have volume reflux; it is less clear that surgery is beneficial for those who achieve poor control with PPIs or who have extraesophageal GERD syndromes, especially in the absence of documented reflux.[5]

Although PPIs are effective in most situations, there are certain problems that are being increasingly recognized. First, although PPIs lead to healing in 88% to 96% of patients with mild erosive esophagitis over 8 weeks, the overall efficacy in symptom control is suboptimal. With 4 weeks of standard dose PPI therapy, the pooled symptom response rate was only 36.7% in patients with nonerosive reflux disease (NERD) and 55.5% in those with erosive esophagitis.[6] Among those on long-term PPIs, 59% of patients with GERD, 40% of those with NERD, and 40% of those with extraesophageal disease have persistent symptoms on standard once a day PPI therapy.[7,8] Thus, PPI failure is a common problem whose causes need to be identified and addressed. Identified causes of PPI failure include poor compliance, low bioavailability, rapid metabolism, lack of sustained acid suppression, presence of duodenogastric reflux, delayed gastric emptying, hiatus hernia, visceral hypersensitivity, and psychological comorbidities. Second, the pharmacokinetic and pharmacodynamic profiles of currently available PPIs are suboptimal, leading to lack of sustained acid suppression, delay in onset of effect, nocturnal breakthrough symptoms, and requirement of intake at an appropriate time relative to meals to maximize benefit. Third, although PPIs target acid secretion to treat GERD, increased acid production is not the key underlying pathogenetic mechanism. The key pathophysiological mechanisms for GERD such as frequent transient lower esophageal sphincter relaxations (TLESRs), esophageal and gastric dysmotility, and visceral hypersensitivity are not addressed by PPI therapy. Fourth, because GERD is a chronic condition, the overall costs of management are substantial. Fifth, there are increasing concerns about harms from long-term PPI therapy or acid suppression, such that the US Food and Drug Administration (http://www.fda.gov) and the UK Medicines and Healthcare products Regulatory Agency (http://www.mcha.gov.uk) have recently issued public warnings and changed labeling recommendations for these drugs. There is, therefore, a need and an opportunity to innovate, rationalize, and individualize therapy for patients with GERD to improve outcomes, including quality of life, to save costs, and to minimize adverse events.

OBJECTIVE OF THIS REVIEW

Improvements over current treatment strategies must be based on an understanding of the pathophysiology of GERD in relation to the potential roles of novel pharmaceutical approaches; this approach will permit therapies targeted at specific pathophysiological mechanisms to lead to rational therapeutic strategies based on symptom assessment and investigations. Recent advances in the fields of GERD pathogenesis and drug development have opened up newer options, which now require exploration. An electronic search was conducted in MEDLINE and EMBASE from January 2009 to October 2012 for key search terms "gastroesophageal reflux and its variants," "esophagitis," "heartburn," or "proton pump inhibitors" to obtain recent relevant articles for review.

PATHOPHYSIOLOGY: IMPLICATIONS FOR MANAGEMENT

Transient relaxation of the lower esophageal sphincter (LES) is a normal physiologic phenomenon that occurs, intermittently, to allow gastric decompression. Under normal physiologic conditions, air, accompanied by varying amounts of acid, may reflux into the esophagus, depending on the mechanical alterations of the gastro-esophageal junction (GEJ).[9] In health, refluxed acid and gastric contents are cleared rapidly by esophageal peristalsis, complemented by neutralization of residual acid by saliva and local mucous secretions. GERD occurs when the defensive factors that protect the esophagus (antireflux barrier, esophageal clearance, squamous epithelial resistance, mucus and bicarbonate secretion, as well as saliva and salivary bicarbonate) are overwhelmed by aggressive factors (volume, frequency, and constituents of gastroesophageal reflux [GER]).

Role of Acid and Pepsin

Gastric acid and pepsin, activated at pH less than 4, are the key components of the refluxate implicated in the causation of esophagitis. Although acid or pepsin alone can cause mucosal injury, it is the presence of acid and acid-activated pepsin that results in significant tissue injury. Acid suppression not only renders the refluxate benign but also reduces the number of reflux episodes because it decreases the overall gastric volume. However, acid suppression does, also, compromise the detection of reflux episodes using current pH monitoring techniques and diagnostic criteria. Despite the central role of acid in the pathogenesis of GER-related injury and symptoms, gastric acid secretion per se is not increased in most individuals with GERD.[10]

Role of the Proximal "Acid Pocket"

Recent studies have demonstrated a proximal "acid pocket" extending from the gastric cardia to the distal esophagus in normal subjects and in patients with

GERD. The mean pH in this pocket can be as low as 1.6, and the acid in this pocket is unbuffered by meals.[11,12] This pocket has been found to play a key role in postprandial acid reflux and in severe reflux disease.[11,12]

Role of Gastric Contents

Gastric distension triggers the occurrence of TLESRs, which permit GER. Delayed gastric emptying has been noted in 40% of patients with GERD.[13] Diabetic gastroparesis, gastric outlet obstruction, and gastric dysmotility are all associated with prolonged gastric emptying and, in some cases, with persistent dyspeptic symptoms despite adequate acid suppressive therapy, and it is tempting to postulate that prokinetic agents and measures to relieve delayed gastric emptying will have a role in relieving reflux symptoms in this subgroup of patients. Patients with hypersecretory states such as Zollinger-Ellison syndrome are likely to produce large volumes of acid, and they will, often, require potent high-dose antisecretory agents to control acid-related symptoms, including those of GERD.

Role of Duodenal Contents

In patients with increased duodenogastroesophageal reflux (DGER), bile salts and pancreatic enzymes can cause esophageal injury. Although conjugated bile acids are more injurious in the presence of acid and pepsin, deconjugated bile acids and trypsin can cause damage even at neutral pH. With the advent of technology to measure bilirubin levels in addition to esophageal luminal pH levels, reflux episodes can now be characterized, with some accuracy, as acidic, weakly acidic, alkaline, or bile reflux. The finding of DGER in 95% of patients with Barrett's esophagus, 79% of those with erosive esophagitis, and 50% of those with NERD, and data implicating DGER in the pathogenesis of esophageal adenocarcinoma, suggest that bile reflux is a marker for more severe GERD[14] and that this might allow better targeting of therapy. However, although aggressive acid suppression may reduce bile-mediated injury, it does not eliminate it; other potential methods to reduce DGER include agents that can increase gastroduodenal motility, target mucosal protection or, like cholestyramine and rikkunshito, sequester bile acids.[15] This approach to treating severe GERD will require the development of effective therapeutic strategies and a better understanding of the potential benefit for reducing the severity and complications of GERD.

Role of Antireflux Barrier

The principal component of the defense mechanism is the antireflux barrier, a high pressure zone, created by the LES and the crural diaphragm. The functional integrity of the GEJ depends on the tone and alignment of these 2 muscular structures. During a TLESR, the tone of both LES and crural diaphragm is inhibited to allow belching. TLESRs account for all reflux episodes in healthy individuals and nearly 80% of reflux episodes in patients with GERD. Thus, agents that inhibit TLESR, such as γ-aminobutyric acid (GABA) agonists, glutamate antagonists, cholecystokinin (CCK) antagonists, anticholinergic agents, nitric oxide (NO) inhibitors, and serotonin (5-hydroxytryptamine [5-HT$_3$] or 5-HT$_4$) agonists or antagonists may have a role to play in the management of GERD.[16–21] A wide range of agents that may reduce TLESR are currently in various stages of investigation.

Recent understanding of the dynamics of the GEJ suggests that hiatus hernia is indeed a major risk factor for GERD. In patients with hiatus hernia, the mechanism of reflux is complex. The 2 muscular structures, LES and crural diaphragm, are not aligned. Thus, reflux occurs not only with TLESRs but also during deglutitive LES relaxation and with isolated LES hypotension.[11,12,22] The intrathoracic position of the GEJ (negative pressure) in the presence of a hiatus hernia results in a greater pressure gradient during LES relaxation resulting in more reflux. Also, the compliance of GEJ is increased, leading to a larger cross-sectional area at a given pressure gradient and, hence, to increased volume of refluxate. Moreover, if reflux occurs, the refluxate is often acidic because of entrapment of the acid pocket in the hiatal hernia.[23] Patients with a hiatus hernia may require repair using surgical or endoscopic techniques if their disease does not respond to optimal pharmacologic measures.

Recently, patients with GERD have been found to have an altered microbial profile in the distal esophagus, characterized by an increase in gram-negative flora and a decrease in gram-positive flora. The lipopolysaccharide released by the gram-negative bacteria may perpetuate local inflammation and also cause LES relaxation by inducing nitric oxide synthase and delaying gastric emptying via the cyclooxygenase-2 pathway.[24] Probiotic administration has been found to enhance gastric emptying and decrease regurgitation in infants.[25] Further understanding of the role of microbial flora in the causation or perpetuation of GERD may pave the way for using probiotics and antibiotics in the management of GERD.

Role of Esophageal Acid Clearance

The clearance of acid by esophagus has 2 main components: mechanical clearance and chemical neutralization. Reflux of gastric contents may result in esophageal distension and secondary peristalsis, thereby returning refluxed material to the stomach. Patients with esophageal dysmotility have defective clearance resulting in significant mucosal injury because of persistent exposure of the mucosa to noxious agents. Although prokinetic agents have a theoretical role to play in the management of GERD, their overall efficacy in the clinical setting has been relatively disappointing.[26,27]

Residual acid, which persists after peristaltic volume clearance, is neutralized by saliva and bicarbonate-rich secretions from the submucosal glands of the esophagus. Use of oral lozenges, bethanechol, and smoking cessation are associated with increasing salivation, which helps in improving GER symptoms. Hyposalivation during sleep contributes to prolonged nocturnal reflux episodes. Raising the bed head may be helpful in controlling nocturnal or recumbent GER, but it would be helpful if esophageal clearance could be improved pharmacologically.

Role of Tissue Resistance

Tissue resistance is a function of the buffering capacity of mucus secreted by the submucosal glands, intercellular tight junctions, intracellular defense mechanisms against acidification, frequent cell turnover, and local blood supply. Dilated intercellular spaces (DIS) in the esophageal epithelium is considered an early morphologic marker of acid damage in patients with GERD.[28] DIS is thought to allow passage of water and hydrogen ions, with or without other noxious agents, into the esophageal epithelium, resulting in direct tissue injury as well as activation of the chemosensitive nerve endings located within the mucosa.[29] Recent novel imaging techniques such as narrow band imaging and confocal laser endomicroscopy demonstrate these early changes even in patients who have no obvious damage on standard white light endoscopy.[30]

Role of Visceral Hypersensitivity

Noxious luminal agents as well as inflammatory mediators can stimulate nerve endings that play a key role in visceral hypersensitivity. In some individuals with functional heartburn or NERD and in those with underlying psychological morbidity, symptoms may occur even in the absence of frankly acidic reflux. In these patients, even small quantities of noxious agents are thought to penetrate the DIS and stimulate chemosensitive nociceptors.[31] In these cases, symptoms may be secondary to peripheral sensitization or to central mechanisms resulting in esophageal hyperalgesia. Psychological stress has been shown to increase DIS in the esophageal epithelium, promoting cell injury and chemosensitization.[32] Consequently, various pain modulators are being studied for the management of pain and other symptoms in patients with GERD.

NOVEL PHARMACEUTICAL APPROACHES

Two key facts have emerged from decades of research and clinical practice. First, acid inhibition has been the single most successful approach to the management of GERD. Second, current acid inhibition strategies do not deliver the 3 key outcomes of interest in all patients: symptom relief, mucosal healing, and prevention of complications. Thus, novel strategies must explore the role of drugs for improving acid suppression and for targeting other pathophysiological mechanisms to provide complete symptom relief, mucosal healing, and absence of complications (**Fig. 1**).

TARGETING ACID SUPPRESSION
Traditional PPIs

The traditional delayed-release PPIs—omeprazole, lansoprazole, pantoprazole, and rabeprazole—are prodrugs that are activated by conversion to the sulfenamide form in the acidic environment of the secretory canaliculus. The activated sulfenamide then forms a covalent disulfide bond with a cysteine moiety in the proton pump, blocking the H^+K^+ ATPase exchange pathway. All traditional PPIs are acid labile as prodrugs, and they, therefore, require enteric coating to delay release, with subsequent absorption in the small bowel. After absorption, they are metabolized rapidly, with a short half-life of only 1 to 1.5 hours; fortunately, PPIs bind irreversibly to the proton pump so their effect extends well beyond their plasma residence time. However, because proton pumps are regenerated continuously, acid secretion capacity increases steadily through the day allowing nocturnal acid breakthrough. In addition, traditional PPIs do not achieve maximal acid suppression immediately, generally requiring at least 5 days for peak effect. Acid suppression is optimized if the action of the PPI on the proton pump is maximized by synchronizing ingestion with meal-stimulated acid secretion. Ideally, therefore, a PPI should be taken within 15 to 60 minutes before the first meal of the day. Compliance with this recommendation is adhered to by less than 10% of patients and emphasized by only one-third of the physicians at the time of prescription. Also, the efficacy of the drug depends on the rate of metabolism of the drug by the hepatic cytochrome system. Rapid metabolizers have lower drug levels, translating into reduced acid suppression. These shortcomings of traditional PPIs have resulted in incomplete efficacy, poor compliance, and increasing costs of care.

Newer PPIs

In the past decade, novel pharmacologic approaches have been taken to improve existing molecules or to discover newer agents that might enhance or prolong acid suppression and overcome some of the shortcomings of traditional PPIs (**Tables 1** and **2**).

Stereoisomers
Isomers of traditional PPIs have been developed to improve bioavailability and efficacy. The common preparations in this category are esomeprazole, dexlansoprazole,

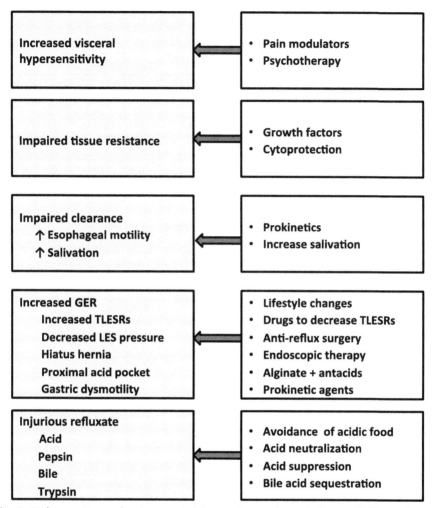

Fig. 1. Pathogenetic mechanisms underlying gastroesophageal disease (*left*) matched to potential therapeutic interventions (*right*).

dexrabeprazole, and S-pantoprazole. Of these, esomeprazole and dexlansoprazole have been studied in clinical trials and used extensively in routine clinical practice.[33,34] In general, they have been found to be clinically more effective than their parent racemic formulations, albeit at higher doses, while maintaining similar safety profiles.[35,36]

Extended-release PPIs

Dexlansoprazole MR (modified release) is an isomeric PPI that, also, has a dual delayed-release delivery system that releases the drug at 2 different pH levels, resulting in absorption over a longer period and sustained serum levels for up to 6.4 hours. As a result, dexlansoprazole MR, 90 mg, has been found to be somewhat more effective than lansoprazole, 30 mg daily.[33] In addition, the effect of dexlansoprazole is not affected significantly by the time of ingestion, relative to food intake, with the potential for greater flexibility in drug dosing.

Table 1
Novel agents for improved acid inhibition

Drug/Type of Modification	Status	Modification	Modified Action
Selective isomeric formulation			
Esomeprazole	Approved	S-enantiomer	Greater bioavailability
Dexlansoprazole MR	Approved	R-enantiomer	Increased area under plasma
Dexrabeprazole	Approved	R-enantiomer	concentration–time curve
S-pantoprazole	Phase 3	S-enantiomer	Lesser interindividual variability
Extended-release formulations			
ER-rabeprazole	Approved	Slow release	Greater plasma residence time
CMA-omeprazole (AGN201904-Z)	Approved	Chemically metered release	Increased area under plasma concentration-time curve
Dexlansoprazole MR (TAK 390 MR)	Approved	Dual release	
Immediate-release preparations			
IR omeprazole	Approved	No enteric coating	Rapid onset and sustained
IR esomeprazole	Approved	Combined with NaHCO$_3$	action
Modified site of action			
Revaprazan	Discontinued	PCABs)	Higher pK_a
Soraprazan	Discontinued	Act on K$^+$ channel	Greater concentration in
Linaprazan (AZD0865)	Discontinued		secretory canaliculus
TAK-438	Phase 2		
YH4808	Phase 2		
Modified chemical structure			
Tenatoprazole (TU-199)	Phase 3	Modified imidopyridine	Prolonged $t_{1/2}$ Increased area under plasma
Ilaprazole	Phase 2	Modified benzimidazole	concentration–time curve
Combined with another agent			
4VB101	Phase 2b	PPI with pentagastrin	Meal-independent secretory effect
NMI-826	Phase 2	PPI with NO-releasing moiety	Mucosal protection
OX17	Phase 2	PPI with H$_2$RA	Enhances acid suppression
H$_2$RA	Patented	Tenatoprazole with H$_2$RA	Better nocturnal acid suppression
Alginate	Phase 3	PPI with alginate	Reduces reflux from acid pocket

Abbreviation: PCAB, potassium-competitive acid blockers.

Extended-release (ER) rabeprazole is designed to release the drug throughout the lower gastrointestinal tract. It contains a combination of standard enteric-coated delayed-release tablets and pulsatile-release tablets. Rabeprazole is released from the former in the proximal small intestine and from the latter in the distal gut. In a combined analysis of 2 studies, in patients with moderate to severe erosive esophagitis, ER rabeprazole was reported not to be inferior to esomeprazole, 40 mg daily, with respect to esophagitis healing and symptom relief.[37]

Table 2
Overcoming limitations of traditional proton pump inhibitors

Problem with Traditional PPI	Potential Solution	Drug	Mechanism of Action	Remarks
Slow onset (5 d to achieve peak action)	Rapid onset	IR omeprazole IR esomeprazole TAK-438	Rapid absorption and action PCABs	Useful for rapid relief of symptoms
Meal-dependent antisecretory effect	Meal-independent antisecretory effect	Pantoprazole Tenatoprazole Dexlansoprazole IR omeprazole IR esomeprazole Vecam (PPI + VB101)	Action relatively independent of meal timing Gastrin agonist	Meal-independent administration may improve compliance
Short half-life (1–2 h)	Sustained action	Tenatoprazole (TU199) Ilaprazole ER-rabeprazole Dexlansoprazole CMA-omeprazole	Prolonged half-life (9 h) Prolonged half-life (6 h) Enteric-coated extended release Dual pH-dependent release Pro-PPI	Useful for chronic symptoms Provides better symptom relief
Nocturnal breakthrough	Nocturnal acid suppression Prolonged action, see above	Add night dose Add H$_2$-RA Tenatoprazole IR omeprazole	Suppresses nighttime acid secretion	Nocturnal symptoms and for extraesophageal manifestations
Breakthrough symptoms	Therapy on pro re nata basis	Step-up dose Add antacids (pro re nata)	Better acid suppression	Rapid short-term symptom relief
Rapid metabolizers	Use alternatives or increase dose of PPI in use	Esomeprazole Rabeprazole	Inhibits CYP2C19 Alternate metabolic pathway	In those with cytochrome P450 variant alleles
Drug interactions	PPI metabolized by pathways other than P450	Pantoprazole Rabeprazole Ilaprazole	Alternate metabolic pathway Alternate metabolic pathway Alternate metabolic pathway	Possible role in patients with suspected drug interactions

Chemically metered absorption omeprazole (CMA-omeprazole/AGN 201904-Z) is a slowly absorbed acid-stable prodrug, which is converted into the active drug after absorption. This prodrug is absorbed throughout the length of the small intestine, resulting in a steady and prolonged serum residence time. In a phase I study, it was found to be better than esomeprazole in producing acid suppression at nighttime.[38]

Immediate-release PPIs

Immediate-release (IR) formulations are nonenteric-coated PPIs that are combined with sodium bicarbonate to protect the drug from acid-induced degradation. The uncoated PPI is then rapidly absorbed, from the proximal intestine, resulting in rapid onset of action. In addition, the antacid-induced rise in gastric pH value itself stimulates acid secretion, which facilitates uptake of the PPI prodrug by the activated parietal cell and formation of the active sulfenamide derivative in the secretory canaliculi. As a result, the IR formulation's efficacy is likely to be less affected by administration before a meal. IR omeprazole and IR esomeprazole have been found to offer a rapid onset of action and sustained acid suppression, associated with decreased nocturnal acid breakthrough, compared with traditional PPIs.[7]

Newer PPIs

Tenatoprazole is an imidazopyridine derivative unlike traditional PPIs, which are benzimidazole derivatives. Tenatoprazole too is a prodrug that requires conversion into the active agent in the acidic environment of the secretory canaliculus of the parietal cell, where it binds at the Cys813 and Cys822 residues of the proton pump. Tenatoprazole has a long half-life of 8.7 ± 2.6 hours, which translates into prolonged acid suppression. Like other traditional PPIs, tenatoprazole is a racemic mixture of 2 stereoisomers, of which the S-isomer has been selected for further development. In addition, it was determined that the sodium salt of S-tenatoprazole offered better solubility and bioavailablity than the free form of S-tenatoprazole. In another phase 1 study, S-tenatoprazole-Na produced significantly greater and more prolonged dose-dependent 24-hour and nocturnal acid suppression than esomeprazole.[39] In a meta-analysis of individual patient data, S-tenatoprazole sodium, 60 mg once a day, was found to be more effective in producing acid suppression than esomeprazole at standard doses (40 mg once a day), its acid suppression being equivalent to that of esomeprazole given twice daily.[40] The efficacy of tenatoprazole is consistent with our current understanding that the antisecretory effect of PPIs is proportional to the area under the curve of plasma drug levels. Given its pharmacologic characteristics, S-tenatoprazole-Na may provide greater clinical efficacy compared with current PPIs for patients in whom once-daily therapy is ineffective.[40]

Ilaprazole is a new substituted benzimidazole PPI that has been reported to produce higher gastric acid suppression and has a more prolonged half-life and a better safety profile than omeprazole. Reports that the metabolism of ilaprazole may differ from that of other PPIs suggests that it may be useful in patients at risk of drug interactions or in those with CYP2C19 variants. Recent studies of ilaprazole in healing gastroduodenal ulcers are promising, but there are no published clinical trials on its use in GERD.[41]

Potassium-competitive acid blockers (PCABs)

PCABs are members of a new class of drugs that specifically target the potassium-binding region of the H^+K^+ ATPase. PCABs are lipophilic weak bases that are stable at low pH values; this feature allows them to concentrate in acidic environment, resulting in 100,000-fold higher levels in the parietal cell canaliculus. The differences from traditional PPIs are highlighted in the **Table 3**, which has been modified from the review article by Scarpignato and Hunt.[40] These agents block the H^+K^+ ATPase in

Table 3
Differences between traditional proton pump inhibitors and potassium-competitive acid blockers

Characteristics	PPI	PCAB	Implications for PCAB Therapy
Drug	Prodrug	Active form	More rapid onset of action
Concentration in parietal cell compared with plasma	1000-fold higher	100,000 fold	More potent acid suppression
Binding to H^+K^+ ATPase	Covalent binding and irreversible	Competitive and reversible	More potent acid inhibition
Factor on which the duration of effect depends	Half-life of sulfenamide–enzyme complex	Half-life of drug in plasma and the pH of secretory canaliculus	More sustained action
Peak effect	After repeated dosing	After first dose	More rapid onset

Data from Scarpignato C, Hunt RH. Proton pump inhibitors: the beginning of the end or the end of the beginning? Curr Opin Pharmacol 2008;8:682.

a competitive reversible manner resulting in rapid and sustained acid inhibition. Drugs in this class, including revaprazan, soraprazan, linaprazan (AZD0865), and TAK 438, share the same final mechanism of action, but they belong to 4 different chemical classes, namely, imidazopyridines, pyrimidines, imidazonaphthyridines, and quinolones, respectively. Despite excellent pharmacokinetic and pharmacodynamic properties, most of these agents have been discontinued because of safety concerns or because they were not demonstrably superior to standard PPIs in clinical studies. However, evaluation of TAK 438 is still underway and the results of phase 3 trials are awaited.

Drug metabolism
CYP2C19 hepatic enzyme systems are involved in the metabolism of not only PPIs but also 10% of all medications in clinical use. As a result of variant alleles, 75% of patients of Asian ethnic origin are slow metabolizers, leading to higher drug levels.[42] PPI dose adjustment based on the nature of the polymorphism may help in individualizing therapy and reducing drug interactions, but this requires knowledge of the patients' metabolizer status. Recent insights into the drug metabolic pathways and genetic variation have improved our understanding of PPI failure and drug interactions. Developing drugs that may be metabolized slowly by alternate pathways may potentially be useful in increasing PPI bioavailability and reducing drug interactions.[43]

Combinations of PPI with other agents
VB101 VB101 has pentagastrin-like activity that activates the parietal cell and stimulates proton pump activity. When administered with a PPI, it facilitates the antisecretory effect and, potentially, reduces the effect of meal timing on PPI activity. Studies in rats have shown that this combination augments PPI-induced acid inhibition.[44] Recently, VECAM, a combination of VB101 and omeprazole, has been under phase 3 trial for evaluation of its efficacy (ClinicalTrials.gov identifier: NCT01059383).

Nitric-oxide-enhanced PPI NO has been recognized, recently, as an important mediator of gastrointestinal mucosal defense; it modulates mucosal blood flow and mucus production and helps in mucosal repair, thereby exerting a "cytoprotective" effect. The role of an NO-enhanced PPI (NMI-826) is under evaluation[45]; it is reported to be more effective than a PPI alone in the healing of gastric ulcers (90% vs 50%).[40,45,46]

PPI–H$_2$RA combination The combination of PPI and H$_2$RA may be useful because up to 79% of patients with GERD have nocturnal symptoms that may respond to greater nocturnal acid suppression. Addition of a bedtime H$_2$RA to a twice-daily PPI regimen resulted in 70% improvement in nocturnal reflux symptoms.[47] This result has led to resurgence of interest in combining H$_2$RAs with a PPI into a single formulation. Recently, *OX17*, a fixed-dose combination of omeprazole and famotidine, has undergone a phase 2 clinical trial. The time with gastric pH value above 4 during the first 12 hours after dosing was, on an average, 60% longer with OX17 than with omeprazole alone (*P*<.05). After 14 days treatment, the time with gastric pH value above 4 was twice as long as after treatment with famotidine. (http://www.orexo.com/en/Investor-Relations/Press-releases/?guid=341021) In addition, tenatoprazole has been combined with a standard H$_2$RA to form a novel combination that has been patented recently (patent number 20120122919).[40]

PPI–alginate combination The combination of PPI and alginate has garnered increased interest after the recent discovery of an acid pocket in the proximal part of the stomach. Alginates are natural polysaccharides that polymerize when exposed to acid, forming gel matrices that are further stabilized by Ca^{++} ions.[11,12,48] An alginate–antacid combination was found to be effective in preventing reflux from the acid pocket, thereby providing a rationale for its use in GERD.[48] In a recent study, omeprazole, 20 mg once a day, and alginate, 30 mL 4 times a day, was compared with omeprazole alone in patients with NERD. Complete resolution of heartburn for at least 7 consecutive days was significantly more common in the combination arm than in the PPI alone arm (56.7% vs 25.7%; *P*<.05).[49] Future studies are needed to evaluate the role of a PPI–alginate combination.

PPI–prokinetic combination Although there is a theoretical rationale for this approach, the combination of a prokinetic with a PPI has demonstrated only limited benefit in clinical trials, to date. Mosapride, 5 mg 3 times a day, in combination with pantoprazole, 40 mg once daily, is reported to provide better symptom relief in a subgroup of patients with erosive esophagitis (95% vs 46%; *P* = .003)[50] and to improve esophageal contractility and lower intrabolus pressure in patients with GERD. Furthermore, mosapride and esomeprazole cotherapy tended to yield better response in patients with concomitant dyspepsia and to improve symptoms in a subgroup of patients with NERD who had delayed gastric emptying and dyspepsia.[51–55]

LOWER ESOPHAGEAL SPHINCTER RELAXATION
TLESR Inhibitors

Despite double-dose acid suppression therapy, persistent acid reflux has been reported in 16% patients with GERD,[56] and in a cross-sectional survey of 726 patients receiving long-term PPI therapy, reflux symptoms persisted in 59% of the patients.[8] Reflux symptoms may be due to frankly acidic reflux, weakly acidic reflux, weakly alkaline reflux, or duodenogastroesophageal reflux. TLESRs are considered to be the major mechanism underlying pathologic gastroesophageal reflux, and the inhibition of TLESRs would, therefore, have the potential to reduce all forms of reflux. The only therapy that has been shown, consistently, to decrease TLESR is surgery, but because a surgical approach is not appropriate for all patients with GERD, there is still a need for effective pharmaceutical approaches.

TLESRs occur in response to a vagovagal reflex, triggered by gastric distension and stimulation of gastric mechanoreceptors, relayed via the brainstem to vagal efferent neurons. LES relaxation is mediated by the nonadrenergic/noncholinergic neurons whose main neurotransmitters are vasoactive intestinal peptide and NO. GABA is an inhibitory neurotransmitter in the central nervous system (CNS) and GABA$_B$ receptors are present on vagal afferents in the dorsal medulla. The 2 dominant neurotransmitters involved in the modulation of this signaling pathway are GABA and glutamate[57]; however, there are other potential targets for modulating TLESRs including cannabinoid (CB) receptors, nitric oxide synthase inhibitors, CCK receptors, and muscarinic and opioid receptors.[19] Various novel agents targeting mechanisms other than acid suppression are outlined in **Table 4**. Although many animal experiments and fewer human trials have been performed using these agents, most have not been found to be useful in a clinical setting except for baclofen, a GABA$_B$ receptor agonist.

GABA Agonists

Baclofen, a GABA$_B$ receptor agonist, used clinically in the management of spasticity was also found to reduce GER.[58] This agent can reduce TLESRs by 60%, can increase basal LES pressure, and is effective in reducing acid reflux, weakly acidic reflux, and bile reflux. In 2 placebo-controlled randomized studies, monotherapy with baclofen was found to be effective in reducing GER. However, poor tolerability, because of CNS side effects (dizziness, somnolence, nausea, and vomiting), has significantly limited its use in routine clinical practice. Moreover, baclofen requires frequent dosing up to 3 to 4 times per day, which reduces compliance. Recently, other GABA$_B$ receptor agonists, lesogaberan, arbaclofen placarbil (XP19986), and AZD9343, have been studied in clinical trials.[59–62]

Lesogaberan (AZD3355) was designed as a GABA$_B$ agonist without CNS side effects, and it was found to reduce TLESRs by 36% and acid reflux by 44% in healthy volunteers. In a phase 2 randomized control trial, 16% of the patients with GERD who failed PPI responded in contrast to only 8% in the control arm. Lesogaberan was found to achieve a significant response only at a dose of 240 mg twice daily. The response, however, even at this high dose was only modest (26% vs 18%).[60,61] It was concluded that the response was not clinically important enough to make further development of this drug worthwhile.

Arbaclofen placarbil (XP19986) is a prodrug of the pharmacologically active R isomer of baclofen. This prodrug is a sustained release formulation that is absorbed throughout the gut, resulting in sustained plasma levels of the drug and a favorable tolerability profile. At a dose of 60 mg/d, it reduced acid reflux episodes by 35% and heartburn episodes by 49% compared with placebo. The subgroup that most benefited was the one that had a history of partial response to PPI therapy.[59,63,64]

Although these modifications of baclofen have been found to reduce reflux and to have lower CNS side effects than baclofen, their toxicity and overall poor efficacy have precluded further development.[65] However, this should not hinder future studies to identify a subset of patients in whom these drugs may offer benefit.

Metabotropic Glutamate Receptor Antagonists

These agents have the potential to reduce TLESRs by modulating the mechanosensitivity of vagal afferents.[19] Transmission of signals from vagal afferent terminals in the nucleus tractus solitarius is mainly glutaminergic; suppression of this activity modulates the frequency of TLESRs. ADX10059, a negative allosteric modulator of mGluR5 in a phase 2 trial, at a dose of 250 mg 3 times daily, was shown to be effective in reducing acid exposure. However, these promising results were hampered by poor

Table 4
Novel agents targeting nonacid suppression mechanisms

Drug Category	Effects	Side Effects	Limiting Factors	Present Status
Reduce gastroesophageal reflux				
GABA agonists				
Baclofen	48% decrease in reflux	Multiple CNS side effects	Needs multiple dosing	Trials ongoing
AZD9343	—	Multiple CNS side effects	Side effects	Suspended
Lesogaberan	21% response rate	Diarrhea, nausea, increased transaminases	Poor efficacy, side effects	Suspended
Arbaclofen placarbil	50% decrease in reflux	Better tolerated	No efficacy in large trial	Suspended
mGluR5 antagonists				
AZX 10,059	Dose-dependent decrease in reflux	Increased transaminases, hepatic failure	Side effects	Suspended
Riluzole	—	Nausea, diarrhea, hepatitis	Nonspecific action	Suspended
Cholecystokinin antagonists				
Loxiglumide, itriglumide	Only modest effect	—	Poor efficacy	Suspended
NO synthase inhibitors				
L-NAME, L-NMMA	Modest effect	Systemic effect on endothelium	Systemic action	Suspended
CB1 receptor target				
Decrease meal-induced TLESR	Decrease meal-induced TLESR	Vomiting, hypotension, tachycardia	Decrease baseline LES pressures	Suspended

		Side effects		
Rimonabant	Decrease meal-induced TLESR	CNS side effects, major depression		Suspended
Reduce visceral hypersensitivity				
SSRI, TCA, Trazodone	Decrease pain perception	Minimal side effects	In non–mood-altering dose	Used in NERD and functional pain
AZD1386 (TRPV-1 antagonist)	Increase pain threshold	Well tolerated	Promising	Ongoing studies
Increase esophageal clearance				
Prokinetics				
Mosapride	Increase volume clearance	Well tolerated	As add on to PPI	In poor UGI motility
Rikkunshito	Increase volume clearance	Potential multiple side effects	Combination of 8 herbs	Ongoing trials
Erythromycin Azithromycin	Decrease acid/bile reflux Increase emptying	Antibiotic resistance, tachyphylaxis	Used in low doses	Hiatus hernia Proximal acid pocket
Improve mucosal healing				
EGF, MCSF	Increase mucosal healing	Well tolerated	Cost	Under development
Improve mucosal protection				
Rebamipide	Cytoprotective and antiinflammatory	Well tolerated	Limited efficacy	Preliminary clinical studies
NO-releasing moieties	Increase mucosal healing	Pharmacologic challenges	Decrease LES pressure (?)	Under development

Abbreviations: EGF, epidermal growth factor; L-NAME, L-nitroarginine methyl ester; L-NMMA, L-NG-monomethylarginine; MCSF, macrophage colony stimulating factor; SSRI, selective serotonin reuptake inhibitor; TCA, tricyclic antidepressant; UGI, upper gastrointestinal.

tolerability, mainly because of dizziness and nausea. A modified-release formulation with altered absorption characteristics was better tolerated when used in a phase 2 randomized double-blind placebo-controlled trial in 103 patients with GERD. Monotherapy with this agent at a dose of 120 mg twice daily consistently improved GERD symptoms and reduced reflux episodes by 25%.[66,67] However, it was not effective in refractory GERD. ADX10059 is no longer being developed because long-term use in patients with migraine was associated with hepatotoxicity. Riluzole, another mGluR5 antagonist, was ineffective and also poorly tolerated, leading to frequent nausea, diarrhea, and hepatitis. Recently, AZD2066, another mGluR5 antagonist, has been found to be well tolerated and efficacious in a small study of 13 healthy patients; however, these results need further confirmation.[66,67]

Cannabinoid Receptor Agonists

The active substance in cannabis is delta-9-tetrahydrocannabinol, a cannabinoid (CB) receptor agonist. A study in dogs followed by a study in human volunteers showed that CB receptor agonist reduced meal-induced TLESRs. However, it was associated with significant nausea and vomiting, precluding further drug development.[18] Rimonabant, a CB1 receptor antagonist, tested in 12 volunteers at a dose of 20 mg/d increased basal LES pressure by 45%, decreased TLESRs by 61%, and decreased postprandial reflux by 78% compared with placebo. However, it has since been withdrawn because of the side effect of depression.[68]

ESOPHAGEAL CLEARANCE
Prokinetics

Prokinetic agents have multiple potential mechanisms whereby they might reduce GER or esophageal exposure to gastroesophageal refluxate. These agents may increase basal LES pressure, improve esophageal peristalsis, enhance esophageal acid clearance and, also, promote gastric emptying. As an isolated therapy, all prokinetic agents have been found to be inferior to PPI for the treatment of GERD. However, they may have a limited role for short-term use in select subgroup of patients with associated gastric dysmotility. Metoclopramide, a dopamine receptor antagonist and cholinomimetic, has been used in patients with GERD in conjunction with acid suppression; however, the poor efficacy and frequent CNS adverse events limit its use.[69] Domperidone, a dopamine receptor antagonist, may be a useful adjunct to acid suppression therapy, but tachyphylaxis and side effects limit routine long-term use.[7,70] Cisapride, previously indicated for treatment of GERD, has been withdrawn from the market because of the risk of fatal cardiac arrhythmias. Mosapride citrate has 5-HT$_4$ receptor agonist and 5-HT$_3$ receptor antagonist actions and has been reported to be an effective adjunct to PPI therapy.[71] Itopride, an acetylcholine esterase inhibitor and dopamine receptor antagonist, improves symptoms and decreases esophageal acid exposure in patients with mild erosive esophagitis.[72] However, neither itopride nor mosapride has been approved for GERD therapy in North America.[72,73]

Macrolides

Prokinetic agents such as macrolides increase gastric emptying, proximal stomach tone, and LES pressure, presumably via a cholinergic pathway mediated by motilin receptors or, possibly, by serotonin receptors.[74] Erythromycin has been reported to improve the amplitude and duration of esophageal peristalsis, significantly, and to increase basal LES pressure.[74] In a recent human study, azithromycin was found to reduce acid reflux episodes, hiatal hernia size, and esophageal acid exposure.[75] As such, this drug might decrease the proximal gastric acid pocket in patients with severe GERD, but this potential mechanism awaits confirmation. Alemcinal and mitemcinal are modifications of macrolide antibiotics with enhanced motilin agonist effect but no antibacterial activity.[76] These drugs have been found to be effective in diabetic gastroparesis,[77] but their role in GERD needs to be evaluated.

Rikkunshito

Rikkunshito is a Japanese traditional medicine composed of 8 herbs used to treat heartburn symptoms. This drug decreases esophageal acid exposure, enhances gastric emptying, and binds to bile acids.[15] In a recent, randomized multicenter study, addition of rikkunshito to standard rabeprazole therapy was found to be equivalent to doubling the dose of rabeprazole.[78] However, further studies are required to establish its mode of action, efficacy, and safety.

GASTRIC EMPTYING

In theory, accelerated gastric emptying should reduce GER but there are no data to confirm therapeutic benefit with currently available approaches using prokinetic agents or endoscopic injection of botulinum toxin at the pyloric sphincter.[79]

VISCERAL HYPERSENSITIVITY

Visceral hypersensitivity plays a key role in perception of GER.[80] Patients on effective acid suppressive therapy may still have persistent symptoms because of weakly acidic reflux as well as esophageal distension. Dilation of intercellular spaces (DIS) in the esophagus, resulting in stimulation of free nerve endings by luminal contents, may induce peripheral sensitization to pain[31]; in addition, somatic hyperalgesia has been demonstrated in patients with NERD, suggesting a role for central sensitization. In this context, putative visceral pain modulators such as low-dose antidepressants have been found to be effective.[80] Recently, the expression of transient receptor potential vanilloid 1 (TRPV-1), a nonselective cation channel, has been found to be upregulated in patients with erosive esophagitis.[31] AZD1386, a TRPV-1 antagonist, has been shown to increase pain thresholds in a proof-of-concept study in 21 healthy volunteers.[81] This agent may, therefore, have potential for use in patients with NERD and refractory GERD.

MUCOSAL PROTECTION

Drugs that enhance mucosal protection are promising as a class of agents in promoting mucosal healing. Sucralfate, an aluminum salt of sulfated disaccharide, binds to the inflamed tissue, prevents acid and pepsin entry into the mucosal break, and stimulates local healing mechanisms. This drug has been found to be useful in healing mild erosive esophagitis and in patients with NERD.[82] Sucralfate requires multiple dosing, leading to poor compliance. This drug is safe during pregnancy and has been found to be modestly effective as a monotherapy.[83] Rebamipide, a cytoprotective antiulcer agent that enhances endogenous prostaglandin production, has been shown to protect gastric and intestinal mucosa from damage induced by nonsteroidal antiinflammatory drugs. In addition, rebamipide reportedly exerts its antiinflammatory function through suppression of IL-8 production and neutrophil infiltration in the esophagus and stomach. Unfortunately, preliminary proof-of-concept studies have not been encouraging.[84]

MUCOSAL HEALING

NO-releasing moieties can enhance mucosal healing[80] but, unfortunately, they may also reduce LES tone, thereby facilitating GER. Moreover, NO is likely to have systemic effects thus limiting its use. Tegaserod was reported to have mucosal healing effects through its action on increasing epidermal growth factor (EGF) and mucus secretion,[80] but the clinical significance of this remains unclear and tegaserod has now been withdrawn from the market. The role of growth factors such as EGF and macrophage colony-stimulating factors although theoretically promising, needs to be evaluated in clinical trials.

AGENTS IN PIPELINE

The following agents are registered under clinicaltrials.gov with respect to the management of GERD:

- AH23844 (lavoltidine: H_2RA, also known as loxtidine) phase 2 study—effect on 24-hour pH value in man. Loxtidine development had, previously, been suspended in 1987, when it was reported to cause carcinoid tumors in rats (NCT00405119).
- AGSPT201 (S-pantoprazole: isomeric PPI) phase 3 study—comparison with pantoprazole in erosive esophagitis (NCT01400945).
- ONO-8539 (prostaglandin EP-1 receptor antagonist) phase 1 studies—effect of ONO-8539 on esophageal pain hypersensitivity to acid perfusion and in NERD (NCT01707901/NCT01705275).
- Rozerem (ramelteon: G-protein-coupled melatonin receptor agonist) phase 3 study—comparison with placebo of the effect on GERD symptoms in chronic insomnia (NCT01128582).
- Secretol, 60 mg once daily, (lansoprazole + omeprazole combination) versus Nexium, 40 mg once daily, phase 1/2 study in severe erosive esophagitis (NCT01129713).
- M0003 (SPD557) serotonin $5\text{-}HT_4$ receptor agonist, 0.5 mg 3 times a day, phase 2 study as adjunct to stable PPI therapy in GERD [NCT01370863].
- SSP-002358 (selective $5\text{-}HT_4$ RA, 0.1 to 2.0 mg 3 times a day and PPI) phase 2 study in GERD (NCT01472939).
- YH4808 (PCAB) phase 2 study—dose ranging compared with esomeprazole in GERD (NCT01538849).
- TAK-438 (PCAB), 10 mg or 20 mg, phase 3 study: dose-ranging placebo-controlled study in NERD (NCT01474369).
- Pantoprazole (20 mg) + domperidone (20 mg) tablet: phase 3 study compared with pantoprazole, 40 mg, or pantoprazole, 20 mg, in patients with GERD (NCT01710462).
- Esomeprazole (40 mg) + sodium bicarbonate (721 mg) (immediate-release PPI): phase 3 study compared with esomeprazole in GERD [NCT01471925].
- Azithromycin 250 mg 3 times per week (motilide: phase 2 study compared with placebo in esophageal hypomotility and GERD [NCT01448993]).

IMPLICATIONS FOR FUTURE RESEARCH

The management of GERD has been revolutionized over the past 20 years by the use of PPIs; even in their original formulations, as "traditional delayed-release" agents, they achieved healing rates of 85% to 90% in erosive esophagitis, albeit with rather lower symptom relief rates. Furthermore, they achieved this with a remarkably low incidence of adverse events, despite the sentiment to the contrary from the burgeoning literature on complications of acid suppression or PPI therapy. The success of PPIs is, arguably, serendipitous. PPIs are prodrugs and are activated and concentrated only in a low pH environment; their main therapeutic target, the gastric parietal cell secretory canaliculus, is the major site where acid secretion occurs. Furthermore, although traditional PPIs have a short serum half-life, they are taken up, activated, and concentrated up to 1000- to 10,000-fold in the secretory canaliculus where they bind, irreversibly, with the proton pump. Clinically, they block the final common pathway in the pathogenesis of acid-related disorders, and although they do not address the pathogenetic mechanisms underlying GERD, they have been proved to be safe and effective in a high proportion of patients who have an increasingly common disease. Thus, as a result of a series of happy accidents, traditional PPIs are highly selective, highly effective in a large proportion of patients, and safe; as such, they have set a very high therapeutic bar, and although they have limitations, it will be very difficult, if not impossible, for any novel therapy to demonstrate superiority in the general population of patients with GERD. The shortcomings of current PPIs with respect to duration of effect may be addressed by the development of agents that have a longer half-life, but this also increases the potential for adverse events related directly to the drug, because of increased plasma residence time, or to prolonged reduction in gastric acidity. Furthermore, it is not clear that refractory GERD symptoms are necessarily attributable to persistent esophageal acid exposure, so increased acid suppression may not produce the expected benefit. This is not to say that there will be no benefit from agents that can increase or prolong acid suppression; however, the benefit is likely to be limited to a subset of patients with GERD who will be difficult to identify specifically for inclusion in clinical trials designed to document the incremental benefit that may accrue from the use of a more-effective acid suppression agent. This is a particularly tall order because patients with refractory GERD will often have a normal endoscopy; it is difficult to know, therefore, whether study subjects have truly refractory GERD, mediated by acid in the esophagus, or whether their symptoms indicate nonacid reflux, esophageal hypersensitivity, central mechanisms, or functional heartburn. Without better tools to identify patients who have refractory acid-mediated symptoms, it will be difficult to document benefit from novel acid suppressants in comparison with current PPIs.

Recognizing that acid inhibitors do not address the mechanisms underlying GER, it is theoretically attractive to consider therapies that will target the causes directly. Unfortunately, the pathogenesis of GERD is multifactorial, encompassing disorders of esophageal and gastric motility, LES control, esophageal epithelial defense and repair, and salivary secretion, in addition to anatomic abnormalities, such as hiatus hernia, that may disrupt the antireflux barrier and dietary and other factors implicated, increasingly, in obesity-related reflux disease. Many, if not all of these potential pathogenetic mechanisms are controlled by multiple redundant processes, and the underlying neural, endocrine, and receptor-mediated mechanisms are widespread, if not ubiquitous throughout the body. Thus, although GABA, serotonin, and mGluR5 receptors may play very important roles in the mechanisms underlying the control of GER, there is considerable redundancy in these control mechanisms and the relative importance of any abnormality may differ between individuals or patients. It is, therefore, a huge challenge to develop a novel agent that can target a specific receptor or mechanism in a susceptible individual such that there are no remote effects on other tissues and, furthermore, demonstrate superiority in an economic, regulatory, and clinical environment in which PPIs have been so successful for a condition that is viewed, by many, as "just heartburn" attributable to an unhealthy lifestyle and readily amenable to nonpharmacologic intervention.

This is not a nihilistic view of the need for novel therapies for reflux disease. Clearly, GERD is a common condition throughout the world, and it is associated with considerable impairment of quality of life, morbidity, mortality, and costs. Equally, refractory GERD or GERD symptoms constitute a significant problem that is not responsive to current therapy, and furthermore, current therapy does not address the underlying pathophysiology. However, it seems highly improbable that any new therapy will be superior to current PPI therapy for the overall general population of patients with GERD. The overwhelming need, therefore, is for a better understanding of the mechanisms causing reflux and for tools to identify those mechanisms that are responsible for disease manifestations in individual patients; in this way, the underlying mechanisms may be targeted appropriately by lifestyle measures, by acid suppression agents with appropriate pharmacologic properties, by antireflux agents, by promotility agents, or by sensory modulators, alone or in combination; then, if necessary, endoscopic or surgical procedures may be considered for those patients in whom anatomic abnormalities are important. If possible, future studies of novel agents should also include standard outcome measures to facilitate comparisons with other agents and pooling of data to help understand the epidemiology and pathogenesis of GERD in different populations. The inclusion of exploratory mechanistic subprotocols would also be important to help understand how and why interventions may have been successful in specific patients or patient groups.

REFERENCES

1. Vakil N, van Zanten SV, Kahrilas P, et al. The Montreal definition and classification of gastroesophageal reflux disease: a global evidence-based consensus. Am J Gastroenterol 2006;101:1900–20.
2. Sandler RS, Everhart JE, Donowitz M, et al. The burden of selected digestive diseases in the United States. Gastroenterology 2002;122:1500–11.
3. Peery AF, Dellon ES, Lund J, et al. Burden of gastrointestinal disease in the United States: 2012 update. Gastroenterology 2012;143:1179–87.
4. Dent J, El-Serag HB, Wallander MA, et al. Epidemiology of gastro-oesophageal reflux disease: a systematic review. Gut 2005;54:710–7.
5. Kahrilas PJ, Shaheen NJ, Vaezi MF. American Gastroenterological Association Institute technical review on the management of gastroesophageal reflux disease. Gastroenterology 2008;135:1392–413.
6. Fass R, Shapiro M, Dekel R, et al. Systematic review: proton-pump inhibitor failure in gastro-oesophageal reflux disease–where next? Aliment Pharmacol Ther 2005;22:79–94.
7. Altan E, Blondeau K, Pauwels A, et al. Evolving pharmacological approaches in gastroesophageal reflux disease. Expert Opin Emerg Drugs 2012;17:347–59.
8. Raghunath AS, Hungin AP, Mason J, et al. Symptoms in patients on long-term proton pump inhibitors: prevalence and predictors. Aliment Pharmacol Ther 2009;29:431–9.
9. Pandolfino JE, Shi G, Trueworthy B, et al. Esophagogastric junction opening during relaxation distinguishes nonhernia reflux patients, hernia patients, and normal subjects. Gastroenterology 2003;125:1018–24.
10. Hirschowitz BI. A critical analysis, with appropriate controls, of gastric acid and pepsin secretion in clinical esophagitis. Gastroenterology 1991;101:1149–58.
11. Herbella FA, Vicentine FP, Silva LC, et al. Postprandial proximal gastric acid pocket and gastroesophageal reflux disease. Dis Esophagus 2012;25:652–5.

12. Kwiatek MA, Roman S, Fareeduddin A, et al. An alginate-antacid formulation (Gaviscon Double Action Liquid) can eliminate or displace the postprandial 'acid pocket' in symptomatic GERD patients. Aliment Pharmacol Ther 2011;34:59–66.
13. Buckles DC, Sarosiek I, McMillin C, et al. Delayed gastric emptying in gastroesophageal reflux disease: reassessment with new methods and symptomatic correlations. Am J Med Sci 2004;327:1–4.
14. Vaezi MF, Richter JE. Role of acid and duodenogastroesophageal reflux in gastroesophageal reflux disease. Gastroenterology 1996;111:1192–9.
15. Araki Y, Mukaisho KI, Fujiyama Y, et al. The herbal medicine rikkunshito exhibits strong and differential adsorption properties for bile salts. Exp Ther Med 2012;3:645–9.
16. Blackshaw LA, Staunton E, Lehmann A, et al. Inhibition of transient LES relaxations and reflux in ferrets by GABA receptor agonists. Am J Physiol 1999;277:G867–74.
17. Keywood C, Wakefield M, Tack J. A proof-of-concept study evaluating the effect of ADX10059, a metabotropic glutamate receptor-5 negative allosteric modulator, on acid exposure and symptoms in gastro-oesophageal reflux disease. Gut 2009; 58:1192–9.
18. Beaumont H, Jensen J, Carlsson A, et al. Effect of delta9-tetrahydrocannabinol, a cannabinoid receptor agonist, on the triggering of transient lower oesophageal sphincter relaxations in dogs and humans. Br J Pharmacol 2009;156:153–62.
19. Rohof WO, Aronica E, Beaumont H, et al. Localization of mGluR5, GABAB, GABAA, and cannabinoid receptors on the vago-vagal reflex pathway responsible for transient lower esophageal sphincter relaxation in humans: an immunohistochemical study. Neurogastroenterol Motil 2012;24:383–92.
20. Hirsch DP, Tiel-Van Buul MM, Tytgat GN, et al. Effect of L-NMMA on postprandial transient lower esophageal sphincter relaxations in healthy volunteers. Dig Dis Sci 2000;45:2069–75.
21. Boeckxstaens GE, Hirsch DP, Fakhry N, et al. Involvement of cholecystokininA receptors in transient lower esophageal sphincter relaxations triggered by gastric distension. Am J Gastroenterol 1998;93:1823–8.
22. Sifrim D, Zerbib F. Diagnosis and management of patients with reflux symptoms refractory to proton pump inhibitors. Gut 2012;61:1340–54.
23. Boeckxstaens GE. Alterations confined to the gastro-oesophageal junction: the relationship between low LOSP, TLOSRs, hiatus hernia and acid pocket. Best Pract Res Clin Gastroenterol 2010;24:821–9.
24. Yang L, Francois F, Pei Z. Molecular pathways: pathogenesis and clinical implications of microbiome alteration in esophagitis and Barrett esophagus. Clin Cancer Res 2012;18:2138–44.
25. Indrio F, Riezzo G, Raimondi F, et al. Lactobacillus reuteri accelerates gastric emptying and improves regurgitation in infants. Eur J Clin Invest 2011;41:417–22.
26. Hsu YC, Lin HJ. Addition of prokinetic therapy to a PPI in reflux diseases. Aliment Pharmacol Ther 2011;33:983–5.
27. Kim YS, Kim TH, Choi CS, et al. Effect of itopride, a new prokinetic, in patients with mild GERD: a pilot study. World J Gastroenterol 2005;11:4210–4.
28. Tobey NA, Carson JL, Alkiek RA, et al. Dilated intercellular spaces: a morphological feature of acid reflux–damaged human esophageal epithelium. Gastroenterology 1996;111:1200–5.
29. Tobey NA, Hosseini SS, Argote CM, et al. Dilated intercellular spaces and shunt permeability in nonerosive acid-damaged esophageal epithelium. Am J Gastroenterol 2004;99:13–22.
30. Chu CL, Zhen YB, Lv GP, et al. Microalterations of esophagus in patients with non-erosive reflux disease: in-vivo diagnosis by confocal laser endomicroscopy

and its relationship with gastroesophageal reflux. Am J Gastroenterol 2012;107: 864–74.

31. Knowles CH, Aziz Q. Visceral hypersensitivity in non-erosive reflux disease. Gut 2008;57:674–83.

32. Farre R, De VR, Geboes K, et al. Critical role of stress in increased oesophageal mucosa permeability and dilated intercellular spaces. Gut 2007;56:1191–7.

33. Sharma P, Shaheen NJ, Perez MC, et al. Clinical trials: healing of erosive oeso-phagitis with dexlansoprazole MR, a proton pump inhibitor with a novel dual delayed-release formulation–results from two randomized controlled studies. Aliment Pharmacol Ther 2009;29:731–41.

34. Kahrilas PJ, Falk GW, Johnson DA, et al. Esomeprazole improves healing and symptom resolution as compared with omeprazole in reflux oesophagitis patients: a randomized controlled trial. The Esomeprazole Study Investigators. Aliment Pharmacol Ther 2000;14:1249–58.

35. Gralnek IM, Dulai GS, Fennerty MB, et al. Esomeprazole versus other proton pump inhibitors in erosive esophagitis: a meta-analysis of randomized clinical trials. Clin Gastroenterol Hepatol 2006;4:1452–8.

36. Edwards SJ, Lind T, Lundell L. Systematic review: proton pump inhibitors (PPIs) for the healing of reflux oesophagitis - a comparison of esomeprazole with other PPIs. Aliment Pharmacol Ther 2006;24:743–50.

37. Laine L, Katz PO, Johnson DA, et al. Randomised clinical trial: a novel rabepra-zole extended release 50 mg formulation vs. esomeprazole 40 mg in healing of moderate-to-severe erosive oesophagitis - the results of two double-blind studies. Aliment Pharmacol Ther 2011;33:203–12.

38. Hunt RH, Armstrong D, Yaghoobi M, et al. Predictable prolönged suppression of gastric acidity with a novel proton pump inhibitor, AGN 201904-Z. Aliment Phar-macol Ther 2008;28:187–99.

39. Hunt RH, Armstrong D, Yaghoobi M, et al. The pharmacodynamics and pharma-cokinetics of S-tenatoprazole-Na 30 mg, 60 mg and 90 mg vs. esomeprazole 40 mg in healthy male subjects. Aliment Pharmacol Ther 2010;31:648–57.

40. Scarpignato C, Hunt RH. Proton pump inhibitors: the beginning of the end or the end of the beginning? Curr Opin Pharmacol 2008;8:677–84.

41. Wang L, Zhou L, Hu H, et al. Ilaprazole for the treatment of duodenal ulcer: a randomized, double-blind and controlled phase III trial. Curr Med Res Opin 2012;28:101–9.

42. Rosemary J, Adithan C. The pharmacogenetics of CYP2C9 and CYP2C19: ethnic variation and clinical significance. Curr Clin Pharmacol 2007;2:93–109.

43. Li XQ, Andersson TB, Ahlstrom M, et al. Comparison of inhibitory effects of the proton pump-inhibiting drugs omeprazole, esomeprazole, lansoprazole, pantopra-zole, and rabeprazole on human cytochrome P450 activities. Drug Metab Dispos 2004;32:821–7.

44. Chowers Y, Atarot T, Kostadinov A, et al. PPI activity is optimized by VB101, a pari-etal cell activator. Gastroenterology 2008;134(Suppl 1):A-172.

45. Sorba G, Galli U, Cena C, et al. A new furoxan NO-donor rabeprazole derivative and related compounds. Chembiochem 2003;4:899–903.

46. Saha JK, Wang T, Stewart R, et al. Enhanced gastroprotective and anti-ulcerogenic activities in rats of a new class of proton pump inhibitor containing nitrosothiol nitric oxide donor. Gastroenterology 2001;120(Suppl 1):A144–5.

47. Rackoff A, Agrawal A, Hila A, et al. Histamine-2 receptor antagonists at night improve gastroesophageal reflux disease symptoms for patients on proton pump inhibitor therapy. Dis Esophagus 2005;18:370–3.

48. Pouchain D, Bigard MA, Liard F, et al. Gaviscon® vs. omeprazole in symptomatic treatment of moderate gastroesophageal reflux. a direct comparative randomised trial. BMC Gastroenterol 2012;23:12–8.
49. Manabe N, Haruma K, Ito M, et al. Efficacy of adding sodium alginate to omeprazole in patients with nonerosive reflux disease: a randomized clinical trial. Dis Esophagus 2012;25:373–80.
50. Madan K, Ahuja V, Kashyap PC, et al. Comparison of efficacy of pantoprazole alone versus pantoprazole plus mosapride in therapy of gastroesophageal reflux disease: a randomized trial. Dis Esophagus 2004;17:274–8.
51. Cho YK, Choi MG, Park EY, et al. Effect of mosapride combined with esomeprazole improves esophageal peristaltic function in patients with gastroesophageal reflux disease: a study using high resolution manometry. Dig Dis Sci 2012. [Epub ahead of print].
52. Ezzat WF, Fawaz SA, Fathey H, et al. Virtue of adding prokinetics to proton pump inhibitors in the treatment of laryngopharyngeal reflux disease: prospective study. J Otolaryngol Head Neck Surg 2011;40:350–6.
53. Futagami S, Iwakiri K, Shindo T, et al. The prokinetic effect of mosapride citrate combined with omeprazole therapy improves clinical symptoms and gastric emptying in PPI-resistant NERD patients with delayed gastric emptying. J Gastroenterol 2010;45:413–21.
54. Miwa H, Inoue K, Ashida K, et al. Randomised clinical trial: efficacy of the addition of a prokinetic, mosapride citrate, to omeprazole in the treatment of patients with non-erosive reflux disease - a double-blind, placebo-controlled study. Aliment Pharmacol Ther 2011;33:323–32.
55. Miyamoto M, Manabe N, Haruma K. Efficacy of the addition of prokinetics for proton pump inhibitor (PPI) resistant non-erosive reflux disease (NERD) patients: significance of frequency scale for the symptom of GERD (FSSG) on decision of treatment strategy. Intern Med 2010;49:1469–76.
56. Karamanolis G, Vanuytsel T, Sifrim D, et al. Yield of 24-hour esophageal pH and bilitec monitoring in patients with persisting symptoms on PPI therapy. Dig Dis Sci 2008;53:2387–93.
57. Dent J. Reflux inhibitor drugs: an emerging novel therapy for gastroesophageal reflux disease. J Dig Dis 2010;11:72–5.
58. Zhang Q, Lehmann A, Rigda R, et al. Control of transient lower oesophageal sphincter relaxations and reflux by the GABA(B) agonist baclofen in patients with gastro-oesophageal reflux disease. Gut 2002;50:19–24.
59. Gerson LB, Huff FJ, Hila A, et al. Arbaclofen placarbil decreases postprandial reflux in patients with gastroesophageal reflux disease. Am J Gastroenterol 2010;105:1266–75.
60. Boeckxstaens GE, Rydholm H, Lei A, et al. Effect of lesogaberan, a novel GABA(B)-receptor agonist, on transient lower oesophageal sphincter relaxations in male subjects. Aliment Pharmacol Ther 2010;31:1208–17.
61. Boeckxstaens GE, Beaumont H, Hatlebakk JG, et al. A novel reflux inhibitor lesogaberan (AZD3355) as add-on treatment in patients with GORD with persistent reflux symptoms despite proton pump inhibitor therapy: a randomised placebo-controlled trial. Gut 2011;60:1182–8.
62. Beaumont H, Smout A, Aanen M, et al. The GABA(B) receptor agonist AZD9343 inhibits transient lower oesophageal sphincter relaxations and acid reflux in healthy volunteers: a phase I study. Aliment Pharmacol Ther 2009;30:937–46.
63. Froestl W. Chemistry and pharmacology of GABAB receptor ligands. Adv Pharmacol 2010;58:19–62.

64. Vakil NB, Huff FJ, Bian A, et al. Arbaclofen placarbil in GERD: a randomized, double-blind, placebo-controlled study. Am J Gastroenterol 2011;106:1427–38.
65. Lehmann A, Jensen JM, Boeckxstaens GE. GABAB receptor agonism as a novel therapeutic modality in the treatment of gastroesophageal reflux disease. Adv Pharmacol 2010;58:287–313.
66. Zerbib F, Keywood C, Strabach G. Efficacy, tolerability and pharmacokinetics of a modified release formulation of ADX10059, a negative allosteric modulator of metabotropic glutamate receptor 5: an esophageal pH-impedance study in healthy subjects. Neurogastroenterol Motil 2010;22:859–65.
67. Rohof WO, Lei A, Hirsch DP, et al. The effects of a novel metabotropic glutamate receptor 5 antagonist (AZD2066) on transient lower oesophageal sphincter relaxations and reflux episodes in healthy volunteers. Aliment Pharmacol Ther 2012; 35:1231–42.
68. Scarpellini E, Blondeau K, Boecxstaens V, et al. Effect of rimonabant on oesophageal motor function in man. Aliment Pharmacol Ther 2011;33:730–7.
69. Fass R. Healing erosive esophagitis with a proton pump inhibitor: the more the merrier? Am J Gastroenterol 2012;107:531–3.
70. Hershcovici T, Fass R. Pharmacological management of GERD: where does it stand now? Trends Pharmacol Sci 2011;32:258–64.
71. Curran MP, Robinson DM. Mosapride in gastrointestinal disorders. Drugs 2008; 68:981–91.
72. Scarpellini E, Vos R, Blondeau K, et al. The effects of itopride on oesophageal motility and lower oesophageal sphincter function in man. Aliment Pharmacol Ther 2011;33:99–105.
73. Fass R. Therapeutic options for refractory gastroesophageal reflux disease. J Gastroenterol Hepatol 2012;27(Suppl 3):3–7.
74. Koutsoumbi P, Epanomeritakis E, Tsiaoussis J, et al. The effect of erythromycin on human esophageal motility is mediated by serotonin receptors. Am J Gastroenterol 2000;95:3388–92.
75. Rohof WO, Bennink RJ, de Ruigh AA, et al. Effect of azithromycin on acid reflux, hiatus hernia and proximal acid pocket in the postprandial period. Gut 2012;61: 1670–7.
76. Ozaki K, Monnai M, Onoma M, et al. Effects of mitemcinal (GM-611), an orally active erythromycin-derived prokinetic agent, on delayed gastric emptying and postprandial glucose in a new minipig model of diabetes. J Diabetes Complications 2008;22:339–47.
77. Takanashi H, Cynshi O. Motilides: a long and winding road: lessons from mitemcinal (GM-611) on diabetic gastroparesis. Regul Pept 2009;155:18–23.
78. Tominaga K, Iwakiri R, Fujimoto K, et al. Rikkunshito improves symptoms in PPI-refractory GERD patients: a prospective, randomized, multicenter trial in Japan. J Gastroenterol 2012;47:284–92.
79. Bai Y, Xu MJ, Yang X, et al. A systematic review on intrapyloric botulinum toxin injection for gastroparesis. Digestion 2010;81:27–34.
80. Zerbib F, Simon M. Novel therapeutics for gastro-esophageal reflux symptoms. Expert Rev Clin Pharmacol 2012;5:533–41.
81. Krarup AL, Ny L, Astrand M, et al. Randomised clinical trial: the efficacy of a transient receptor potential vanilloid 1 antagonist AZD1386 in human oesophageal pain. Aliment Pharmacol Ther 2011;33:1113–22.
82. Simon B, Ravelli GP, Goffin H. Sucralfate gel versus placebo in patients with non-erosive gastro-oesophageal reflux disease. Aliment Pharmacol Ther 1996;10: 441–6.

83. Fass R. Alternative therapeutic approaches to chronic proton pump inhibitor treatment. Clin Gastroenterol Hepatol 2012;10:338–40.
84. Adachi K, Furuta K, Miwa H, et al. A study on the efficacy of rebamipide for patients with proton pump inhibitor-refractory non-erosive reflux disease. Dig Dis Sci 2012;57:1609–17.

Surgical Management of Gastroesophageal Reflux Disease

Candice L. Wilshire, MD, Thomas J. Watson, MD*

KEYWORDS

- Gastroesophageal reflux disease • Antireflux surgery • Laparoscopic fundoplication
- High-resolution manometry • Impedance-pH monitoring

KEY POINTS

- Antireflux surgery has become a well-established therapy for gastroesophageal reflux disease and its complications.
- Minimally invasive surgical techniques have revolutionized the use of fundoplication.
- Surgical outcomes are highly dependent on appropriate and thorough preoperative patient evaluation.
- Foregut diagnostics and surgical techniques continue to be refined.
- Laparoscopic fundoplication has compared favorably to medical therapy long term.
- Laparoscopic fundoplication remains the gold standard to which evolving endoscopic and surgical technologies for control of gastroesophageal reflux disease must be compared.

INTRODUCTION

Over half a century has passed since Rudolph Nissen first reported the use of fundoplication for the treatment of gastroesophageal reflux disease (GERD).[1] In the ensuing years, antireflux operations by a variety of methods have proven effective and durable in the control of GERD and its various manifestations. Surgical therapy for GERD was subsequently revolutionized by the introduction and popularization of minimally invasive operative techniques in the early 1990s.[2,3] Today, laparoscopic Nissen fundoplication (LNF) is the most commonly performed antireflux procedure (ARP) and remains the "gold standard" against which other operative interventions are compared.

The indications for surgery, preoperative evaluation, and techniques of fundoplication have been refined, leading to favorable outcomes as assessed by both subjective and objective parameters in most appropriately selected candidates. The availability of a laparoscopic approach to fundoplication, coupled with the excellent long-term

Division of Thoracic and Foregut Surgery, Department of Surgery, University of Rochester School of Medicine and Dentistry, 601 Elmwood Avenue, Rochester, NY 14642, USA
* Corresponding author. Division of Thoracic and Foregut Surgery, Department of Surgery, University of Rochester School of Medicine and Dentistry, 601 Elmwood Avenue, Box Surgery, Rochester, NY 14642.
E-mail address: Thomas_Watson@urmc.rochester.edu

Gastroenterol Clin N Am 42 (2013) 119–131
http://dx.doi.org/10.1016/j.gtc.2012.11.005
0889-8553/13/$ – see front matter © 2013 Elsevier Inc. All rights reserved.

control of symptoms afforded by such procedures, has made antireflux surgery an attractive alternative for the management of GERD. On the other hand, surgery has the potential for morbidity, is costly, and can be associated with a suboptimal outcome in a minority of patients. Recent data suggest that the peak use of antireflux surgery in the United States occurred in 1999, with an estimated 15.7 cases per 100,000 adults at that time.[4] Since then, the frequency of antireflux surgery has declined, such that an estimated 11 ARPs were performed per 100,000 adults in 2003, a 30% reduction. In a separate analysis of the National Inpatient Sample database, the use of antireflux operations decreased 40% between 2000 and 2006.[5] These declines may reflect the widespread use of prescription medications, over-the-counter proton pump inhibitors (PPIs) and other acid suppressive medications, as well as concerns about both the durability of surgical repair and the potential for long-term postoperative side effects. Given the various treatment options for GERD, each with their potential advantages and shortcomings, accurate and current data regarding outcomes of antireflux surgery are necessary as a basis against which other established and novel therapies must be judged. The purpose of this article is to review the contemporary literature regarding the optimal work-up and patient selection for antireflux surgery, as well as to assess the data regarding both short-term and long-term symptomatic and objective outcomes.

INDICATIONS

In the era of "open" surgery before 1990, the need for a laparotomy or thoracotomy limited the use of fundoplication to patients manifesting only the most severe complications of GERD, such as refractory esophagitis, esophageal stricture, or repetitive aspiration. The introduction of less invasive surgical approaches brought an expansion of the indications for operative repair to include patients with longstanding symptoms and no complications seeking an alternative to life-long acid suppression therapy. A medical position statement on the management of GERD published by the American Gastroenterological Association in 2008 recommended that antireflux surgery be considered an option (1) when a patient with an esophageal GERD syndrome is responsive to, but intolerant of, acid suppressive therapy (grade A recommendation); (2) for patients with an esophageal GERD syndrome who have persistent troublesome symptoms, especially troublesome regurgitation, despite PPI therapy (grade B recommendation); (3) for patients with an extraesophageal GERD syndrome with persistent troublesome symptoms despite PPI therapy (grade C recommendation).[6]

The evaluation for antireflux surgery commences with a thorough history emphasizing the patient's reflux symptoms and response to antisecretory and promotility therapy. The presence of both "typical" reflux symptoms, such as heartburn, regurgitation, or dysphagia, as well as "atypical" symptoms that might be attributable to GERD, such as cough, wheezing, hoarseness, shortness of breath, or sore throat, is noted. Because there are fewer potential mechanisms for their generation, typical symptoms are more likely to be secondary to pathologic gastroesophageal reflux than are atypical symptoms. The patient must be made aware of the relatively diminished probability of success of antireflux surgery when atypical symptoms are the primary factors driving intervention, in that other contributors may persist. Also relevant is the longer time frame anticipated for respiratory symptoms to improve after surgery compared with typical symptoms.

Symptomatic response to acid suppression medications is of importance as it can predict relief following surgery.[7] A paradox of patient referral for an ARP is that patients well controlled on medical therapy, who may be among the best candidates for surgery, often are not sent for a surgical opinion. On the other hand, those patients who do not respond to medical therapy and, therefore, may not respond well to surgery, frequently are referred for surgical therapy. A detailed objective evaluation for the presence of pathologic gastroesophageal reflux is particularly important in the latter group, as well as a careful determination of whether the patient's main complaints are reflux-related. The surgeon needs to be aware of primary symptoms, such as nausea, early satiety, epigastric pain or bloating, that may be indicative of foregut pathologic abnormality and may even occur in the presence of excessive esophageal acid exposure, although may not be caused by gastroesophageal reflux per se. Persistent symptoms despite PPI use, PPI dose escalation, young age with concerns over chronic PPI use, nocturnal regurgitation, and chronic cough are common reasons for surgical referral.

Other historical factors of interest include the presence of asthma, other pulmonary disease (eg, recurrent aspiration/pneumonia, "idiopathic" pulmonary fibrosis, or interstitial lung disease), concomitant cardiac disease, exercise tolerance, and prior surgical procedures involving the abdomen, chest, or neck. Physical examination should include the patient's body habitus and weight, detailed assessment of the lungs, documentation of surgical scars, as well as an overall assessment of functional status. Obesity and extensive prior upper abdominal surgery are relative indications for a transthoracic approach to fundoplication in the hands of some surgeons, whereas a thoracotomy is generally avoided in elderly persons or in a patient of poor functional status.[8] In the setting of morbid obesity, whether fundoplication or a bariatric procedure such as Roux-en-Y gastric bypass is the preferable operation to control reflux is a matter of ongoing study. Many surgeons favor the latter option because of the questionable durability of a fundoplication in the setting of morbid obesity as well as the multiple non-GERD-related health benefits derived from weight loss following gastric bypass.[9–11]

Anatomic Factors

In addition to patients who are severely symptomatic from GERD, other individuals commonly referred for consideration of antireflux surgery are those with a paraesophageal hernia (PEH) and intrathoracic stomach. The traditional recommendation, dating back to a landmark article by Skinner and Belsey[12] from 1967, had been to repair all such large hernias at the time of diagnosis. In that report, the risk of fatal complications from an untreated, minimally symptomatic PEH was found to be 29% over the patient's lifetime, a rate thought high enough to justify operative intervention.

With increasing experience, however, the observation has been made that the risk of leaving asymptomatic or minimally symptomatic PEHs uncorrected is not nearly that high.[13] In addition, the repair of such hernias is not without risk of morbidity or mortality, especially in light of the demographics of this condition. Patients presenting with PEH are commonly elderly, kyphotic and possessing significant comorbidities.[14] Finally, the long-term success rate after repair of large hernias is not as good as following repair of smaller, sliding hiatal hernias or after operation for GERD without an associated hiatal hernia. This fact deserves emphasis, in that the outcomes of all patients undergoing fundoplication tend to be lumped together and, perhaps, has been a mitigating factor against referral of patients for fundoplication to control GERD. Many centers, including ours, are seeing an increasing proportion of patients with PEH referred for fundoplication, a trend that may negatively impact overall surgical outcomes.

Another point worthy of emphasis is that most studies of novel endoscopic or alternative minimally invasive therapies for GERD have excluded cohorts of patients with symptomatic, functional, or anatomic factors that might preclude effective reflux control through such approaches. Clinical trials of investigational antireflux therapies have, by and large, included only study subjects with uncomplicated GERD and typical symptoms of heartburn and regurgitation that have responded to medical therapy. Patients with severe anatomic derangements, such as esophageal strictures, persistent esophagitis, Barrett's esophagus, or sizable hiatal hernias, as well as those with severe motility disorders or significant comorbidities, are excluded from such investigations. Similarly, patients who have demonstrated a poor response to medical therapy and those with primarily extraesophageal manifestations of GERD have not been studied. These factors must be kept in mind as one compares outcomes following a fundoplication to those reported for novel endoscopic or surgical therapies; the patients expected to have the worst outcomes generally are excluded from trials of the latter.

PREOPERATIVE EVALUATION

An appropriate and thorough evaluation of patients considered for antireflux surgery is of paramount importance. The proof of pathologic gastroesophageal reflux, as well as the characterization of associated abnormalities in foregut structure and function, is critical to a successful surgical outcome. Likewise, inadequate or inaccurate preoperative evaluation can be a major contributor to a poor outcome following an antireflux repair. Three factors have emerged as being most predictive of a successful symptomatic outcome after antireflux surgery: the presence of typical symptoms of GERD (heartburn or regurgitation), symptomatic improvement in response to acid suppression therapy before surgery, and an abnormal score on ambulatory esophageal pH monitoring, with an abnormal score on ambulatory esophageal pH monitoring being of greatest importance.[7] Each of these factors helps to establish that GERD is, indeed, the cause of the patient's symptoms, although they have little relationship to the severity of the underlying disease.

The goals of preoperative evaluation for potential antireflux surgery are provided in **Box 1**. The most common preoperative diagnostic studies include the following:

1. Video esophagography;
2. Flexible upper gastrointestinal endoscopy;

Box 1
Goals of preoperative evaluation

1. Elucidation of all symptoms that might be attributable to GERD, as well as symptoms potentially attributable to associated foregut abnormalities;

2. Assessment of comorbidities that might impact candidacy for surgery, the surgical approach, and perioperative complications;

3. Objective confirmation of the presence of GERD;

4. Appreciation of associated anatomic abnormalities (eg, Barrett's esophagus, shortened esophagus, esophageal stricture, large sliding or paraesophageal hiatal hernia);

5. Assessment of associated functional abnormalities of the foregut;

6. Estimation of the probability of a successful symptomatic response to surgical therapy;

7. Planning the type of fundoplication, the operative approach (laparoscopic, open transabdominal, or transthoracic), and the likelihood of needing to perform an esophageal lengthening procedure (Collis gastroplasty).

3. Stationary esophageal manometry;
4. Ambulatory esophageal pH monitoring.

Further investigations, in particular, gastric-emptying scans or impedance monitoring, are added depending on the findings of standard testing and the presence of symptoms that warrant additional study.

Most of the preoperative studies have been well described and are established in common clinical practice. A few newer technologies have emerged that deserve emphasis in terms of their applicability to patients being considered for an ARP.

High-Resolution Manometry

The introduction of high-resolution manometry (HRM) into clinical practice in 2000 (ManoScan[360]; Given Imaging, Duluth, GA), along with the development of sophisticated algorithms to display the expanded data set as esophageal pressure topography plots, has transformed conventional esophageal manometry from an analysis of wave tracings to an image-based paradigm assisted with color enhancements (**Fig. 1**).[15] Just as high-definition television has made standard-definition broadcasting seem antiquated, HRM has made conventional manometry (CM) seem obsolete.

Several advantages exist for HRM over the CM systems currently available. The HRM catheter is 4.2 mm in diameter and consists of 36 solid-state circumferential sensors spaced at 1-cm increments, compared with the standard 3- to 5-cm spacing of traditional water-perfused or solid-state catheters. The tighter spacing allows for a more thorough assessment of esophageal function. Given the density and span of transducers across the length of the catheter, the upper esophageal sphincter, esophageal body, and lower esophageal sphincter can be assessed simultaneously without moving the catheter. Thus, the study can be performed more quickly and with improved patient comfort compared with CM in that multiple repositionings of the catheter are not required to complete the evaluation. The experience from the authors' laboratory has been that HRM takes, on average, only 8 minutes to complete, whereas CM with a solid-state catheter takes over 24 minutes.[16] In addition, the color-coded

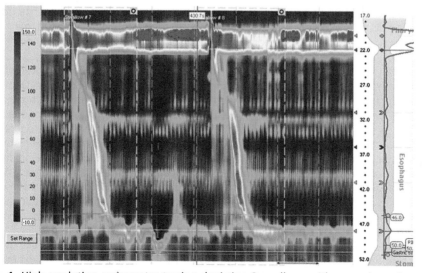

Fig. 1. High-resolution manometry tracing depicting 2 swallows with normal esophageal structure and function.

readouts allow for a better, more intuitive, graphic description of the motor activity of the esophagus, the characteristics of the lower esophageal sphincter, and the presence of a hiatal hernia compared with the other technologies. The catheter, however, is expensive with a high replacement cost should it break. With increasing experience and further study, the pros and cons of this new technology will continue to be elucidated.

Relative to decisions about antireflux surgery, manometry provides several types of useful information. An esophageal motility disorder, such as achalasia, masquerading as GERD or occurring in the setting of GERD, can be ruled out. Most surgeons will perform a total or 360° fundic wrap (Nissen) for control of GERD in the setting of normal or near-normal esophageal body peristaltic function. In the setting of severe peristaltic dysfunction, concerns exist over the potential for such a wrap to cause an esophageal outflow obstruction; a partial anterior or posterior fundic wrap (Dor, Toupet, or Belsey procedure) is typically chosen in such situations. The degree of peristaltic dysfunction required to abandon a Nissen fundoplication in favor of a partial wrap is not clearly defined from the available data, although studies suggest that once the wave amplitudes in the distal esophagus drop below 20 to 30 mm Hg, a Nissen should be avoided.[17]

Manometry can also be useful in evaluating the patient with dysphagia after fundoplication. Preliminary data from the authors' institution using HRM show that impaired lower esophageal sphincter relaxation, as determined by the presence of an elevated 4-second integrated relaxation pressure, correlates with the presence of dysphagia and may imply a technical abnormality of a fundoplication leading to esophageal outflow obstruction.[18]

Ambulatory pH and Combined Impedance–pH Monitoring

Ambulatory pH monitoring is the "gold standard" for the assessment of pathologic esophageal acid exposure. Present technology includes transnasal catheter-based pH probes and an implantable capsule (Bravo pH system; Given Imaging) placed under endoscopic control. Several limitations exist, however, to standard pH monitoring: nonacid reflux events are not detected, the height and quantity of refluxate above the gastroesophageal junction are not defined, and the physical nature of the refluxed material (ie, liquid, gas or a mixture) cannot be differentiated.[19] It has been well-established that reflux symptoms such as regurgitation and cough may be present in the absence of demonstrable reflux of acid. Thus, improved modalities for detection of non–acid refluxate may be clinically important.

New technology has been introduced into clinical practice that allows for detection of both acid reflux and non–acid reflux. The Sleuth system (Sandhill Scientific, Denver, Colorado) combines pH monitoring and intraluminal impedance measurements using a single catheter. The technology identifies refluxate via changes in impedance caused by the presence of a bolus in the esophagus. The event can be categorized as acid or non-acid by the contemporaneous measurement of intraluminal pH. Esophageal impedance has been validated as an appropriate method for the evaluation of gastrointestinal function and reflux.[20] All episodes of gastroesophageal reflux now can be detected without regard to their chemical composition. Studies using this technology have shown that, in normal subjects, PPI therapy does not alter the number of reflux episodes, but rather, simply converts the refluxate to a neutral pH.[21] This observation may have important implications in the treatment of GERD.

Combined impedance–pH monitoring has been used to select patients, with both typical and atypical manifestations of GERD and who are resistant to medical treatment, for fundoplication.[22] Patients with a positive symptom index, as assessed by combined impedance-pH testing while on PPI therapy, were noted to respond well to surgery. Another recent trial demonstrated that combined impedance–pH testing is more accurate for the preoperative assessment of GERD in patients off of PPI therapy compared with pH monitoring alone.[23]

OUTCOMES

Much has been written about results following antireflux surgery. Any discussion regarding fundoplication outcomes should include the following:

1. Perioperative morbidity and mortality;
2. Control of typical and atypical symptoms;
3. Objective relief from excessive esophageal acid exposure;
4. Side effects;
5. Anatomic rates of failure, such as recurrent hiatal herniation or slippage, and the need for reoperation.

Perioperative Morbidity/Mortality

Laparoscopic fundoplication is a safe procedure in experienced hands and in appropriately selected patients. A recent review of the American College of Surgeons National Surgical Quality Improvement Program (ACS NSQIP) database from 2005 to 2009 identified a total of 7531 fundoplications.[24] Thirty-day mortality was rare in patients less than 70 years of age, occurring in 1 of 2000 (0.05%). Mortality increased to 0.8% for patients older than 70 years, although this cohort likely underwent fundoplication mainly for treatment of PEH rather than for GERD. Complications occurred in 2.2% of patients younger than 50 years of age, 3.8% of those 50 to 69 years of age, and 7.3% of patients older than 69 years of age. Serious complications occurred in 0.8% of patients under 50 years of age, 1.8% in patients 50 to 69 years of age, and 3.9% of those older than 69 years of age.

Similar analyses of ACS NSQIP data have been undertaken for appendectomy and cholecystectomy.[25,26] Despite commonly being perceived as a more invasive and potentially riskier intervention, laparoscopic fundoplication is associated with morbidity (appendectomy 4.46%, cholecystectomy 3.1%) and 30-day mortality (appendectomy 0.07%, cholecystectomy 0.27%) equivalent to these other commonly performed operations.

Relief of Primary Symptoms

Multiple retrospective series have demonstrated relief of heartburn and regurgitation in approximately 90% of patients at follow-up intervals of 2 to 3 years, and 80% to 90% at 5 years, following both laparoscopic and open antireflux surgery.[27–31] As LNF was first reported in 1991,[2,3] outcomes data after 10 or more years of follow-up have only recently appeared in the literature.

A review from a single center in Belgium, where the first LNF was performed, showed that of 100 consecutive patients undergoing an LNF in 1993, 93% were free of significant reflux symptoms at 5 years after surgery and 89.5% were still symptom-free at 10 years.[32]

Two reviews of single-center experiences from the United States were recently reported. In the first review, outcomes were assessed from 239 patients undergoing LNF at least 10 years prior.[33] Eighty-five percent of patients reported their preoperative GERD symptoms to be almost completely resolved or greatly improved after surgery, and 85% reported that they would undergo LNF again if given the choice. In the second review, results more than 6 years after surgery were available on

166 patients with a median follow-up of 11.1 years.[34] All GERD-related symptoms were significantly improved with the largest benefits noted in control of heartburn and regurgitation. Ninety-three percent of patients stated they would have the procedure again and 70% no longer took daily antireflux medications, although only 22% of patients with recurrent symptoms were demonstrated to have evidence of fundoplication failure or pathologic reflux.

Although several reports, including one highly publicized Veterans Administration study,[35] have suggested that a significant percentage of patients resume taking acid suppressive medications after an ARP, other reports have shown contrary results or that most of such patients do not, in fact, have recurrent GERD.[36–38] Resumption of medications, therefore, should not be equated to the failure of surgery or the return of GERD.

The ability to control the "atypical" or extraesophageal manifestations of GERD tends to be somewhat less reliable following antireflux surgery, given the variety of triggers other than GERD that are potentially etiologic. Multiple prospective and retrospective, randomized, and nonrandomized studies suggest an approximately 70% rate of success at improving cough, asthma, or laryngitis following an ARP.[39–42]

Objective Outcomes

Objective outcomes following fundoplication have been assessed in different manners. The "gold standard" for assessment of reflux control, ambulatory esophageal pH monitoring, is difficult to obtain in the postoperative setting, in that satisfied and asymptomatic patients after fundoplication generally are reluctant to undergo the study. In a Swedish study comparing LNF and open fundoplication (OF), pH data were available on 16 patients undergoing LNF and 22 patients undergoing OF at both 6 months and 5 years after surgery.[43] Esophageal acid exposure returned to normal at both time points in all patients tested, with no significant difference between the 2 groups. In a multicenter trial from the Netherlands, pathologic esophageal acid exposure was found in 12.5% of patients following LNF and 4.1% following OF at 5 years after surgery.[44]

An important and often underemphasized point is that the rate of failure of fundoplication is largely dependent on the size of the hiatal hernia being repaired. Repair of large sliding and paraesophageal hiatal hernias is associated with a higher risk of recurrent hiatal herniation compared with fundoplication for GERD in the setting of no or small hiatal hernias. Multiple potential explanations exist to explain this differential, including the presence of weakened or attenuated crural fibers that must be brought together under tension, the coexistence of esophageal body shortening, and the generally older and frailer nature of patients with a PEH.

The need for reoperation after fundoplication for GERD is only approximately 5% over the lifetime of a patient, whereas the risk of recurrent herniation tends to be greater and can run as high as 40% to 60% after repair of a giant PEH.[45,46] Some surgeons routinely add a Collis gastroplasty as an esophageal lengthening procedure in the setting of fundoplication for giant PEH given the high incidence of acquired esophageal body shortening associated with this condition. Methods to reduce the risk of recurrent hiatal herniation following repair of giant PEH, such as gastroplasty, mesh reinforcement, extensive esophageal mobilization, or use of open surgical approaches rather than laparoscopy, are areas of active ongoing investigation.

COMPARISONS OF MEDICAL AND SURGICAL THERAPY FOR CONTROL OF GERD

Although several randomized clinical trials comparing acid suppression therapy to laparoscopic antireflux surgery for control of GERD have been published, 2 trials are particularly noteworthy. The first study, from Sweden, was initially reported with a follow-up at 5 years,[47] whereas a later update provided follow-up of at least 7 years.[48] The proportion of patients in whom treatment did not fail during the 7 years was significantly higher in the surgical arm (66.7%) than in the medical arm (46.7%). A smaller difference in outcomes was noted, however, after dose adjustment in the medical group. More patients in the surgical cohort, however, complained of side effects, such as dysphagia, inability to belch or vomit, and hyperflatulence. Disease control was stable between 5 and 7 years of follow-up. The authors concluded that surgery was more effective in controlling overall GERD symptoms, although postfundoplication side effects were a concern.

The second study was the LOTUS trial, a multi-institutional study conducted in 11 European countries and published in 2011.[49] Five-hundred fifty-four patients with chronic GERD initially responsive to medical therapy were randomized to undergo an LNF performed by a standardized protocol or to medical therapy with esomeprazole. Relief of GERD symptoms at 5 years was higher in the esomeprazole group (92%) than in the surgical cohort (85%), although the difference did not reach statistical significance after accounting for study dropout. Surgery was better at controlling the symptom of regurgitation (2% vs 13%, $P<.001$), although leading to a higher incidence of dysphagia (11% vs 5%, $P<.001$), bloating (40% vs 28%, $P<.001$), and flatulence (57% vs 40%, $P<.001$), compared with medical therapy. Of note, nearly a quarter (23%) of patients in the medical arm required dose escalation of PPI therapy to maintain symptom relief. The authors concluded that both antireflux surgery and medical therapy with esomeprazole were effective means to control chronic GERD.

SURGICAL ALTERNATIVES TO NISSEN FUNDOPLICATION

Although LNF has been the most widely used antireflux operation, several other procedures are within the surgical armamentarium and are worth noting. Open fundoplication, by either laparotomy or thoracotomy, continues to play a role, particularly in the redo setting. Several reports have demonstrated the utility of Roux-en-Y gastric bypass procedures, with or without associated distal gastrectomy, for both redo operations and patients with morbid obesity or associated foregut dysmotility, such as in scleroderma.[9–11,50–52] The role of partial fundoplication (Dor, Toupet, or Belsey procedures), as compared with a total Nissen wrap, has been studied with data suggesting a better side effect profile, but slightly less durable control of GERD, with the former.[53] Laparoscopic or open Hill repair has been performed with outcomes similar to LNF and remains a viable surgical alternative in experienced hands.[54] Given the variety of effective surgical options, the esophageal surgeon is advised to be well versed in several different operative approaches and to tailor the procedure to the specific circumstances of the individual patient.

SUMMARY

Antireflux surgery has become a well-established therapy for GERD and its complications. The popularization of minimally invasive surgical techniques has brought about a revolution in the use of fundoplication for the long-term management of GERD. The outcome of antireflux surgery, however, is only as good as the evaluation to document the presence of pathologic reflux and associated abnormalities in the foregut, as well as the determination that the patient's main symptoms or complications are, in fact, reflux related. Established and novel foregut diagnostics continue to be refined and aid in the preoperative investigation of GERD. Surgical techniques similarly continue to be refined as the understanding of both short-term and long-term symptomatic and objective outcomes matures. Laparoscopic fundoplication has been proven an effective and durable treatment of GERD and has compared favorably to medical therapy over the long term. Despite this fact, the use of fundoplication continues to be questioned and novel therapies continue to arise. As with all operative interventions, successful results depend on an experienced surgeon and the proper conduct of the procedure; the patient is well-advised to choose a surgical specialist with extensive experience performing antireflux operations. A reliable and objective understanding of the outcomes following fundoplication is important for all physicians treating GERD, so that informed decisions can be made regarding the optimal treatment strategy for a given patient. As new endoscopic and surgical therapies emerge, their efficacy and limitations must be judged against the favorable and generally durable reflux control afforded by surgery under the full spectrum of clinical presentations of GERD. With ongoing study, the appropriate indications for surgical intervention among the array of potential antireflux therapies will continue to be elucidated.

REFERENCES

1. Nissen R. A simple operation for control of reflux esophagitis. Schweiz Med Wochenschr 1956;86:590–2.
2. Dallemagne B, Weerts JM, Jehaes C. Laparoscopic Nissen fundoplication: preliminary report. Surg Laparosc Endosc 1991;1:138–43.
3. Geagea T. Laparoscopic Nissen fundoplication: preliminary report on 10 cases. Surg Endosc 1991;5:170–3.
4. Finks JF, Wei Y, Birkmeyer JD. The rise and fall of antireflux surgery in the United States. Surg Endosc 2006;20:1698–701.
5. Wang YR, Dempsey DT, Richter JE. Trends and perioperative outcomes of inpatient antireflux surgery in the United States, 1993-2006. Dis Esophagus 2011;24: 215–23.
6. Kahrilas PJ, Shaheen NJ, Vaezi MF, et al. American Gastroenterological Association medical position statement on the management of gastroesophageal reflux disease. Gastroenterology 2008;135:1383–91.
7. Campos GM, Peters JH, DeMeester TR, et al. Multivariate analysis of factors predicting outcome after laparoscopic Nissen fundoplication. J Gastrointest Surg 1999;3:292–300.
8. Watson TJ, DeMeester TR. Collis-Belsey antireflux procedure. Dis Esophagus 1995;8:222–8.
9. Prachand VN, Alverdy JC. Gastroesophageal reflux disease and severe obesity: fundoplication or bariatric surgery? World J Gastroenterol 2010;16:3757–61.
10. Madalosso CA, Gurski RR, Callegari-Jacques SM, et al. The impact of gastric bypass on gastroesophageal reflux disease in patients with morbid obesity: a prospective study based on the Montreal consensus. Ann Surg 2010;251: 244–8.
11. Nelson LG, Gonzalez R, Haines K, et al. Amelioration of gastroesophageal reflux symptoms following Roux-en-Y gastric bypass for clinically significant obesity. Am Surg 2005;71:950–3.
12. Skinner DB, Belsey RH. Surgical management of esophageal reflux and hiatus hernia: long-term results with 1,030 patients. J Thorac Cardiovasc Surg 1967; 53:33–54.
13. Stylopoulos N, Gazelle GS, Rattner DW. Paraesophageal hernias: operation or observation? Ann Surg 2002;236:492–501.

14. Polomsky M, Siddall KA, Salvador R, et al. Association of kyphosis and spinal skeletal abnormalities with intrathoracic stomach: a link toward understanding its pathogenesis. J Am Coll Surg 2009;208:562–9.

15. Clouse RE, Staiano A, Alrakawi A, et al. Application of topographical methods to clinical esophageal manometry. Am J Gastroenterol 2000;95:2720–30.

16. Salvador R, Dubecz A, Polomsky M, et al. A new era in esophageal diagnostics: the image-based paradigm of high-resolution manometry. J Am Coll Surg 2009; 208:1035–44.

17. Roman S, Lin Z, Kwiatek MA, et al. Weak peristalsis in esophageal pressure topography: classification and association with dysphagia. Am J Gastroenterol 2011;106:349–56.

18. Wilshire CL, Niebisch S, Watson TJ, et al. Dysphagia post-fundoplication: more commonly hiatal outflow resistance than poor esophageal body motility. Surgery 2012;152:584–94.

19. Balaji NS, Blom D, DeMeester TR, et al. Redefining gastroesophageal reflux (GER): detection using multichannel intraluminal impedance in healthy volunteers. Surg Endosc 2003;17:1380–5.

20. Tutuian R, Vela MF, Shay SS, et al. Multichannel intraluminal impedance in esophageal function testing and gastroesophageal reflux monitoring. J Clin Gastroenterol 2003;37:206–15.

21. Vela MF, Camacho-Lobato L, Srinivasan R, et al. Simultaneous intraesophageal impedance and pH measurement of acid and nonacid gastroesophageal reflux: effect of omeprazole. Gastroenterology 2001;120:1599–606.

22. Mainie I, Tutuian R, Agrawal A, et al. Combined multichannel intraluminal impedance-pH monitoring to select patients with persistent gastro-oesophageal reflux for laparoscopic Nissen fundoplication. Br J Surg 2006;93:1483–7.

23. Gruebel C, Linke G, Tutuian R, et al. Prospective study examining the impact of multichannel intraluminal impedance on antireflux surgery. Surg Endosc 2008;22: 1241–7.

24. Niebisch S, Fleming FJ, Galey KM, et al. Perioperative risk of laparoscopic fundoplication: safer than previously reported—analysis of the American College of Surgeons National Surgical Quality Improvement Program 2005 to 2009. J Am Coll Surg 2012;215:61–9.

25. Ingraham AM, Cohen ME, Bilimoria KY, et al. Comparison of outcomes after laparoscopic versus open appendectomy for acute appendicitis at 222 ACS NSQIP hospitals. Surgery 2010;148:625–35.

26. Ingraham AM, Cohen ME, Ko CY, et al. A current profile and assessment of North American cholecystectomy: results from the American College of Surgeons National Surgical Quality Improvement Program. J Am Coll Surg 2010;211: 176–86.

27. Peters JH, DeMeester TR, Crookes P, et al. The treatment of gastroesophageal reflux disease with laparoscopic Nissen fundoplication: prospective evaluation of 100 patients with "typical" symptoms. Ann Surg 1998;228:40.

28. Hinder RA, Filipi CJ, Wetscher G, et al. Laparoscopic Nissen fundoplication is an effective treatment for gastroesophageal reflux disease. Ann Surg 1994;220:472.

29. DeMeester TR, Bonavina L, Albertucci M. Nissen fundoplication for gastroesophageal reflux disease— evaluation of primary repair in 100 consecutive patients. Ann Surg 1986;204:9.

30. Granderath FA, Kamolz T, Schweiger UM, et al. Long-term results of laparoscopic antireflux surgery: surgical outcomes and analysis of failure after 500 laparoscopic antireflux procedures. Surg Endosc 2002;16:753.

31. Catarci M, Gentileschi P, Papi C, et al. Evidence-based appraisal of antireflux fundoplication. Ann Surg 2004;239:325.
32. Dallemagne B, Weerts J, Markiewicz S, et al. Clinical results of laparoscopic fundoplication at ten years after surgery. Surg Endosc 2006;20:159–65.
33. Cowgill SM, Gillman R, Kraemer E, et al. Ten-year follow up after laparoscopic Nissen fundoplication for gastroesophageal reflux disease. Am Surg 2007;73: 748–53.
34. Morgenthal CB, Shane MD, Stival A, et al. The durability of laparoscopic Nissen fundoplication: 11-year outcomes. J Gastrointest Surg 2007;11:693–700.
35. Spechler SJ, Lee E, Ahnen D, et al. Long-term outcome of medical and surgical therapies for gastroesophageal reflux disease: follow-up of a randomized controlled trial. JAMA 2001;18:2331–8.
36. Lord RV, Kaminski A, Oberg S, et al. Absence of gastroesophageal reflux disease in a majority of patients taking acid suppression medications after Nissen fundoplication. J Gastrointest Surg 2002;6:3–10.
37. Thompson SK, Jamieson GG, Myers JC, et al. Recurrent heartburn after laparoscopic fundoplication is not always recurrent reflux. J Gastrointest Surg 2007;11: 642–7.
38. Bonatti H, Bammer T, Achem SR, et al. Use of acid suppressive medications after laparoscopic antireflux surgery: prevalence and clinical indications. Dig Dis Sci 2007;52:267–72.
39. Larrain A, Carrasco E, Galleguillos F, et al. Medical and surgical treatment of nonallergic asthma associated with gastroesophageal reflux. Chest 1991;99: 1330–5.
40. Sontag SJ, O'Connell S, Khandelwal S, et al. Asthmatics with gastroesophageal reflux: long term results of a randomized trial of medical and surgical antireflux therapies. Am J Gastroenterol 2003;98:987–99.
41. Vaezi MF, Hicks DM, Abelson TI, et al. Laryngeal signs and symptoms and gastroesophageal reflux disease (GERD): a critical assessment of cause and effect association. Clin Gastroenterol Hepatol 2003;1:333–44.
42. DeMeester TR, Bonavina L, Iascone C, et al. Chronic respiratory symptoms and occult gastroesophageal reflux. A prospective clinical study and results of surgical therapy. Ann Surg 1990;211:337–45.
43. Nilsson G, Wenner J, Larsson S, et al. Randomized clinical trial of laparoscopic versus open fundoplication for gastro-esophageal reflux. Br J Surg 2004;91: 552–9.
44. Draaisma WA, Rijnhart-de Jong HG, Broeders IA, et al. Five-year subjective and objective results of laparoscopic and conventional Nissen fundoplication: a randomized trial. Ann Surg 2006;244:34–41.
45. Hashemi M, Peters JH, DeMeester TR, et al. Laparoscopic repair of large type III hiatal hernia: objective follow-up reveals high recurrence rate. J Am Coll Surg 2000;190:553–60.
46. Dallemagne B, Kohnen L, Perretta S, et al. Laparoscopic repair of paraesophageal hernia. Long-term follow-up reveals good clinical outcome despite high radiological recurrence rate. Ann Surg 2011;253:291–6.
47. Lundell L, Miettinen P, Myrvold HE, et al. Continued (5-year) followup of a randomized clinical study comparing antireflux surgery and omeprazole in gastroesophageal reflux disease. J Am Coll Surg 2001;192:172–81.
48. Lundell L, Miettinen P, Myrvold HE, et al. Seven-year follow-up of a randomized clinical trial comparing proton-pump inhibition with surgical therapy for reflux oesophagitis. Br J Surg 2007;94:198–203.

49. Galmiche JP, Hatlebakk J, Attwood S, et al. Laparoscopic antireflux surgery vs esomeprazole treatment for chronic GERD: the LOTUS randomized clinical trial. JAMA 2011;305:1969–77.
50. Williams VA, Watson TJ, Gellersen O, et al. Gastrectomy as a remedial operation for failed fundoplication. J Gastrointest Surg 2007;11:29–35.
51. Awais O, Luketich J, Tam J, et al. Roux-en-Y gastric near esophagojejunostomy for intractable gastroesophageal reflux after antireflux surgery. Ann Thorac Surg 2008;85:1954–9.
52. Stefanidis D, Navarro F, Augenstein VA, et al. Laparoscopic fundoplication takedown with conversion to Roux-en-Y gastric bypass leads to excellent reflux control and quality of life after fundoplication failure. Surg Endosc 2012;26(12):3521–7.
53. Broeders JA, Roks DJ, Jamieson GG, et al. Five-year outcome after laparoscopic anterior partial versus Nissen fundoplication: four randomized trials. Ann Surg 2012;25:637–42.
54. Aye RW, Swanstrom LL, Kapur S, et al. A randomized multiinstitution comparison of the laparoscopic Nissen and Hill repairs. Ann Thorac Surg 2012;94:9541–86.

Eosinophilic Esophagitis

Evan S. Dellon, MD, MPH

KEYWORDS

- Eosinophilic esophagitis • Diagnosis • Treatment • Epidemiology • Endoscopy
- Allergy

KEY POINTS

- Over the past 10 years, eosinophilic esophagitis (EoE) has become a major cause of gastrointestinal symptoms, including dysphagia and food impaction in adolescents and adults, and feeding intolerance, failure to thrive, regurgitation, heartburn, and vomiting in children.
- EoE is a clinicopathologic condition, so the entire clinical and histologic picture must be considered in making a diagnosis; no single feature is diagnostic on its own.
- EoE is now diagnosed based on consensus guidelines requiring symptoms of esophageal dysfunction, at least 15 eosinophils per high-power microscopy field on esophageal biopsy, and eosinophilia limited to the esophagus with other causes of esophageal eosinophilia (including proton-pump inhibitor–responsive esophageal eosinophilia) excluded.
- Effective first-line treatment strategies include topical steroids, such as swallowed fluticasone or budesonide, or dietary therapy with an elemental formula, a 6-food elimination diet, or a targeted elimination diet.

INTRODUCTION

Eosinophilic esophagitis (EoE) is currently defined as a chronic immune-mediated condition whereby infiltration of eosinophils into the esophageal mucosa leads to symptoms of esophageal dysfunction.[1] Although the first case was described in the late 1970s,[2] the disease as it is now recognized was reported in children and adults in the early 1990s.[3–5] EoE was initially thought to be rare, but data from multiple centers now show that the incidence and prevalence are increasing rapidly and have outpaced the increased recognition of the disease.[6–12] In fact, over the past

This work was supported in part by NIH award number 1K23 DK090073-01.

Disclosures: There are no conflicts of interested pertaining to this article. Dr Dellon has received research support from AstraZeneca, Meritage Pharma, Olympus, NIH, ACG, AGA, and CURED Foundation. Dr Dellon has been a consultant for Oncoscope.

Center for Esophageal Diseases and Swallowing; Division of Gastroenterology and Hepatology, Department of Medicine, Center for Gastrointestinal Biology and Disease, University of North Carolina School of Medicine, CB#7080, Bioinformatics Building, 130 Mason Farm Road, UNC-CH, Chapel Hill, NC 27599-7080, USA

E-mail address: edellon@med.unc.edu

10 years EoE has become an important and frequent cause of upper gastrointestinal symptoms in both children and adults.[13,14] More than 6% of patients undergoing upper endoscopy for any reason, and more than 15% having the procedure for an indication of dysphagia, will be diagnosed with EoE.[15–17] The prevalence of EoE has been estimated to range between 43 to 52 per 100,000 in the general population,[10,18,19] a level that is beginning to approach the population prevalence of inflammatory bowel disease.[20]

The increasing recognition and evolving epidemiology of EoE has led to an explosion of research interest. Although many questions related to EoE remain unanswered, there has been substantial progress toward understanding the pathogenesis and genetic basis of the disease,[21–23] the clinical presentation, and effective treatment strategies. This review discusses clinical, endoscopic, and histologic features of EoE, presents the most recent guidelines for the diagnosis of EoE and selected diagnostic dilemmas, and highlights evidence to support both pharmacologic and nonpharmacologic treatment.

PATIENT HISTORY

EoE has been described throughout the world including North America, Europe, South America, Australia, and Asia, but the prevalence appears to be highest in the United States and Western Europe in comparison with Japan and China.[9,10,19,24–26] It also occurs in patients of all ages,[1,27,28] but is more frequent in children and adults younger than 40 years.[27–29] For reasons that are not understood, EoE is seen 3 to 4 times more frequently in males than in females, and is also more common in whites.[1,8,9,16,17,28,30] However, as centers accrue more experience and report data from larger populations of subjects from more diverse areas, racial minorities have also been found to have EoE.[31–34]

The clinical presentation of EoE varies by patient age.[1,6,8,35,36] In infants and toddlers symptoms are nonspecific, and can include failure to thrive, fussiness, poor growth, feeding intolerance or food aversion, abdominal pain, nausea, vomiting, and regurgitation.[29,35,37] By contrast, dysphagia is the most characteristic symptom in adolescents and adults, and in some studies this symptom is nearly universal.[8,15,17,28,29] For patients who present to an emergency department with a food impaction, EoE is the cause at least 50% of the time.[38–40] Of importance is that patients can minimize symptoms of dysphagia by avoiding solid foods, lubricating foods, drinking copious liquids during meals, and chewing carefully, so asking about these dietary modifications is necessary. Heartburn can affect patients with EoE of any age, and in 1% to 8% of those with proton-pump inhibitor (PPI) refractory reflux symptoms, EoE is the cause.[15,17,29,41–44] Because of the many potential symptoms and because no single symptom is specific for EoE, there is often a delay in making the diagnosis.[45]

EoE is also strongly associated with atopic diseases such as asthma, allergic rhinitis and sinusitis, atopic dermatitis, and food allergies. This relationship was first reported in children, up to 80% of whom can have atopy, and helped to support the allergic etiology of EoE.[29,37,46,47] Although fewer adults with EoE have atopy, it is still a prominent feature in this population.[8,48,49] There have been several reports of seasonal variation in the diagnosis of EoE as well as variation based on climate zone.[8,9,50,51]

ENDOSCOPIC FEATURES

Upper endoscopy is required for evaluation of clinical symptoms of EoE, assessment for other possible causes, and performance of esophageal biopsies. Multiple characteristic endoscopic findings of EoE have been reported,[1,52–54] but in up to 10% of cases the esophageal mucosa can appear normal, and biopsies are required or the diagnosis will be missed.[55] These findings have a fair to good interobserver and intraobserver reliability,[56,57] and efforts are under way to standardize reporting and scoring of endoscopic findings in EoE.[58]

Typical endoscopic findings of EoE are presented in **Fig. 1**, and include:

- Esophageal rings: these can be fixed (previously referred to as esophageal trachealization or corrugation) or transient (sometimes termed felinization).
- Narrow-caliber esophagus: this can be difficult to appreciate on visual inspection alone, but there can be resistance to the scope passage without seeing a clear stricture.
- Focal esophageal strictures.
- Linear furrows: grooves in the esophageal mucosa that run parallel to the axis of the esophagus.
- White plaques or exudates: punctate white spots on the esophageal mucosa that can be confused for esophageal candidiasis.
- Decreased vascularity: here the normal mucosal vascular pattern is lost and the esophagus appears pale, congested, or edematous.
- Crêpe-paper mucosa: a manifestation of mucosal fragility in EoE whereby the mucosa tears with passage of the endoscope, but a focal stricture or resistance is not appreciated.

These features can occur in isolation, but more commonly occur together. There are some data to suggest that younger children tend to have more inflammatory features such as linear furrows, white plaques, and decreased vasculature, whereas adults (particularly those with symptoms of long duration) tend to have more fibrotic features such as rings and strictures.[8,59,60]

It is important to be aware that the endoscopic findings of EoE are not pathognomonic, and a recent meta-analysis found that the sensitivity, specificity, and predictive values of endoscopic findings in EoE were not high enough to be the basis for diagnostic decisions.[55] This finding emphasizes the importance obtaining esophageal biopsies when EoE is suspected clinically. This tenet is reiterated in recent guidelines, which recognize that the eosinophilic infiltrate in EoE is patchy and that increasing numbers of biopsies increase diagnostic sensitivity.[61–64] Therefore, it is recommended for the endoscopist to obtain 2 to 4 biopsies from the distal esophagus and an additional 2 to 4 samples from the proximal esophagus.[1]

HISTOLOGIC FEATURES

Infiltration of the esophageal mucosa with eosinophils is the histologic hallmark of EoE.[65,66] At present, finding at least 15 eosinophils per high-power microscopy field (eos/hpf) is suggestive of EoE.[1] However, as discussed in more detail later, the finding of esophageal eosinophilia on biopsy is not specific for EoE. When biopsy samples are examined, in addition to the eosinophil count, which by convention represents the peak value in the most highly inflamed area on the biopsy, other features are also present (**Fig. 2**).[1,65,66] Eosinophils are often found toward the apical aspect of the epithelium, and clusters of eosinophils can form eosinophilic microabscesses. Because eosinophils are activated in EoE, they degranulate, and the granule proteins can be seen extracellularly. There is also basal layer hypertrophy whereby the cells in the basal layer expand and the rete pegs elongate. Spongiosis, also termed dilated intracellular spaces, is frequently observed. Finally, if the biopsy sample is deep enough to contain lamina propria, fibrosis of this area can be noted.

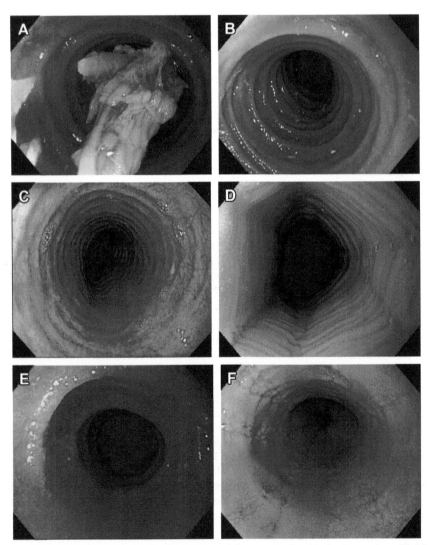

Fig. 1. The range of endoscopic findings in EoE. (*A*) An acute food-bolus impaction. (*B*) After the bolus is cleared, fixed esophageal rings are noted. (*C*) Less prominent esophageal rings. (*D*) Felinization of the esophageal with rings that are transiently present. Congestion and loss of vascular marking area also noted. (*E*) A narrow-caliber esophagus, which prevented passage of an adult upper endoscope. Rings, congestion, and decreased vasculature are also present. (*F*) Linear furrows in the distal esophagus, associated subtle rings, and decreased vasculature. (*G*) Prominent white plaques and exudates, as well as subtle rings and furrows. In this patient, brushings were negative for *Candida* and biopsies showed multiple eosinophilic microabscesses. (*H*) Crêpe-paper mucosa. This tear was noted after uneventful passage of the endoscope. The mucosa is also congested with decreased vascularity. (*I*) Multiple findings of rings, furrows, decreased vascularity, narrow-caliber esophagus, and crêpe-paper mucosa.

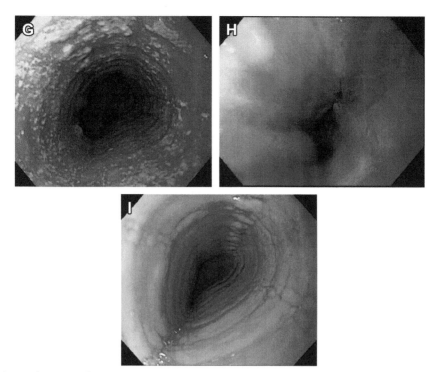

Fig. 1. (*continued*)

DIAGNOSTIC CRITERIA
Consensus Guidelines

Because of heterogeneity in disease definition and reporting of data pertaining to EoE,[28,67,68] an initial set of diagnostic guidelines was proposed in 2007 and represented a major step forward for the field.[69] These guidelines have been recently updated after taking into account advances in understanding and complexities related to diagnosis.[1] In this most recent document, EoE is defined conceptually as a "chronic immune/antigen-mediated esophageal disease characterized clinically by symptoms

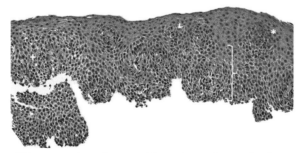

Fig. 2. Esophageal biopsy specimen in EoE. This specimen shows a brisk eosinophilic infiltration in the esophageal epithelium, as well as spongiosis (*plus sign*), eosinophil degranulation (*arrowhead*), basal-zone hyperplasia (*bracket*), and an eosinophilic microabscess (*asterisk*). (hematoxylin-eosin, original magnification ×40).

related to esophageal dysfunction and histologically by eosinophil-predominant inflammation." Three specific criteria were required to diagnose EoE:

- Symptoms related to esophageal dysfunction
- A peak eosinophil count of at least 15 eos/hpf on esophageal biopsy, with few exceptions
- Eosinophilia limited to the esophagus with other causes of esophageal eosinophilia excluded

Taken together, the conceptual definition and the diagnostic criteria emphasize that EoE is a clinicopathologic condition. Specifically, the entire clinical and histologic picture must be considered to make a diagnosis, and no single feature is diagnostic on its own.

Diagnostic Dilemmas

Despite having a set of diagnostic guidelines, the ability to characterize patients clinically and endoscopically, well-defined histologic findings with a marker, and the eosinophil count, which is reliable and reproducible if approached systematically,[70] diagnosis of EoE can still be challenging.

Just as symptoms of dysphagia and findings of esophageal rings on endoscopy are not specific for EoE, there is a differential diagnosis for esophageal eosinophilia on biopsy.[1,69] Several conditions that have been reported to cause or be associated with esophageal eosinophilia, such as achalasia, infections (fungal, viral, parasitic), connective-tissue disease, graft-versus-host disease, Crohn disease, adrenal insufficiency, hypereosinophilic syndrome, and eosinophilic gastroenteritis, have their own distinct clinical presentations and can typically be diagnosed with a focused history and physical examination with limited supplemental evaluation. However, 2 conditions, gastroesophageal reflux disease (GERD) and PPI-responsive esophageal eosinophilia (PPI-REE), deserve special attention when attempting to diagnose EoE.

There is substantial overlap between GERD and EoE, including symptoms of heartburn, chest pain, and dysphagia, and biopsy findings of eosinophilia; even very high eosinophil counts, do not distinguish the two conditions.[44,71] In the 2007 EoE diagnostic guidelines, exclusion of GERD, either with a high-dose PPI trial or with pH monitoring, was required before definitively diagnosing EoE.[69] As more clinical experience was gained, it was clear that there were some patients who had coexisting EoE and GERD and that the relation between the two conditions was complicated.[71]

In addition, there was the observation that some patients who appeared to have EoE would have a clinical and histologic response to PPI therapy. This finding was first reported in a case series by Ngo and colleagues,[72] and since then several studies have reported that one-third or more of patients with esophageal eosinophilia have a response to PPIs.[73–78] This phenomenon has been termed PPI-REE.[1] It is not currently known whether this is a distinct clinical entity, a subtype of GERD, or a phenotype of EoE, but its role must currently be addressed in the diagnostic algorithm for EoE. Specifically, when esophageal eosinophilia is found on biopsy in a clinical setting where there is suspicion for EoE, a high-dose PPI trial (20–40 mg twice daily of any of the available agents for 8 weeks) is necessary. If a patient responds to this regimen, additional clinical evaluation can be performed to determine if GERD was the cause of the esophageal eosinophilia or if the patient has PPI-REE. If a patient has persistent symptoms of EoE and there are still at least 15 eos/hpf on esophageal biopsy, EoE can be diagnosed.

Because of these challenges and the somewhat rudimentary way in which EoE is diagnosed, there is active research aimed at identifying better ways to diagnose

EoE. Some methods under investigation include clinical scoring systems,[8,79,80] endoscopic imaging techniques,[56,81,82] functional luminal assessment of the esophagus,[83] biomarker measurements on esophageal biopsies,[84–88] radiolabeling of esophageal biopsies,[89] noninvasive assessment of esophageal cytokines,[90] noninvasive serum biomarkers,[91–93] and genetic testing.[21,94] Although these techniques are promising, none have been validated or are ready to be used in clinical practice.

TREATMENT

There are now several evidence-based treatment options for EoE. Pharmacologic agents are commonly used, but nonpharmacologic approaches such as dietary elimination therapy and endoscopy dilation are also effective. Of note, there are currently no medications for EoE approved by the Food and Drug Administration, so all pharmacologic treatment options are off-label. The overall goal of treating patients with EoE is to improve symptoms and normalize the esophageal mucosa without adversely affecting quality of life, although specific end points have been difficult to define in clinical trials.[95] Because EoE is chronic, when medications or dietary therapy are stopped, symptoms will recur for the majority of patients.[96–98] For this reason, in patients with severe, frequent, or recurrent symptoms, or in patients who have had complications such as esophageal strictures, food impactions requiring emergency evaluation for endoscopy and bolus clearance, or esophageal perforations, long-term treatment may be required.

Pharmacologic Treatment

Corticosteroids
Corticosteroid medications are an effective and commonly used treatment for EoE (**Fig. 3**). Initially systemic steroids were administered with good effect,[96,99] but because of concerns about side effects, this class was not a viable option for long-term used. Instead, a topical method of administration of steroids was developed.[100]

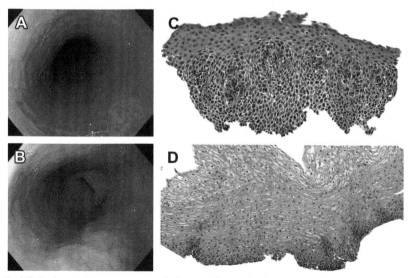

Fig. 3. (*A*) Endoscopic appearance of the esophagus before topical steroid therapy, with rings, furrows, and degreased vascularity noted. (*B*) Appearance has completely normalized after topical steroid therapy. A similar improvement is noted on this patient's biopsies before (*C*) and after (*D*) treatment. (hematoxylin-eosin, original magnification ×40).

Patients were instructed to use asthma medication preparations, either in a multidose inhaler (MDI) or aqueous-solution formulations, and instead of inhaling the medications they swallowed them to coat the esophagus. With this technique, several studies showed that agents such as fluticasone, budesonide, mometasone, beclomethasone, and ciclesonide all effectively decreased esophageal eosinophil counts and improved clinical symptoms.[100–108] In addition, a randomized controlled trial (RCT) by Schaefer and colleagues[109] that compared topical fluticasone with prednisone showed that the 2 agents were equivalent for improving symptoms and eosinophil counts.

The 2 most commonly used topical steroids are fluticasone and budesonide. The first placebo-controlled RCT in EoE was conducted in children by Konikoff and colleagues.[110] Using fluticasone, they showed that 50% of the 21 subjects receiving fluticasone had complete histologic remission (defined as ≤ 1 eos/hpf) compared with 9% of the 15 subjects receiving placebo. Recently, a similar study was conducted in adults by Alexander and colleagues.[111] Here, 62% of the 21 adults treated with fluticasone had a greater than 90% decrease in eosinophil counts, compared with 0% of the 15 subjects in the placebo arm. When used clinically the typical dose of fluticasone is 880 to 1760 μg/d, administered twice daily, with the final dose determined by the patient's age or size.

Topical budesonide has also been studied. Here, the aqueous formulation of the medication is typically mixed with a sugar substitute such as sucralose, and the resultant slurry (which has been termed oral viscous budesonide, or OVB) is swallowed.[105,112] In the first RCT in children, Dohil and colleagues[113] reported that 87% of the 15 subjects who received OVB had a histologic response (≤ 6 eos/hpf), whereas none of the 9 patients in the placebo group had this response. The marked histologic response seen with budesonide was confirmed in a larger placebo-controlled dose-finding trial of 80 children, but in this study the symptoms significantly improved in both the active-therapy and placebo arms, making the results somewhat difficult to interpret and highlighting a trend that has been seen in some other recent trials.[114] There have also been 2 RCTs of budesonide in adults. Straumann and colleagues[115] compared a nebulized and then swallowed protocol for budesonide with placebo, and found that budesonide was highly effective for improving symptoms and decreasing eosinophil counts. The second study compared OVB with the nebulized/swallowed budesonide administration protocol, and showed that OVB was more effective.[116] When used clinically, the typical dose of budesonide is 1 to 2 mg/d, mixed with 5 g of sucralose and administered twice daily, with the final dose determined by the patient's age or size.

Topical steroids are generally considered safe and well tolerated. Adrenal suppression has not been reported with an initial course of treatment,[111,113,114,116] but longer-term safety data are needed.[1] The main adverse effect with topical steroids is local. The rate of candidal esophagitis ranges from 0% to 32% in prospective studies, although many of these cases were detected incidentally on follow-up endoscopy.[109–111,113–116] There is also a case report of herpes esophagitis complicating topical steroid use.[117]

Biological agents

There has been burgeoning interest in nonsteroid treatment modalities for eosinophilic esophagitis, and biological agents targeting key factors in the pathogenesis of EoE are intriguing options. To date, however, these are either still in the experimental phase or have not been shown to be effective.

Mepolizumab and reslizumab are monoclonal anti–interleukin-5 antibodies. A small series showed that mepolizumab had some efficacy for EoE, so these agents were subsequently studied in 3 RCTs, 1 in adults and 2 in children.[118–120] There was a mild to moderate improvement in eosinophil counts, but the medications did not tend to improve symptoms in the active treatment arms compared with placebo, and primary end points of resolution of eosinophilia and symptoms were not met. These agents are not available clinically at present.

Infliximab, an anti–tumor necrosis factor antibody frequently used in inflammatory bowel disease, was examined in a small case series of steroid-refractory EoE patients, but did not improve symptoms or histology.[121]

Omalizumab, a monoclonal antibody against immunoglobulin E and used for allergic asthma, was studied in a placebo-controlled RCT by Fang and colleagues[122] in 30 adults with EoE. There was no difference in any of the outcomes between the groups, and this agent is not recommended for use in EoE.

Other agents

Given the strong association between EoE and allergic diseases, leukotriene antagonists have been studied, but the data are conflicting. In an initial report in adults by Atwood and colleagues,[123] high doses of montelukast (20–40 mg/d) were effective, though associated with nausea and vomiting. Two additional studies, one in adults and one in children, were less encouraging,[124,125] and this agent is not routinely used in EoE.

Mast-cell stabilizers such as cromolyn have also been examined, but were not effective.[29] There are currently no data in EoE for ketotifen, an antihistamine with anti–mast cell properties.

Immunomodulators such as azathioprine and 6-mercaptopurine have been studied in a single series of 3 patients with steroid-dependent EoE.[126] Although the medication was effective for improving eosinophilic counts and maintaining symptom control, given the potential toxicity and paucity of data, this medication is not recommended for routine use in EoE.

Several investigations into novel agents to treat EoE are ongoing. For example, anti–interleukin-13 and anti–eotaxin-3 antibodies are under development,[1] and pilot data were recently presented on a T-helper type 2 cell prostaglandin D2 receptor antagonist, which represents a potentially new medication class for EoE.[127] With the increasing understanding of pathways involved in the pathogenesis of EoE, it is likely that a wide variety of therapeutic modalities will be studied over the coming years.

Nonpharmacologic Treatment

There are 2 major strategies for nonpharmacologic treatment of EoE. The first is dietary elimination, whereby specific foods or groups of foods are removed from the diet to identify potential food allergens that trigger EoE. Similar to pharmacologic therapy, dietary restriction reduces esophageal eosinophilia. The second is endoscopic dilation whereby strictures, rings, or a narrow-caliber esophagus are stretched to relieve symptoms of dysphagia. This technique does not affect the underlying inflammation in the esophagus.

Dietary elimination

There are 3 approaches to dietary elimination for treatment of EoE. First is a completely allergen-free elemental formula, composed of only amino acids, medium-chain triglycerides, and simple carbohydrates. This treatment was initially used in one of the early reports of EoE in which 10 children responded within weeks of starting the formula.[5] In a study of 51 children, Markowitz and colleagues[128] found that 96% of subjects had near-complete resolution of esophageal eosinophilia and symptoms within 1 to 2 weeks, and other studies have reported similar results.[29,129] Until recently, all of the data on elemental diets were in children, but a study by Peterson and colleagues[130] confirms the short-term utility of this approach in adults as well, if they can tolerate the formulation. Although elemental diets are very effective for EoE treatment, they are unpalatable, expensive, sometimes require gastrostomy tubes for administration, and may not be feasible for many patients with EoE.

The second approach, the so-called 6-food elimination diet (SFED), addresses the difficulty with compliance found with the elemental diet. In the SFED, the 6 most highly allergenic food groups, dairy, egg, wheat, soy, nuts, and seafood, are removed from the diet. This approach compares favorably with the elemental diet in children, with three-quarters of subjects having resolution of esophageal eosinophilia and almost all having improvement in symptoms.[129,131,132] Gonsalves and colleagues[133] have now shown that the SFED is equally effective in adult patients as well.

Third is a targeted elimination diet whereby foods are removed based on reactivity on allergy testing. This method is less restrictive than either elemental or SFED diets, but the efficacy is also somewhat less, likely because allergy testing itself is not completely reliable for detecting food triggers.[1,129,134] Several studies have explored this approach, and the overall response rate ranges between 50% and 75% in children and lower in adults, depending on the center and the methods of allergy testing used.[29,129,135–139]

When selecting dietary modification as the treatment modality for a patient with EoE, it is important to have a multidisciplinary approach with collaboration between gastroenterologists, allergists, and nutritionists. This approach ensures not only that patients are having their nutrition requirements met, but also that they have enough information about food choices and potential sources of contamination to maximize the likelihood of success of the elimination diet.

Endoscopic dilation

Endoscopic dilation is an effective way to treat dysphagia caused by strictures or narrow-caliber esophagus in patients with EoE (**Fig. 4**). When the technique was first reported, however, there were high rates of complications such as esophageal perforation, mucosal rents, and hospitalization for postprocedural chest pain, and safety was a significant concern.[52,53,140–143] As more experience with dilation in EoE patients has accumulated, however, the technique seems safer than originally believed, and a cautious approach has been endorsed.[1] In several recently published studies and 2 systematic reviews[144–152] the overall perforation rate is 0.3%, which is similar to the cited rate for upper endoscopy with dilation in patients who do not have EoE.[153]

Dilation is also consistently reported to improve symptoms of dysphagia, even though the underlying eosinophilic inflammation is not affected.[148,149,151,152] In one study by Schoepfer and colleagues,[148] after one dilation session and in the absence of other medical or dietary treatments, the symptom response after dilation persisted for 1 year in 46% and for 2 years in 41%. This same study also observed that if patients are asked prospectively, approximately three-quarters will report postdilation chest discomfort.

There are few data on the timing of dilation. Unless there is a critical stricture noted on the first endoscopy, dilation of a narrow-caliber esophagus is typically postponed until the follow-up endoscopy assessing the effect of medical or dietary therapy.[1,69] There are also few data on the specific dilation technique, and both balloon and bougie dilation have been reported to be effective.[149,154,155] Therefore, regardless of the equipment choice, dilation should be approached with caution, care should be taken in choosing the initial dilator size, dilator size should not be increased after

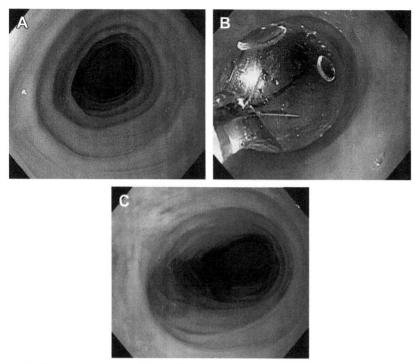

Fig. 4. Dilation for treatment of EoE. (*A*) Endoscopic appearance of an esophageal narrowing with a tight series of rings, as well as mucosal pallor, congestion, and decreased vasculature. (*B*) Through-the-scope balloon deployed and inflated to 10 mm. (*C*) Desired postdilation effect with mucosal disruption.

a mucosal rent is created, and patients should be informed about the risks, benefits, and likelihood of discomfort after the procedure.

TREATMENT NONRESPONSE

Whereas most patients respond to medical or dietary therapy, there are some who remain refractory to therapy. In these cases, a systematic assessment should be made to identify the reason for nonresponse, specifically determining whether ongoing esophageal eosinophilia is the cause of symptoms or if there are other contributing factors. Potential reasons for nonresponse include:

- Nonadherence to the prescribed treatment.
- Inadequate dosing of a topical steroid.
- Candidal esophagitis complicating steroid therapy. In these cases, the eosinophilic inflammation has typically improved, but the infection causes dysphagia and odynophagia.
- Persistent esophageal stricture or narrowing. Here the eosinophilic inflammation has also resolved, but fibrotic changes in the esophagus remain and require dilation therapy for symptom improvement. Many times, subtle narrowing can be difficult to appreciate on endoscopic examination.
- Superimposed motility disorders. Although there is no single characteristic pattern of esophageal dysmotility in EoE, esophageal longitudinal muscle

dysfunction has been reported in a subset of patients with EoE,[156–158] and the esophagus is also less compliant in EoE patients.[83]

- Persistent esophageal eosinophilia that is truly refractory to therapy. This situation could be the result of failure to respond to adequate doses of steroid medications, or be due to persistent (or inadvertent) allergen exposure. In this situation, if patients have failed topical steroid therapy, they should be tried on dietary elimination. Conversely, if they have failed dietary therapy, they should be placed on topical steroids.

SUMMARY

EoE is a chronic allergen-mediated disorder defined by symptoms of esophageal dysfunction and epithelial eosinophilia on biopsy. It has rapidly emerged as an important cause of upper gastrointestinal morbidity in patients of all ages, and is encountered in a substantial proportion of patients undergoing diagnostic upper endoscopy.

Diagnosis of EoE is based on consensus guidelines, but can be challenging because none of the symptoms, endoscopic findings, or histologic features are specific for EoE on their own. From a practical standpoint, EoE is suspected when a patient presents with symptoms of dysphagia, food impaction, or in children with feeding intolerance, abdominal pain, or vomiting. There are often concomitant atopic disorders present. On endoscopic evaluation typical findings include rings, furrows, white plaques or exudates, decreased vascularity or congestion, esophageal narrowing or strictures, and mucosal fragility. When biopsies reveal at least 15 eos/hpf, EoE is a diagnostic consideration. However, other causes of eosinophilia must be considered, and in particular PPI-REE must be excluded with a PPI trial for 8 weeks and a repeat endoscopy. If symptoms persist and biopsies continue to show a peak of at least 15 eos/hpf after the PPI trial, EoE is diagnosed.

For treatment, either swallowed topical corticosteroids or dietary elimination therapy are reasonable first-line options. The choice will depend on both patient preference and local expertise. In cases where there are severe esophageal strictures, dilation is also performed. After an initial trial of treatment for 8 weeks, a follow-up endoscopy is useful in assessing the mucosal response to the antieosinophil treatment and in determining whether further endoscopic dilation is required. For patients who do not respond to either dietary or medical treatment there are limited options, but several new agents are under investigation and will likely change the treatment algorithm in the future.

REFERENCES

1. Liacouras CA, Furuta GT, Hirano I, et al. Eosinophilic esophagitis: updated consensus recommendations for children and adults. J Allergy Clin Immunol 2011;128:3–20.e6.
2. Landres RT, Kuster GG, Strum WB. Eosinophilic esophagitis in a patient with vigorous achalasia. Gastroenterology 1978;74:1298–301.
3. Attwood SE, Smyrk TC, Demeester TR, et al. Esophageal eosinophilia with dysphagia. A distinct clinicopathologic syndrome. Dig Dis Sci 1993;38:109–16.
4. Straumann A, Spichtin HP, Bernoulli R, et al. Idiopathic eosinophilic esophagitis: a frequently overlooked disease with typical clinical aspects and discrete endoscopic findings. Schweiz Med Wochenschr 1994;124:1419–29 [in German].
5. Kelly KJ, Lazenby AJ, Rowe PC, et al. Eosinophilic esophagitis attributed to gastroesophageal reflux: improvement with an amino acid-based formula. Gastroenterology 1995;109:1503–12.

6. Noel RJ, Putnam PE, Rothenberg ME. Eosinophilic esophagitis. N Engl J Med 2004;351:940–1.
7. Straumann A, Simon HU. Eosinophilic esophagitis: escalating epidemiology? J Allergy Clin Immunol 2005;115:418–9.
8. Dellon ES, Gibbs WB, Fritchie KJ, et al. Clinical, endoscopic, and histologic findings distinguish eosinophilic esophagitis from gastroesophageal reflux disease. Clin Gastroenterol Hepatol 2009;7:1305–13.
9. Prasad GA, Alexander JA, Schleck CD, et al. Epidemiology of eosinophilic esophagitis over three decades in Olmsted County, Minnesota. Clin Gastroenterol Hepatol 2009;7:1055–61.
10. Hruz P, Straumann A, Bussmann C, et al. Escalating incidence of eosinophilic esophagitis: a 20-year prospective, population-based study in Olten County, Switzerland. J Allergy Clin Immunol 2011;128:1349–1350.e5.
11. Cherian S, Smith NM, Forbes DA. Rapidly increasing prevalence of eosinophilic oesophagitis in Western Australia. Arch Dis Child 2006;91:1000–4.
12. van Rhijn BD, Verheij J, Smout AJ, et al. Rapidly increasing incidence of eosinophilic esophagitis in a large cohort. Neurogastroenterol Motil 2012. [Epub ahead of print].
13. Katzka DA. Eosinophilic esophagitis: from rookie of the year to household name. Clin Gastroenterol Hepatol 2009;7:370–1.
14. Kidambi T, Toto E, Ho N, et al. Temporal trends in the relative prevalence of dysphagia etiologies from 1999-2009. World J Gastroenterol 2012;18:4335–41.
15. Prasad GA, Talley NJ, Romero Y, et al. Prevalence and predictive factors of eosinophilic esophagitis in patients presenting with dysphagia: a prospective study. Am J Gastroenterol 2007;102:2627–32.
16. Mackenzie SH, Go M, Chadwick B, et al. Clinical trial: eosinophilic esophagitis in patients presenting with dysphagia: a prospective analysis. Aliment Pharmacol Ther 2008;28:1140–6.
17. Veerappan GR, Perry JL, Duncan TJ, et al. Prevalence of eosinophilic esophagitis in an adult population undergoing upper endoscopy: a prospective study. Clin Gastroenterol Hepatol 2009;7:420–6.
18. Spergel JM, Book WM, Mays E, et al. Variation in prevalence, diagnostic criteria, and initial management options for eosinophilic gastrointestinal diseases in the United States. J Pediatr Gastroenterol Nutr 2011;52:300–6.
19. Sealock RJ, Rendon G, El-Serag HB. Systematic review: the epidemiology of eosinophilic oesophagitis in adults. Aliment Pharmacol Ther 2010;32:712–9.
20. Kappelman MD, Rifas-Shiman SL, Kleinman K, et al. The prevalence and geographic distribution of Crohn's disease and ulcerative colitis in the United States. Clin Gastroenterol Hepatol 2007;5:1424–9.
21. Blanchard C, Wang N, Stringer KF, et al. Eotaxin-3 and a uniquely conserved gene-expression profile in eosinophilic esophagitis. J Clin Invest 2006;116:536–47.
22. Rothenberg ME, Spergel JM, Sherrill JD, et al. Common variants at 5q22 associate with pediatric eosinophilic esophagitis. Nat Genet 2010;42:289–91.
23. Sherrill JD, Rothenberg ME. Genetic dissection of eosinophilic esophagitis provides insight into disease pathogenesis and treatment strategies. J Allergy Clin Immunol 2011;128:23–32. [quiz: 33–4].
24. Fujishiro H, Amano Y, Kushiyama Y, et al. Eosinophilic esophagitis investigated by upper gastrointestinal endoscopy in Japanese patients. J Gastroenterol 2011;46:1142–4.
25. Kinoshita Y, Furuta K, Ishimaura N, et al. Clinical characteristics of Japanese patients with eosinophilic esophagitis and eosinophilic gastroenteritis. J Gastroenterol 2012. [Epub ahead of print].

26. Shi YN, Sun SJ, Xiong LS, et al. Prevalence, clinical manifestations and endo-scopic features of eosinophilic esophagitis: a pathological review in China. J Dig Dis 2012;13:304–9.
27. Kapel RC, Miller JK, Torres C, et al. Eosinophilic esophagitis: a prevalent disease in the United States that affects all age groups. Gastroenterology 2008;134:1316–21.
28. Dellon ES, Aderoju A, Woosley JT, et al. Variability in diagnostic criteria for eosin-ophilic esophagitis: a systematic review. Am J Gastroenterol 2007;102:2300–13.
29. Liacouras CA, Spergel JM, Ruchelli E, et al. Eosinophilic esophagitis: a 10-year experience in 381 children. Clin Gastroenterol Hepatol 2005;3:1198–206.
30. Franciosi JP, Tam V, Liacouras CA, et al. A case-control study of sociodemo-graphic and geographic characteristics of 335 children with eosinophilic esoph-agitis. Clin Gastroenterol Hepatol 2009;7:415–9.
31. Sperry SL, Woosley JT, Shaheen NJ, et al. Influence of race and gender on the presentation of eosinophilic esophagitis. Am J Gastroenterol 2012;107:215–21.
32. Bohm M, Malik Z, Sebastiano C, et al. Mucosal eosinophilia: prevalence and racial/ethnic differences in symptoms and endoscopic findings in adults over 10 years in an urban hospital. J Clin Gastroenterol 2012;46:567–74.
33. Sharma HP, Mansoor DK, Sprunger AC, et al. Racial disparities in the presentation of pediatric eosinophilic esophagitis. J Allergy Clin Immunol 2011;127:AB110.
34. Moawad FJ, Veerappan GR, Dias JA, et al. Race may play a role in the clinical presentation of eosinophilic esophagitis. Am J Gastroenterol 2012;107:1263.
35. Putnam PE. Evaluation of the child who has eosinophilic esophagitis. Immunol Allergy Clin North Am 2009;29:1–10.
36. Straumann A. Clinical evaluation of the adult who has eosinophilic esophagitis. Immunol Allergy Clin North Am 2009;29:11–8.
37. Spergel JM, Brown-Whitehorn TF, Beausoleil JL, et al. 14 years of eosinophilic esophagitis: clinical features and prognosis. J Pediatr Gastroenterol Nutr 2009; 48:30–6.
38. Desai TK, Stecevic V, Chang CH, et al. Association of eosinophilic inflammation with esophageal food impaction in adults. Gastrointest Endosc 2005;61:795–801.
39. Kerlin P, Jones D, Remedios M, et al. Prevalence of eosinophilic esophagitis in adults with food bolus obstruction of the esophagus. J Clin Gastroenterol 2007; 41:356–61.
40. Sperry SL, Crockett SD, Miller CB, et al. Esophageal foreign-body impactions: epidemiology, time trends, and the impact of the increasing prevalence of eosin-ophilic esophagitis. Gastrointest Endosc 2011;74:985–91.
41. Foroutan M, Norouzi A, Molaei M, et al. Eosinophilic esophagitis in patients with refractory gastroesophageal reflux disease. Dig Dis Sci 2010;55:28–31.
42. Garcia-Compean D, Gonzalez Gonzalez JA, Marrufo Garcia CA, et al. Preva-lence of eosinophilic esophagitis in patients with refractory gastroesophageal reflux disease symptoms: a prospective study. Dig Liver Dis 2011;43:204–8.
43. Poh CH, Gasiorowska A, Navarro-Rodriguez T, et al. Upper GI tract findings in patients with heartburn in whom proton pump inhibitor treatment failed versus those not receiving antireflux treatment. Gastrointest Endosc 2010;71:28–34.
44. Rodrigo S, Abboud G, Oh D, et al. High intraepithelial eosinophil counts in esophageal squamous epithelium are not specific for eosinophilic esophagitis in adults. Am J Gastroenterol 2008;103:435–42.
45. Garrean CP, Gonsalves N, Hirano I. Epidemiologic implications of symptom onset in adults with eosinophilic esophagitis. Gastroenterology 2009;136(Suppl 1): AB S1875.

46. Assa'ad AH, Putnam PE, Collins MH, et al. Pediatric patients with eosinophilic esophagitis: an 8-year follow-up. J Allergy Clin Immunol 2007;119:731–8.
47. Chehade M, Aceves SS. Food allergy and eosinophilic esophagitis. Curr Opin Allergy Clin Immunol 2010;10:231–7.
48. Penfield JD, Lang DM, Goldblum JR, et al. The role of allergy evaluation in adults with eosinophilic esophagitis. J Clin Gastroenterol 2010;44:22–7.
49. Roy-Ghanta S, Larosa DF, Katzka DA. Atopic characteristics of adult patients with eosinophilic esophagitis. Clin Gastroenterol Hepatol 2008;6:531–5.
50. Almansa C, Devault KR, Achem SR. A comprehensive review of eosinophilic esophagitis in adults. J Clin Gastroenterol 2011;45:658–64.
51. Hurrell JM, Genta RM, Dellon ES. Prevalence of esophageal eosinophilia varies by climate zone in the United States. Am J Gastroenterol 2012;107:698–706.
52. Straumann A, Rossi L, Simon HU, et al. Fragility of the esophageal mucosa: a pathognomonic endoscopic sign of primary eosinophilic esophagitis? Gastrointest Endosc 2003;57:407–12.
53. Vasilopoulos S, Murphy P, Auerbach A, et al. The small-caliber esophagus: an unappreciated cause of dysphagia for solids in patients with eosinophilic esophagitis. Gastrointest Endosc 2002;55:99–106.
54. Straumann A, Spichtin HP, Bucher KA, et al. Eosinophilic esophagitis: red on microscopy, white on endoscopy. Digestion 2004;70:109–16.
55. Kim HP, Vance RB, Shaheen NJ, et al. The prevalence and diagnostic utility of endoscopic features of eosinophilic esophagitis: a meta-analysis. Clin Gastroenterol Hepatol 2012;10:988–996.e5.
56. Peery AF, Cao H, Dominik R, et al. Variable reliability of endoscopic findings with white-light and narrow-band imaging for patients with suspected eosinophilic esophagitis. Clin Gastroenterol Hepatol 2011;9:475–80.
57. Moy N, Heckman MG, Gonsalves N, et al. Inter-observer agreement on endoscopic esophageal findings in eosinophilic esophagitis. Gastroenterology 2011;140(Suppl 1):S236 (Ab Sa1146).
58. Hirano I, Moy N, Heckman MG, et al. Endoscopic assessment of the oesophageal features of eosinophilic oesophagitis: validation of a novel classification and grading system. Gut 2012. [Epub ahead of print].
59. Toto E, Kern E, Moy N, et al. Duration of dysphagia is associated with increased frequency of dysphagia and food impaction in adults with eosinophilic esophagitis. Gastroenterology 2010;138(Suppl 1):AB S1088.
60. Schoepfer A, Safroneeva E, Bussmann C, et al. Fixed rings and strictures in eosinophilic esophagitis develop due to continuing inflammation over time. Gastroenterology 2012;142(Suppl 2):AB 1032.
61. Saffari H, Peterson KA, Fang JC, et al. Patchy eosinophil distributions in an esophagectomy specimen from a patient with eosinophilic esophagitis: implications for endoscopic biopsy. J Allergy Clin Immunol 2012;130:798–800.
62. Dellon ES, Speck O, Woodward K, et al. The patchy nature of esophageal eosinophilia in eosinophilic esophagitis: insights from pathology samples from a clinical trial. Gastroenterology 2012;142(Suppl 2):Ab Su1129.
63. Gonsalves N, Policarpio-Nicolas M, Zhang Q, et al. Histopathologic variability and endoscopic correlates in adults with eosinophilic esophagitis. Gastrointest Endosc 2006;64:313–9.
64. Shah A, Kagalwalla AF, Gonsalves N, et al. Histopathologic variability in children with eosinophilic esophagitis. Am J Gastroenterol 2009;104:716–21.
65. Collins MH. Histopathologic features of eosinophilic esophagitis. Gastrointest Endosc Clin N Am 2008;18:59–71, viii–ix.

66. Odze RD. Pathology of eosinophilic esophagitis: what the clinician needs to know. Am J Gastroenterol 2009;104:485–90.
67. Peery AF, Shaheen NJ, Dellon ES. Practice patterns for the evaluation and treatment of eosinophilic oesophagitis. Aliment Pharmacol Ther 2010;32:1373–82.
68. Sperry SL, Shaheen NJ, Dellon ES. Toward uniformity in the diagnosis of eosinophilic esophagitis (EoE): the effect of guidelines on variability of diagnostic criteria for EoE. Am J Gastroenterol 2011;106:824–32 [quiz: 33].
69. Furuta GT, Liacouras CA, Collins MH, et al. Eosinophilic esophagitis in children and adults: a systematic review and consensus recommendations for diagnosis and treatment. Gastroenterology 2007;133:1342–63.
70. Dellon ES, Fritchie KJ, Rubinas TC, et al. Inter- and intraobserver reliability and validation of a new method for determination of eosinophil counts in patients with esophageal eosinophilia. Dig Dis Sci 2010;55:1940–9.
71. Spechler SJ, Genta RM, Souza RF. Thoughts on the complex relationship between gastroesophageal reflux disease and eosinophilic esophagitis. Am J Gastroenterol 2007;102:1301–6.
72. Ngo P, Furuta GT, Antonioli DA, et al. Eosinophils in the esophagus–peptic or allergic eosinophilic esophagitis? Case series of three patients with esophageal eosinophilia. Am J Gastroenterol 2006;101:1666–70.
73. Dranove JE, Horn DS, Davis MA, et al. Predictors of response to proton pump inhibitor therapy among children with significant esophageal eosinophilia. J Pediatr 2009;154:96–100.
74. Sayej WN, Patel R, Baker RD, et al. Treatment with high-dose proton pump inhibitors helps distinguish eosinophilic esophagitis from noneosinophilic esophagitis. J Pediatr Gastroenterol Nutr 2009;49:393–9.
75. Moawad FJ, Dias JA, Veerappan GR, et al. Comparison of aerosolized swallowed fluticasone to esomeprazole for the treatment of eosinophilic esophagitis. Am J Gastroenterol 2011;S12 (AB 30).
76. Molina-Infante J, Ferrando-Lamana L, Ripoll C, et al. Esophageal eosinophilic infiltration responds to proton pump inhibition in most adults. Clin Gastroenterol Hepatol 2011;9:110–7.
77. Peterson KA, Thomas KL, Hilden K, et al. Comparison of esomeprazole to aerosolized, swallowed fluticasone for eosinophilic esophagitis. Dig Dis Sci 2010;55:1313–9.
78. Dellon ES, Speck O, Woodward K, et al. Prospective determination of the prevalence of PPI-responsive esophageal eosinophilia in patients with dysphagia undergoing upper endoscopy [abstract]. Am J Gastroenterol 2012;107(Suppl 1):S9 (AB 20).
79. Aceves SS, Newbury RO, Dohil MA, et al. A symptom scoring tool for identifying pediatric patients with eosinophilic esophagitis and correlating symptoms with inflammation. Ann Allergy Asthma Immunol 2009;103:401–6.
80. von Arnim U, Wex T, Rohl FW, et al. Identification of clinical and laboratory markers for predicting eosinophilic esophagitis in adults. Digestion 2011;84:323–7.
81. Yoo H, Kang D, Katz AJ, et al. Reflectance confocal microscopy for the diagnosis of eosinophilic esophagitis: a pilot study conducted on biopsy specimens. Gastrointest Endosc 2011;74:992–1000.
82. Safdarian N, Liu Z, Zhou X, et al. Quantifying human eosinophils using three-dimensional volumetric images collected with multiphoton fluorescence microscopy. Gastroenterology 2012;142:15–20.e1.
83. Kwiatek MA, Hirano I, Kahrilas PJ, et al. Mechanical properties of the esophagus in eosinophilic esophagitis. Gastroenterology 2011;140:82–90.

84. Protheroe C, Woodruff SA, de Petris G, et al. A novel histologic scoring system to evaluate mucosal biopsies from patients with eosinophilic esophagitis. Clin Gastroenterol Hepatol 2009;7:749–755.e11.
85. Kephart GM, Alexander JA, Arora AS, et al. Marked deposition of eosinophil-derived neurotoxin in adult patients with eosinophilic esophagitis. Am J Gastroenterol 2010;105:298–307.
86. Blanchard C, Stucke EM, Rodriguez-Jimenez B, et al. A striking local esophageal cytokine expression profile in eosinophilic esophagitis. J Allergy Clin Immunol 2011;127:208–17, 217.e1–7.
87. Dellon ES, Chen X, Miller CR, et al. Tryptase staining of mast cells may differentiate eosinophilic esophagitis from gastroesophageal reflux disease. Am J Gastroenterol 2011;106:264–71.
88. Dellon ES, Chen X, Miller CR, et al. Diagnostic utility of major basic protein, eotaxin-3, and leukotriene enzyme staining in eosinophilic esophagitis. Am J Gastroenterol 2012;107:1503–11.
89. Saffari H, Gleich GJ, Pease L, et al. A new approach to image and enhance diagnosis of EoE: radiolobeled contrast agents. Gastroenterology 2012;142(Suppl 2):AB Sa1836.
90. Furuta GT, Kagalwalla AF, Lee JJ, et al. The oesophageal string test: a novel, minimally invasive method measures mucosal inflammation in eosinophilic oesophagitis. Gut 2012. [Epub ahead of print].
91. Gupta SK, Fitzgerald JF, Kondratyuk T, et al. Cytokine expression in normal and inflamed esophageal mucosa: a study into the pathogenesis of allergic eosinophilic esophagitis. J Pediatr Gastroenterol Nutr 2006;42:22–6.
92. Konikoff MR, Blanchard C, Kirby C, et al. Potential of blood eosinophils, eosinophil-derived neurotoxin, and eotaxin-3 as biomarkers of eosinophilic esophagitis. Clin Gastroenterol Hepatol 2006;4:1328–36.
93. Subbarao G, Rosenman MB, Ohnuki L, et al. Exploring potential noninvasive biomarkers in eosinophilic esophagitis in children. J Pediatr Gastroenterol Nutr 2011;53:651–8.
94. Blanchard C, Mingler MK, Vicario M, et al. IL-13 involvement in eosinophilic esophagitis: transcriptome analysis and reversibility with glucocorticoids. J Allergy Clin Immunol 2007;120:1292–300.
95. Hirano I. Therapeutic end points in eosinophilic esophagitis: is elimination of esophageal eosinophils enough? Clin Gastroenterol Hepatol 2012;10:750–2.
96. Liacouras CA, Wenner WJ, Brown K, et al. Primary eosinophilic esophagitis in children: successful treatment with oral corticosteroids. J Pediatr Gastroenterol Nutr 1998;26:380–5.
97. Helou EF, Simonson J, Arora AS. 3-yr-follow-up of topical corticosteroid treatment for eosinophilic esophagitis in adults. Am J Gastroenterol 2008;103:2194–9.
98. Straumann A, Conus S, Degen L, et al. Long-term budesonide maintenance treatment is partially effective for patients with eosinophilic esophagitis. Clin Gastroenterol Hepatol 2011;9:400–409.e1.
99. Picus D, Frank PH. Eosinophilic esophagitis. AJR Am J Roentgenol 1981;136:1001–3.
100. Faubion WA Jr, Perrault J, Burgart LJ, et al. Treatment of eosinophilic esophagitis with inhaled corticosteroids. J Pediatr Gastroenterol Nutr 1998;27:90–3.
101. Teitelbaum JE, Fox VL, Twarog FJ, et al. Eosinophilic esophagitis in children: immunopathological analysis and response to fluticasone propionate. Gastroenterology 2002;122:1216–25.

102. Arora AS, Perrault J, Smyrk TC. Topical corticosteroid treatment of dysphagia due to eosinophilic esophagitis in adults. Mayo Clin Proc 2003;78:830–5.
103. Noel RJ, Putnam PE, Collins MH, et al. Clinical and immunopathologic effects of swallowed fluticasone for eosinophilic esophagitis. Clin Gastroenterol Hepatol 2004;2:568–75.
104. Remedios M, Campbell C, Jones DM, et al. Eosinophilic esophagitis in adults: clinical, endoscopic, histologic findings, and response to treatment with fluticasone propionate. Gastrointest Endosc 2006;63:3–12.
105. Aceves SS, Bastian JF, Newbury RO, et al. Oral viscous budesonide: a potential new therapy for eosinophilic esophagitis in children. Am J Gastroenterol 2007; 102:2271–9.
106. Lucendo AJ, Pascual-Turrion JM, Navarro M, et al. Endoscopic, bioptic, and manometric findings in eosinophilic esophagitis before and after steroid therapy: a case series. Endoscopy 2007;39:765–71.
107. Bergquist H, Larsson H, Johansson L, et al. Dysphagia and quality of life may improve with mometasone treatment in patients with eosinophilic esophagitis: a pilot study. Otolaryngol Head Neck Surg 2011;145:551–6.
108. Schroeder S, Fleischer DM, Masterson JC, et al. Successful treatment of eosinophilic esophagitis with ciclesonide. J Allergy Clin Immunol 2012;129: 1419–21.
109. Schaefer ET, Fitzgerald JF, Molleston JP, et al. Comparison of oral prednisone and topical fluticasone in the treatment of eosinophilic esophagitis: a randomized trial in children. Clin Gastroenterol Hepatol 2008;6:165–73.
110. Konikoff MR, Noel RJ, Blanchard C, et al. A randomized, double-blind, placebo-controlled trial of fluticasone propionate for pediatric eosinophilic esophagitis. Gastroenterology 2006;131:1381–91.
111. Alexander JA, Jung KW, Arora AS, et al. Swallowed fluticasone improves histologic but not symptomatic responses of adults with eosinophilic esophagitis. Clin Gastroenterol Hepatol 2012;10:742–749.e1.
112. Aceves SS, Dohil R, Newbury RO, et al. Topical viscous budesonide suspension for treatment of eosinophilic esophagitis. J Allergy Clin Immunol 2005;116: 705–6.
113. Dohil R, Newbury R, Fox L, et al. Oral viscous budesonide is effective in children with eosinophilic esophagitis in a randomized, placebo-controlled trial. Gastroenterology 2010;139:418–29.
114. Gupta SK, Collins MH, Lewis JD, et al. Efficacy and safety of oral budesonide suspension (obs) in pediatric subjects with eosinophilic esophagitis (EoE): results from the double-blind, placebo-controlled PEER Study. Gastroenterology 2011;140(Suppl 1):S179.
115. Straumann A, Conus S, Degen L, et al. Budesonide is effective in adolescent and adult patients with active eosinophilic esophagitis. Gastroenterology 2010;139:1526–37, 37.e1.
116. Dellon ES, Sheikh A, Speck O, et al. Viscous topical is more effective than nebulized steroid therapy for patients with eosinophilic esophagitis. Gastroenterology 2012;143:321–324.e1.
117. Lindberg GM, Van Eldik R, Saboorian MH. A case of herpes esophagitis after fluticasone propionate for eosinophilic esophagitis. Nat Clin Pract Gastroenterol Hepatol 2008;5:527–30.
118. Straumann A, Conus S, Grzonka P, et al. Anti-interleukin-5 antibody treatment (mepolizumab) in active eosinophilic oesophagitis: a randomised, placebo-controlled, double-blind trial. Gut 2010;59:21–30.

119. Assa'ad AH, Gupta SK, Collins MH, et al. An antibody against IL-5 reduces numbers of esophageal intraepithelial eosinophils in children with eosinophilic esophagitis. Gastroenterology 2011;141:1593–604.
120. Spergel JM, Rothenberg ME, Collins MH, et al. Reslizumab in children and adolescents with eosinophilic esophagitis: results of a double-blind, randomized, placebo-controlled trial. J Allergy Clin Immunol 2012;129:456–63, 63.e1–3.
121. Straumann A, Bussmann C, Conus S, et al. Anti-TNF-alpha (infliximab) therapy for severe adult eosinophilic esophagitis. J Allergy Clin Immunol 2008;122: 425–7.
122. Fang JC, Hilden K, Gleich GJ, et al. A pilot study of the treatment of eosinophilic esophagitis with omalizumab. Gastroenterology 2011;140(Suppl 1):AB Sa1143.
123. Attwood SE, Lewis CJ, Bronder CS, et al. Eosinophilic oesophagitis: a novel treatment using montelukast. Gut 2003;52:181–5.
124. Stumphy J, Al-Zubeidi D, Guerin L, et al. Observations on use of montelukast in pediatric eosinophilic esophagitis: insights for the future. Dis Esophagus 2011; 24:229–34.
125. Lucendo AJ, De Rezende LC, Jimenez-Contreras S, et al. Montelukast was inefficient in maintaining steroid-induced remission in adult eosinophilic esophagitis. Dig Dis Sci 2011;56:3551–8.
126. Netzer P, Gschossmann JM, Straumann A, et al. Corticosteroid-dependent eosinophilic oesophagitis: azathioprine and 6-mercaptopurine can induce and maintain long-term remission. Eur J Gastroenterol Hepatol 2007;19:865–9.
127. Straumann A, Bussmann C, Perkins MC, et al. Treatment of eosinophilic esophagitis with the CRTH2-antagonist OCT000459: a novel therapeutic principle. Gastroenterology 2012;142(Suppl 2):AB 856.
128. Markowitz JE, Spergel JM, Ruchelli E, et al. Elemental diet is an effective treatment for eosinophilic esophagitis in children and adolescents. Am J Gastroenterol 2003;98:777–82.
129. Henderson CJ, Abonia JP, King EC, et al. Comparative dietary therapy effectiveness in remission of pediatric eosinophilic esophagitis. J Allergy Clin Immunol 2012;129:1570–8.
130. Peterson K, Clayton F, Vinson LA, et al. Utility of an elemental diet in adult eosinophilic esophagitis. Gastroenterology 2011;140(Suppl 1):AB 1080.
131. Kagalwalla AF, Sentongo TA, Ritz S, et al. Effect of six-food elimination diet on clinical and histologic outcomes in eosinophilic esophagitis. Clin Gastroenterol Hepatol 2006;4:1097–102.
132. Kagalwalla AF, Shah A, Li BU, et al. Identification of specific foods responsible for inflammation in children with eosinophilic esophagitis successfully treated with empiric elimination diet. J Pediatr Gastroenterol Nutr 2011;53:145–9.
133. Gonsalves N, Yang GY, Doerfler B, et al. Elimination diet effectively treats eosinophilic esophagitis in adults; food reintroduction identifies causative factors. Gastroenterology 2012;142:1451–1459.e1.
134. Spergel JM, Brown-Whitehorn T, Beausoleil JL, et al. Predictive values for skin prick test and atopy patch test for eosinophilic esophagitis. J Allergy Clin Immunol 2007;119:509–11.
135. Spergel JM, Beausoleil JL, Mascarenhas M, et al. The use of skin prick tests and patch tests to identify causative foods in eosinophilic esophagitis. J Allergy Clin Immunol 2002;109:363–8.
136. Spergel JM, Brown-Whitehorn TF, Cianferoni A, et al. Identification of causative foods in children with eosinophilic esophagitis treated with an elimination diet. J Allergy Clin Immunol 2012;130:461–467.e5.

137. Spergel JM, Andrews T, Brown-Whitehorn TF, et al. Treatment of eosinophilic esophagitis with specific food elimination diet directed by a combination of skin prick and patch tests. Ann Allergy Asthma Immunol 2005;95:336–43.
138. Molina-Infante J, Martin-Noguerol E, Alvarado-Arenas M, et al. Selective elimination diet based on skin testing has suboptimal efficacy for adult eosinophilic esophagitis. J Allergy Clin Immunol 2012;130(5):1200–2.
139. Simon D, Straumann A, Wenk A, et al. Eosinophilic esophagitis in adults—no clinical relevance of wheat and rye sensitizations. Allergy 2006;61:1480–3.
140. Croese J, Fairley SK, Masson JW, et al. Clinical and endoscopic features of eosinophilic esophagitis in adults. Gastrointest Endosc 2003;58:516–22.
141. Kaplan M, Mutlu EA, Jakate S, et al. Endoscopy in eosinophilic esophagitis: "feline" esophagus and perforation risk. Clin Gastroenterol Hepatol 2003;1:433–7.
142. Potter JW, Saeian K, Staff D, et al. Eosinophilic esophagitis in adults: an emerging problem with unique esophageal features. Gastrointest Endosc 2004;59:355–61.
143. Cohen MS, Kaufman AB, Palazzo JP, et al. An audit of endoscopic complications in adult eosinophilic esophagitis. Clin Gastroenterol Hepatol 2007;5:1149–53.
144. Gonsalves N, Karmali K, Hirano I. Safety and response of esophageal dilation in adults with eosinophilic esophagitis: a single center experience of 81 patients. Gastroenterology 2007;132(Suppl 2):A607.
145. Schoepfer AM, Gschossmann J, Scheurer U, et al. Esophageal strictures in adult eosinophilic esophagitis: dilation is an effective and safe alternative after failure of topical corticosteroids. Endoscopy 2008;40:161–4.
146. Straumann A, Bussmann C, Zuber M, et al. Eosinophilic esophagitis: analysis of food impaction and perforation in 251 adolescent and adult patients. Clin Gastroenterol Hepatol 2008;6:598–600.
147. Dellon ES, Gibbs WB, Rubinas TC, et al. Esophageal dilation in eosinophilic esophagitis: safety and predictors of clinical response and complications. Gastrointest Endosc 2010;71:706–12.
148. Schoepfer AM, Gonsalves N, Bussmann C, et al. Esophageal dilation in eosinophilic esophagitis: effectiveness, safety, and impact on the underlying inflammation. Am J Gastroenterol 2010;105:1062–70.
149. Bohm M, Richter JE, Kelsen S, et al. Esophageal dilation: simple and effective treatment for adults with eosinophilic esophagitis and esophageal rings and narrowing. Dis Esophagus 2010;23:377–85.
150. Jung KW, Gundersen N, Kopacova J, et al. Occurrence of and risk factors for complications after endoscopic dilation in eosinophilic esophagitis. Gastrointest Endosc 2011;73:15–21.
151. Jacobs JW Jr, Spechler SJ. A systematic review of the risk of perforation during esophageal dilation for patients with eosinophilic esophagitis. Dig Dis Sci 2010;55:1512–5.
152. Bohm ME, Richter JE. Review article: oesophageal dilation in adults with eosinophilic oesophagitis. Aliment Pharmacol Ther 2011;33:748–57.
153. Egan JV, Baron TH, Adler DG, et al. Esophageal dilation. Gastrointest Endosc 2006;63:755–60.
154. Madanick RD, Shaheen NJ, Dellon ES. A novel balloon pull-through technique for esophageal dilation in eosinophilic esophagitis (with video). Gastrointest Endosc 2011;73:138–42.
155. Ally MR, Dias J, Veerappan GR, et al. Safety of dilation in adults with eosinophilic esophagitis. Dis Esophagus 2012. [Epub ahead of print].

156. Korsapati HR, Babaei A, Bhargava V, et al. Dysfunction of the longitudinal muscles of the esophagus in eosinophilic esophagitis. Gut 2009;58:1056–62.
157. Nurko S, Rosen R, Furuta GT. Esophageal dysmotility in children with eosinophilic esophagitis: a study using prolonged esophageal manometry. Am J Gastroenterol 2009;104:3050–7.
158. Roman S, Hirano I, Kwiatek MA, et al. Manometric features of eosinophilic esophagitis in esophageal pressure topography. Neurogastroenterol Motil 2011;23:208–14. e111.

Screening and Risk Stratification for Barrett's Esophagus

How to Limit the Clinical Impact of the Increasing Incidence of Esophageal Adenocarcinoma

Massimiliano di Pietro, MD, Rebecca C. Fitzgerald, MD*

KEYWORDS

- Esophageal adenocarcinoma • Barrett's esophagus
- Gastroesophageal reflux disease • Dysplasia • Biomarkers • Screening
- Cost-effectiveness

KEY POINTS

- Esophageal adenocarcinoma (EAC) is the solid malignancy with the fastest increasing incidence in the Western world over the last 3 decades.
- Barrett's esophagus (BE) is the only known precursor to EAC and the strongest risk factor for this type of esophageal cancer.
- Other risk factors for EAC include gastroesophageal reflux disease, obesity, smoking, and male sex.
- Endoscopic screening for BE has the potential to reduce the clinical impact of the changing epidemiology of EAC, but it is not cost-effective.
- Less invasive and more inexpensive modalities (eg, Cytosponge, office-based transnasal endoscopy, and capsule endoscopy) are under investigation, with the aim of making screening feasible in primary care.
- Histologic dysplasia in BE is the only biomarker available in clinical practice; however, it is subject to high interobserver variability among pathologists and sampling error from random biopsies.
- Molecular biomarkers can provide a more objective estimate of the individual cancer risk and are under investigation.

EPIDEMIOLOGY OF ESOPHAGEAL ADENOCARCINOMA

The epidemiology of esophageal adenocarcinoma (EAC) has changed dramatically over the past 50 years in the Western world. Surgical series reported before the 1980s showed that esophageal squamous cell carcinoma (ESCC), which arises

MRC Cancer Cell Unit, Hutchison MRC, Hills Road, Cambridge CB2 0XZ, UK
* Corresponding author.
E-mail address: rcf@hutchison-mrc.cam.ac.uk

Gastroenterol Clin N Am 42 (2013) 155–173
http://dx.doi.org/10.1016/j.gtc.2012.11.006
0889-8553/13/$ – see front matter © 2013 Elsevier Inc. All rights reserved.

gastro.theclinics.com

from the native multilayered squamous epithelium, was the most common malignancy in the esophagus.[1–4] However, subsequent Western case series published 10 to 15 years later indicated that the EAC had become the most common esophageal malignancy, exceeding the number of cases of ESCC.[5–7] A study looking at the relative distribution of these 2 esophageal tumor types over 25 years spanning this transition period showed that this change was statistically significant.[8] Despite a slight decline in the incidence of ESCC, the trend inversion seems to be mostly caused by a dramatic increase in the incidence of EAC during the last 3 to 4 decades, such that in the early years of the twenty-first century EAC has been the fastest rising solid malignancy in the United States.[9–11] This epidemiologic trend for EAC involves mostly Western countries, although there is some geographic variation.[11,12] Between the early 1980s and late 1990s, among all European countries, Ireland and the United Kingdom showed the largest increase in the age-standardized incidence rates (~7% per annum), a trend comparable with the United States and Australia.[11,13] Data have established that this is a true increase in incidence, rather than the effect of histologic reclassification or overdiagnosis associated with technological advancements.[10] Another potential confounding factor is the anatomic classification of adenocarcinomas around the gastroesophageal junction. EAC and gastric cardia adenocarcinoma (GCA) are often grouped together in clinical studies. However, studies looking separately at cancer incidence at these 2 locations between the early 1980s and late 2000s showed that, although incidence of EAC has risen by 6-fold, the incidence of GCA increased initially by 2-fold and declined latterly, remaining overall stable across this temporal period.[10,11] Data from more recent periods show that the overall incidence of EAC continues to increase, although at a slower rate, which is approximately 2% per year.[11]

RISK FACTORS FOR EAC

Table 1 lists the clinical and epidemiologic factors that have been studied in relation to the incidence of EAC.

Gastroesophageal Reflux Disease

Gastroesophageal reflux disease (GERD) and its associated pathologic condition hiatus hernia are well-documented risk factors for the development of EAC.[14,15] A recent meta-analysis that included 5 studies showed that weekly and daily GERD symptoms are associated with an odds ratio (OR) for EAC of 4.92 (95% confidence interval [CI], 3.90–6.22) and 7.4 (95% CI, 4.94–11.1), respectively.[16] Although the pathophysiologic mechanisms of this association are not fully understood, it is believed that oxidative and genotoxic damage provoked by exposure of esophageal epithelium to acid and bile induces genetic and epigenetic changes that support the carcinogenic process.[17,18]

Barrett's Esophagus

GERD is believed to induce esophageal carcinogenesis through the premalignant condition Barrett's esophagus (BE), which is a columnar metaplasia of the distal esophagus generally containing intestinal differentiation.[19] Endoscopic studies have shown that BE can be found in approximately 10% of individuals with reflux disease sufficient to warrant referral for endoscopy.[19–21] Most cases of EACs are believed to develop in this context,[22,23] so that BE is the single strongest risk factor for the development of EAC with a relative risk (RR) of 11.3 (95% CI, 8.8–14.4).[24] The metaplastic conversion to columnar lined epithelium explains how adenocarcinoma can develop in

Table 1
Factors associated with EAC

	Evidence	References
GERD	Weekly symptoms: OR for EAC 4.9 Daily symptoms: OR for EAC 7.4	14–16
BE	Annual risk 0.12%–0.38% for nondysplastic BE Annual risk 0.51%–14.0% for BE with LGD	24–29
Obesity	BMI 25 to <30 kg/m^2: OR for EAC 1.7 BMI >30 kg/m^2: OR for EAC 2.3	30–47
Gender	EAC incidence 6 times higher in men than women EAC risk in male patients with BE 2–3 times higher than female	11,24,26,28
Smoking	Current smokers: OR for EAC 2.3 Ex-smokers: OR for EAC 1.6	55–57
Alcohol	Evidence of lack of association	62,63
Helicobacter pylori	Inverse correlation to EAC (particularly for cytotoxin-associated antigen A-positive strains: OR for EAC 0.4)	66–68
Diet	Weak evidence of positive association with red meat and processed food and inverse association with consumption of fruit and vegetables	69

Abbreviations: BE, Barrett's esophagus; BMI, body mass index; GERD, gastroesophageal reflux disease; LGD, low-grade dysplasia; OR, odds ratio.

an organ normally lined by a squamous epithelial type. Historically, the annual incidence of EAC in patients with BE was believed to be between 0.5% and 1% per year[25–27]; however, more recent population studies and a meta-analysis have set this risk at around 0.12% to 0.38% per year.[24,28,29]

Obesity

Obesity is a risk factor for many types of cancer.[30] Most studies examining the correlation between obesity and EAC have found a positive association.[31–37] Two meta-analyses published in 2006 and 2012 reached similar conclusions, namely that high body mass index (BMI, calculated as weight in kilograms divided by the square of height in meters) is associated with both EAC and GCA, with the strongest effect for EAC.[38,39] The more recent of these meta-analyses found ORs for EAC of 1.7 (95% CI, 1.5–1.96) and 2.34 (95% CI, 1.95–2.81), for a BMI between 25 and 30 kg/m^2 and greater than 30 kg/m^2, respectively.[39] The mechanisms whereby obesity increases EAC risk are likely to be multiple. Obesity leads to increased intra-abdominal pressure,[40] is associated with more frequent transient relaxations of the lower esophageal sphincter,[41] and also correlates with a higher incidence of hiatus hernia.[42] This finding may explain the positive association between obesity and GERD found in many studies and confirmed by a meta-analysis, in which the ORs for GERD symptoms were 1.43 (95% CI, 1.16–1.776) and 1.94 (95% CI, 1.47–2.57), for BMIs between 25 and 30 kg/m^2 and greater than 30 kg/m^2, respectively.[43] However, this correlation also seems to go beyond the simple predisposition to acid reflux.[44–46] It is now clear that the distribution of fat, and visceral adiposity in particular, may play a role in the promotion of BE.[40,44,47] Furthermore, obesity acts not only on the acquisition of the metaplastic precursor but also on the development of genetic abnormalities that drive the transformation to cancer.[48] This situation is likely to be related to the metabolic activity of visceral fat and its ability to produce cytokines, growth factors, and hormones,[48–50] which can alter insulin resistance and lipid metabolism, promoting the condition known as metabolic syndrome.[51] This syndrome has been independently associated with a predisposition to cancer[50] and BE.[52] Overall, it is believed that the increasing prevalence of obesity in Western countries[53,54] is likely to be a significant contributor to the epidemic increase in the incidence of EAC.[9,11]

Smoking

Another risk factor for EAC is tobacco smoking, although to a lesser degree compared with ESCC.[55,56] A recent meta-analysis found a pooled RR for ever-smokers of 1.76 (95% CI, 1.54–2.01), with a direct correlation between the risk of cancer and the dose and the duration of the exposure.[57] The recent decline in smoking in many of the Western countries may account for the slower rate of increase in the incidence of EAC since the late 1990s.[11]

Gender

Male sex is associated with an increased risk of EAC, and 2 recent population studies confirmed this association. Bhat and colleagues[28] showed that the annual cancer incidence in patients with BE with intestinal metaplasia was 0.45% (95% CI, 0.36–0.56) in men and 0.26% (95% CI, 0.18–0.38) in women. Similarly, Hvid-Jensen and colleagues[24] found a significant difference in the cancer incidence between male and female patients. The meta-analysis from Sikkema and colleagues[26] before these studies found an RR associated to male gender of 1.7 (95% CI, 0.6–4.5), whereas a more recent meta-analysis[58] did not perform subgroup analysis related to gender. Independently of a previous diagnosis of BE, EAC incidence is 6-fold to 8-fold higher in men compared with women.[11] The reasons for this gender bias are not entirely clear, although hormonal factors have been proposed.[59]

Alcohol Consumption

Although alcohol is a well-known carcinogen[60] and is a major risk factor for the development of ESCC,[61] alcohol consumption is not associated with an increased risk of EAC and there has been some evidence that a moderate intake may even lead to a slight decreased risk of EAC.[62] Recently a meta-analysis[63] provided definitive evidence of the absence of any association between alcohol consumption and EAC and GCA, even at high doses.

Helicobacter pylori

Helicobacter pylori is a World Health Organization class I carcinogen and is associated with an increased risk of gastric cancer and other gastrointestinal (GI) malignancies.[64,65] However, studies have highlighted an inverse association between *H pylori* gastric colonization and the risk of EAC, such that eradication strategies have been linked to the increased incidence of EAC.[66,67] A meta-analysis of 19 studies on the subject confirmed that *H pylori* infection is inversely associated with EAC risk, with an OR of 0.56 (95% CI, 0.46–0.68), which appeared to relate to cytotoxin-associated antigen A (CagA)-positive strains (OR, 0.41) and not to CagA-negative strains (OR, 1.08).[68]

Diet

There is some evidence that dietary factors can modulate the risk of EAC. Epidemiologic studies suggested a protective effect of high fruit and vegetable intake, whereas red meat and processed food can confer an increased risk for EAC.[69] However, there are substantial obstacles in accurately assessing an individual dietary intake over time, and further research is needed to better estimate the impact of dietary factors on EAC risk.

INTERVENTION TO REDUCE CLINICAL IMPACT OF ESOPHAGEAL CANCER
Modification of Risk Factors

The epidemiologic trends of EAC in the Western world, discussed earlier, have raised concern about this disease amongst public health officials and as a result, there has been a call for clinical and research strategies to limit the impact of this disease.[70–72] Because the modifiable risk factors implicated in the pathogenesis are still not completely understood[73] and because compliance with healthy-living campaigns is poor, it is difficult to promote strategies to change the risk profile at a population level. For example, obesity, which has been related to the increase of incidence of EAC,[39] has been implicated in a variety of diseases for many years[30,74] and social campaigns have been instigated to sensitize the population. However, despite these efforts, obesity is an increasing problem of the modern Western world.[53,54,75] Chemoprevention is an alternative strategy; however, there is lack of robust evidence to support this approach using currently available drugs to control reflux disease[76] or to interfere with inflammatory pathways.[77] However, the results of randomized controlled trials such as AspECT are awaited to shed further light on this. An alternative approach is therefore to focus on early detection.

Screening

The poor survival rates of EAC are mostly related to the fact that symptomatic disease correlates with advanced stage ($\geq$T3N1), whereby only 1 in 7 patients is predicted to be alive at 5 years, despite all the therapeutic efforts to achieve a cure.[78,79] Diagnosis of disease at an earlier stage is therefore paramount and is a distinct possibility, because EAC has a well-established pathologic sequence, whereby it is preceded in most cases by BE. Furthermore, the progression of BE to cancer is gradual and occurs through dysplastic stages, namely low-grade dysplasia (LGD) and high-grade dysplasia (HGD).[70] Several retrospective series[80–82] have shown that a diagnosis of EAC in patients with who were previously in endoscopic surveillance correlates with improved pathologic staging and better survival. However, randomized studies confirming this finding are lacking, and surveillance strategies for BE do not seem to have improved survival from a population perspective. One prime reason for this situation is likely to be that most persons with BE remain undiagnosed in the community, and therefore EAC is more likely to occur de novo in individuals without the benefit of a diagnosis of BE. To overcome this situation, endoscopic screening for BE has been considered for individuals with GERD. Studies on the cost-effectiveness of endoscopic screening have shown a wide range of incremental cost-effectiveness ratios (ICER),[83–85] leaving uncertainty about its feasibility in clinical practice. Moreover, the recent evidence that the cancer risk in BE is significantly lower than previously believed[24,28,58] makes this strategy even less cost-effective. The implications are that an expensive and invasive test (endoscopy) would be used to diagnose a prevalent condition such as BE (about 10% of the GERD population), which carries a relatively low cancer risk (0.12%–0.38% per year[24,28,29]). This large cohort of patients would then need to be monitored with even more expensive and invasive tests (endoscopy + multiple biopsies). This regime is clearly difficult to propose in the current financial climate, and it is also doubtful whether the invasiveness of this approach and the consequent impact on the quality of life could be justified. A solution would therefore require a less costly and invasive alternative. Furthermore, to make this screening strategy more cost-effective, once BE is diagnosed, there needs to be a method for identifying high-risk patients so that surveillance (and treatment) programs can be restricted to those at significant risk for EAC. The recent advent of less invasive endoscopic techniques for the ablation of dysplastic BE fits well into this clinical algorithm,[86,87] in that patients with precancerous conditions and at high risk of progression can be offered ablation therapy for the prevention of cancer.

SCREENING MODALITIES

Table 2 provides a summary of the diagnostic modalities proposed for BE and EAC screening.

Conventional Endoscopy

Conventional endoscopy (CE) is the gold standard for the surveillance of BE, because it allows complete and high-quality visualization of the distal esophagus as well as tissue sampling for histologic diagnosis. CE has been studied as a screening modality for BE and early EAC. Two studies used CE to examine the prevalence of BE in patients undergoing colonoscopy. In the study by Rex and colleagues of 961 individuals,[88] the overall prevalence of BE was 6.8% (5.6% in patients without a previous history of heartburn and 8.3% in patients with a previous history of heartburn, although this difference did not reach significance in the multivariate analysis). Gerson and colleagues[89] detected BE in 27 of 110 asymptomatic veterans (25%). In a further study by this group,[90] BE was detected in 6% of women undergoing either colonoscopy or bariatric surgery. Although these studies investigated a small and selected population of individuals, they suggest that BE, defined as the presence of intestinal metaplasia above the gastroesophageal junction, is a common finding even in the absence of reflux symptoms. Gupta and colleagues[84] analyzed the cost-effectiveness of CE screening in the general population at the time of the screening colonoscopy. Considering that this strategy can lead to diagnosis of any esophageal malignancy (EAC and ESCC) as well as gastric cancer, the scenario of screening endoscopy plus BE surveillance was associated with an ICER of $95,559 per quality-adjusted life-year (QALY), which is comparable with that of other screening interventions performed in the United States, such as mammography for breast cancer or endoscopic surveillance for ulcerative colitis. When considering endoscopic screening as a separate intervention distinct from colonoscopy, most of the studies published so far have assumed a cancer risk that was higher than that indicated by more recent studies, and furthermore, they did not model endoscopic therapies, making the conclusions difficult to

Table 2 Summary of interventions proposed for BE and EAC screening						
	Conventional Endoscopy	Transnasal Endoscopy	Conventional Capsule Endoscopy	Cytosponge	Balloon Cytology	Occult Blood Bead
Patient preference	−	+	++	++	+	++
Accuracy	+++	++	+	+	−	−
Sampling	+++	++	-	++	+	+
Primary care	−	+	++	+++	+	+++
Cost-effective	−	?	−	++	?	?

extrapolate to the current clinical practice.[91] Further studies are therefore needed, and endoscopy cannot be recommended as a screening modality for the general population. However, American societies do suggest discussing the risks and benefits of screening with high-risk patients (white men older than 50 years, with a high BMI and long-standing GERD).[92,93]

Transnasal Endoscopy

Transnasal endoscopy (TNE) has been studied and shown to be a valid alternative to CE for a diagnosis of BE.[94,95] TNE has the advantage that it does not involve contact with the root of the tongue and does not trigger the gag reflex, and as a result, it does not require sedation and is better tolerated than CE. The study from Shariff and colleagues[95] compared CE and TNE using a randomized crossover design and found a similar diagnostic accuracy for both techniques. TNE is now available with office-based technologies that are compatible with a primary care setting, with the advantage of significantly reducing the costs of screening. One of them (EndoSheath, Vision-Sciences, Orangeburg, NY) has been compared with CE in a single-center randomized study in a cohort of 121 patients enriched for BE.[96] This study found that office-based TNE can be used as a screening modality in a tertiary referral center and had a moderate agreement ($\kappa = 0.59$) and a significantly smaller biopsy size when compared with CE. Importantly, 71% of patients preferred TNE over CE. A prospective multicenter study, which enrolled more than 400 individuals, assessed the feasibility of this technique as a screening modality in a primary care setting and found that office-based TNE is feasible and can significantly affect the clinical management of screened individuals, in whom the prevalence of erosive esophagitis and BE was 34% and 4%, respectively.[97] It remains to be established whether a screening approach with this technology in patients with GERD is cost-effective.

Esophageal Capsule Endoscopy

Esophageal capsule endoscopy (ECE) has been extensively investigated as a screening modality in patients with GERD. ECE has the advantage of avoiding intubation and therefore has the potential to be well tolerated. Limitations include the absence of histologic sampling and the smaller number of total frames per centimeter compared with the small bowel capsule endoscopy, which negatively affects the diagnostic accuracy. Initial experience with the first-generation ECE, which had an image quality lower than 10 frames/s, showed a suboptimal sensitivity for BE of between 60% and 67%.[98–100] A small study evaluating a second-generation ECE (18 frames/s)[101] reported 100% sensitivity and 74% specificity for BE, but included only 28 patients. A third-generation ECE that images the esophagus at a rate of 35 frames/s is now available and studies are awaited to assess its diagnostic accuracy in esophageal diseases. The previous limitation of low image frequency has also been addressed with the use of string capsule endoscopy (SCE), to slow the transit through the esophagus. Ramirez and colleagues[102] evaluated SCE in 100 veterans with reflux disease and assessed its diagnostic accuracy. Using the endoscopic diagnosis alone as the gold standard, the sensitivity and specificity of SCE for BE were 78.3% and 82.8%, whereas when SCE was compared with endoscopy with histologic confirmation, the sensitivity and specificity were 93.5% and 78.7%, respectively. Although we look forward to studies evaluating the new-generation ECE, the question of the cost-effectiveness of the ECE remains to be addressed, because a cost-usefulness study performed in 2007[103] showed that ECE and standard esophagogastroduodenoscopy performed similarly, suggesting that in the current context, the ECE may not be cost-effective.

Balloon Cytology

Nonendoscopic devices have been proposed as screening tools for premalignant and early malignant esophageal conditions. Balloon cytology allows collection of superficial cells for cytologic analysis and is cost-effective and better tolerated when compared with endoscopy. However, although cytology from balloon cytology sampling can identify abnormal cells in patients with HGD and EAC, the yield of goblet cells for a reliable diagnosis of BE has been shown to be poor and not adequate for it to be proposed as a screening tool for detecting premalignant lesions.[104,105]

Cytosponge

The Cytosponge coupled to a diagnostic biomarker for BE has recently been proposed as a screening modality. The Cytosponge is a nonendoscopic cell collection device in which a capsule is swallowed and a sponge expands in the proximal stomach over a period of 5 minutes. This sponge samples the gastric cardia, gastroesophageal junction, and distal and proximal esophagus in turn before being pulled out through the mouth. The cytologic specimen is then examined for expression of the biomarker Trefoil factor 3, which was ascertained to be a Barrett's-specific marker from a gene expression profiling experiment that compared gene expression between samples of gastric cardia, BE, and normal squamous esophagus.[106] In a primary care screening study, this test was applied to more than 500 individuals with a history of reflux disease and the diagnosis compared with that obtained from standard endoscopy and biopsies. The primary aims of the study were to determine patient acceptability as well as the feasibility of administering the test in primary care. The prevalence of BE in this population was 3%, and hence there was limited power to determine sensitivity and specificity. Nevertheless, the data were encouraging, with a sensitivity of 73% and 90% for BE segments of at least 1 and 2 cm, respectively, with specificity figures more than 90%.[21] These preliminary data compare well with other screening tests for other conditions such as the fecal occult blood test for colorectal cancer and the prostate specific antigen test for prostate cancer.[107] A cost-usefulness study comparing Cytosponge and endoscopy as screening interventions in patients with GERD found that the 2 did not differ much in terms of the number of QALYs gained; however, the Cytosponge was more cost-effective.[108] Further studies in larger cohorts are needed to confirm this diagnostic accuracy and whether this test can be proposed as a screening tool at a population level.

Occult Blood Bead

Another noninvasive test studied for screening for upper GI malignancy, including EAC, is the occult blood bead, which consists of a blood detector connected to a string that is swallowed by the patient. This test has been studied in large Chinese cohorts at high risk for upper GI malignancy and yielded a positive result in 12% to 24%. Subsequent upper GI endoscopy showed a malignancy in the stomach or esophagus only in a few individuals, leading to a specificity of about 3%.[109,110] Because only people with positive test underwent endoscopy, the sensitivity of the test remains unknown, and in addition, this test is unlikely to detect BE.

MARKERS OF RISK STRATIFICATION IN PATIENTS WITH BE

Once BE is diagnosed, either through screening or as a result of an investigation for upper GI symptoms, surveillance is generally recommended followed by intervention at the point at which HGD or EAC is detected.[111] The recent evidence that the cancer risk in patients with BE is lower than previously believed[24,28,58] has fueled long-standing arguments about whether this approach is justified.[108,112–115] Most patients with BE never develop cancer, and a recent systematic review has found that endoscopic surveillance for all patients with BE with the current technologies is unlikely to be cost-effective.[116] Therefore, there is a pressing need to identify those patients who are at higher risk of cancer progression to tailor management of patients with BE based on their perceived cancer risk.

Dysplasia

Dysplasia is the currently accepted clinical biomarker to determine cancer risk in BE, with evidence from several studies of an increased risk of progression to cancer.[117–119] Two large population studies published recently[24,28] confirmed that patients with LGD have a cancer risk that is approximately 5 times higher than the general BE population. On these grounds, professional societies recommend that the surveillance frequency is increased to every 6 to 12 months in patients with LGD.[93,120,121] However, dysplasia is an inadequate biomarker because it is subject to significant interobserver variability. In a Dutch study,[122] diagnoses of LGD made in community hospitals were subsequently reviewed by 2 expert GI pathologists, and only 15% of dysplasia diagnoses were confirmed. Patients with a confirmed diagnosis of LGD had a striking annual progression rate of 13.4%, compared with 0.49% in the remaining patients (85%), whose LGD was downgraded to nondysplastic BE. These findings were not confirmed in a subsequent American study, in which confirmation of LGD diagnosis by 2 or 3 pathologists did not affect the progression rate.[123] In this latter study, the κ for agreement among pathologists for a diagnosis of LGD was very poor at 0.18%, highlighting the significant subjectivity for diagnosing this pathologic entity. In addition, dysplasia is affected by sampling error, because it relies on random biopsies, which typically represent less than 5% of the entire BE surface.[124]

Molecular Biomarkers

To improve this situation, researchers have been investigating molecular biomarkers (**Table 3**), which have the potential to provide a more objective measure of genetic and epigenetic abnormalities that occur throughout cancer progression.[17] Because it is thought that molecular abnormalities normally precede cytologic and histologic changes reminiscent of cancer, molecular biomarkers also have the potential to give an estimate of the individual's risk of future progression.

DNA ploidy

Galipeau and colleagues[125] and Reid and colleagues[126] have shown that DNA ploidy abnormalities such as aneuploidy and tetraploidy as well as loss of heterozygosity (LOH) at 17p and 9p loci, which affect important tumor suppressor genes (p53 and p16, respectively), occur in BE-related neoplasia. It was shown that these molecular events occur as early as 10 years before the progression to cancer and can be used as a panel to quantify cancer risk; in particular, patients with all 3 abnormalities (aneuploidy/tetraploidy, p53 LOH, and p16 LOH) had an almost 80% risk of cancer at 10 years, with an RR of 38.7 (95% CI, 10.8–138.5).[127] Even although aneuploidy has been assessed in this study by flow cytometry on frozen biopsies, it can now be tested on formalin-fixed paraffin-embedded (FFPE) biopsies by image cytometry, making this test more feasible in standard practice.[128]

Methylation markers

Schulmann and colleagues[129] investigated epigenetic markers and found that methylation at the promoter of 3 genes (HPP1, p16, and RUNX3) strongly correlated with

Table 3
Biomarkers studied to improve risk stratification

Single Biomarkers	Association with Cancer Progression	Reference	Biomarker Panels	Association with Cancer Progression	Reference
DNA ploidy	RR 3.4	127	DNA ploidy,	RR of 38.7 for	127
17p LOH	RR 5.4		17p LOH,	development	
9p LOH	RR 2.4		and 9p LOH	of EAC at 10 y	
p16 methylation	OR 1.74	129	Panel of 8	Prediction of	130
HPP1 methylation	OR 1.77		methylation	cancer	
RUNX3 methylation	OR 1.8		markers	progression at 4 y with 90% sensitivity and 45% specificity	
Cyclin A	OR 7.6	136	AOL, DNA	Incremental OR	138
p53 immunohistochemistry	OR 11.7	132–135	ploidy, and LGD	of 3.9 for cancer	
Aspergillus oryzae lectin	OR 3.79	138		progression for each individual marker positive	

dysplasia. In addition, each of these markers individually associates with an increased risk of progression; furthermore, when used in combination with an additional 5 methylation markers, this panel could predict progression at 2 and 4 years with a specificity of 90% and a sensitivity of approximately 50%.[130]

P53 immunohistochemistry
Immunohistochemical markers have also been studied, because they have the advantage of being easily applicable to clinical practice. Two of them, p53 and cyclin A, seem to be promising. The *p53* gene is known to be mutated in BE-related neoplasia and commonly mutations lead to stabilization and hence overexpression of a nonfunctional protein.[131] Abnormal overexpression of p53 is frequently seen in dysplastic tissue and is recognized by some pathologists as a possible adjunct in the diagnosis of dysplasia.[132–134] p53 overexpression has also been shown by different groups to correlate with the risk of progression in nondysplastic BE.[133,135]

Cyclin A immunohistochemistry
The cell cycle regulator cyclin A is normally expressed at the bottom of the BE crypts; however, expression shifted to the epithelial surface has been shown to correlate with prevalent dysplasia, as well as with an increased cancer risk.[136]

With the exception of p53 immunohistochemistry, these molecular biomarkers have mostly been studied by individual groups in single patient cohorts. A recent population-based nested case-control study on 89 progressors matched 1:3 to non-progressors set out to independently validate some of these previously published biomarkers (LGD, ploidy, cyclin A, and p53) as well as to test an array of novel biomarkers, including surface glycoproteins, which have been shown to change in dysplasia.[137] In this cohort of patients, LGD, ploidy, and *Aspergillus oryzae* lectin independently correlated with the risk of progression.[138] When used as a panel, these 3 biomarkers could predict risk of progression to cancer, with an incremental OR of

3.90 (95% CI, 2.39–6.37) for each individual positive factor. These biomarkers were applied to FFPE tissues collected as part of routine clinical practice and hence should be generalizable. These results are encouraging and show that the experience of individual groups can be combined to generate panels of biomarkers, which can be used more efficiently than single biomarkers to stratify patients with BE according to their risk of progression. Further prospective studies, including a larger array of biomarkers, are awaited to assess which biomarkers outperform others in order to identify the best panel for the risk stratification.

FUTURE PERSPECTIVE

- The economic implications of endoscopic screening within the general population demand the introduction of cheaper and less invasive tests for an early diagnosis of EAC at a presymptomatic stage and identification of patients at higher risk, such as patients with dysplastic or genetically unstable BE.
- Novel endoscopic therapies allow ablation of BE with preventive strategies. Although it is difficult to envisage a scenario in which every single patient with BE undergoes endoscopic therapy, molecular biomarkers may help risk-stratify these patients to concentrate therapeutic efforts on a selected group of individuals with a stronger predisposition to develop cancer and to spare individuals at low risk from repeated surveillance procedures.
- In order for research findings from the field to become implemented as part of routine clinical practice, prospective multicenter studies with appropriate statistical power are required.

REFERENCES

1. Parker EF, Gregorie HB Jr. Combined radiation and surgical treatment of carcinoma of the esophagus. Ann Surg 1965;161:710–22.
2. Parker EF, Marks RD Jr, Kratz JM, et al. Chemoradiation therapy and resection for carcinoma of the esophagus: short-term results. Ann Thorac Surg 1985; 40(2):121–5.
3. Turnbull AD, Goodner JT. Primary adenocarcinoma of the esophagus. Cancer 1968;22(5):915–8.
4. van Andel JG, Dees J, Dijkhuis CM, et al. Carcinoma of the esophagus: results of treatment. Ann Surg 1979;190(6):684–9.
5. Millikan KW, Silverstein J, Hart V, et al. A 15-year review of esophagectomy for carcinoma of the esophagus and cardia. Arch Surg 1995;130(6):617–24.
6. Putnam JB Jr, Suell DM, McMurtrey MJ, et al. Comparison of three techniques of esophagectomy within a residency training program. Ann Thorac Surg 1994; 57(2):319–25.
7. Rice TW, Zuccaro G Jr, Adelstein DJ, et al. Esophageal carcinoma: depth of tumor invasion is predictive of regional lymph node status. Ann Thorac Surg 1998;65(3): 787–92.
8. Ruol A, Castoro C, Portale G, et al. Trends in management and prognosis for esophageal cancer surgery: twenty-five years of experience at a single institution. Arch Surg 2009;144(3):247–54 [discussion: 54].
9. Edgren G, Adami HO, Weiderpass Vainio E, et al. A global assessment of the oesophageal adenocarcinoma epidemic. Gut 2012. [Epub ahead of print].
10. Pohl H, Welch HG. The role of overdiagnosis and reclassification in the marked increase of esophageal adenocarcinoma incidence. J Natl Cancer Inst 2005; 97(2):142–6.

11. Thrift AP, Whiteman DC. The incidence of esophageal adenocarcinoma continues to rise: analysis of period and birth cohort effects on recent trends. Ann Oncol 2012;23(12):3155–62.

12. Botterweck AA, Schouten LJ, Volovics A, et al. Trends in incidence of adenocarcinoma of the oesophagus and gastric cardia in ten European countries. Int J Epidemiol 2000;29(4):645–54.

13. Steevens J, Botterweck AA, Dirx MJ, et al. Trends in incidence of oesophageal and stomach cancer subtypes in Europe. Eur J Gastroenterol Hepatol 2010; 22(6):669–78.

14. Lagergren J, Bergstrom R, Lindgren A, et al. Symptomatic gastroesophageal reflux as a risk factor for esophageal adenocarcinoma. N Engl J Med 1999; 340(11):825–31.

15. Wu AH, Tseng CC, Bernstein L. Hiatal hernia, reflux symptoms, body size, and risk of esophageal and gastric adenocarcinoma. Cancer 2003;98(5):940–8.

16. Rubenstein JH, Taylor JB. Meta-analysis: the association of oesophageal adenocarcinoma with symptoms of gastro-oesophageal reflux. Aliment Pharmacol Ther 2010;32(10):1222–7.

17. di Pietro M, Fitzgerald RC. Barrett's oesophagus: an ideal model to study cancer genetics. Hum Genet 2009;126(2):233–46.

18. Souza RF, Krishnan K, Spechler SJ. Acid, bile, and CDX: the ABCs of making Barrett's metaplasia. Am J Physiol Gastrointest Liver Physiol 2008;295(2): G211–8.

19. Winters C Jr, Spurling TJ, Chobanian SJ, et al. Barrett's esophagus. A prevalent, occult complication of gastroesophageal reflux disease. Gastroenterology 1987; 92(1):118–24.

20. Connor MJ, Weston AP, Mayo MS, et al. The prevalence of Barrett's esophagus and erosive esophagitis in patients undergoing upper endoscopy for dyspepsia in a VA population. Dig Dis Sci 2004;49(6):920–4.

21. Kadri SR, Lao-Sirieix P, O'Donovan M, et al. Acceptability and accuracy of a non-endoscopic screening test for Barrett's oesophagus in primary care: cohort study. BMJ 2010;341:c4372.

22. Cameron AJ, Souto EO, Smyrk TC. Small adenocarcinomas of the esophagogastric junction: association with intestinal metaplasia and dysplasia. Am J Gastroenterol 2002;97(6):1375–80.

23. Lagergren J. Adenocarcinoma of oesophagus: what exactly is the size of the problem and who is at risk? Gut 2005;54(Suppl 1):i1–5.

24. Hvid-Jensen F, Pedersen L, Drewes AM, et al. Incidence of adenocarcinoma among patients with Barrett's esophagus. N Engl J Med 2011;365(15):1375–83.

25. Reid BJ, Levine DS, Longton G, et al. Predictors of progression to cancer in Barrett's esophagus: baseline histology and flow cytometry identify low- and high-risk patient subsets. Am J Gastroenterol 2000;95(7):1669–76.

26. Sikkema M, de Jonge PJ, Steyerberg EW, et al. Risk of esophageal adenocarcinoma and mortality in patients with Barrett's esophagus: a systematic review and meta-analysis. Clin Gastroenterol Hepatol 2010;8(3):235–44 [quiz: e32].

27. Yousef F, Cardwell C, Cantwell MM, et al. The incidence of esophageal cancer and high-grade dysplasia in Barrett's esophagus: a systematic review and meta-analysis. Am J Epidemiol 2008;168(3):237–49.

28. Bhat S, Coleman HG, Yousef F, et al. Risk of malignant progression in Barrett's esophagus patients: results from a large population-based study. J Natl Cancer Inst 2011;103(13):1049–57.

29. Desai TK, Singh J, Samala N, et al. The incidence of esophageal adenocarcinoma in Barrett's esophagus has been overestimated. Am J Gastroenterol 2011;106(7):1364–5 [author reply: 5–6].
30. Calle EE, Rodriguez C, Walker-Thurmond K, et al. Overweight, obesity, and mortality from cancer in a prospectively studied cohort of U.S. adults. N Engl J Med 2003;348(17):1625–38.
31. Brown LM, Swanson CA, Gridley G, et al. Adenocarcinoma of the esophagus: role of obesity and diet. J Natl Cancer Inst 1995;87(2):104–9.
32. Chow WH, Blot WJ, Vaughan TL, et al. Body mass index and risk of adenocarcinomas of the esophagus and gastric cardia. J Natl Cancer Inst 1998;90(2): 150–5.
33. Engel LS, Chow WH, Vaughan TL, et al. Population attributable risks of esophageal and gastric cancers. J Natl Cancer Inst 2003;95(18):1404–13.
34. Lagergren J, Bergstrom R, Nyren O. Association between body mass and adenocarcinoma of the esophagus and gastric cardia. Ann Intern Med 1999; 130(11):883–90.
35. Corley DA, Kubo A, Zhao W. Abdominal obesity and the risk of esophageal and gastric cardia carcinomas. Cancer Epidemiol Biomarkers Prev 2008;17(2): 352–8.
36. Reeves GK, Pirie K, Beral V, et al. Cancer incidence and mortality in relation to body mass index in the Million Women Study: cohort study. BMJ 2007;335(7630):1134.
37. MacInnis RJ, English DR, Hopper JL, et al. Body size and composition and the risk of gastric and oesophageal adenocarcinoma. Int J Cancer 2006;118(10): 2628–31.
38. Kubo A, Corley DA. Body mass index and adenocarcinomas of the esophagus or gastric cardia: a systematic review and meta-analysis. Cancer Epidemiol Biomarkers Prev 2006;15(5):872–8.
39. Turati F, Tramacere I, La Vecchia C, et al. A meta-analysis of body mass index and esophageal and gastric cardia adenocarcinoma. Ann Oncol 2012. [Epub ahead of print].
40. El-Serag HB, Graham DY, Satia JA, et al. Obesity is an independent risk factor for GERD symptoms and erosive esophagitis. Am J Gastroenterol 2005;100(6): 1243–50.
41. O'Brien TF Jr. Lower esophageal sphincter pressure (LESP) and esophageal function in obese humans. J Clin Gastroenterol 1980;2(2):145–8.
42. Wilson LJ, Ma W, Hirschowitz BI. Association of obesity with hiatal hernia and esophagitis. Am J Gastroenterol 1999;94(10):2840–4.
43. Hampel H, Abraham NS, El-Serag HB. Meta-analysis: obesity and the risk for gastroesophageal reflux disease and its complications. Ann Intern Med 2005; 143(3):199–211.
44. Stein DJ, El-Serag HB, Kuczynski J, et al. The association of body mass index with Barrett's oesophagus. Aliment Pharmacol Ther 2005;22(10):1005–10.
45. Smith KJ, O'Brien SM, Smithers BM, et al. Interactions among smoking, obesity, and symptoms of acid reflux in Barrett's esophagus. Cancer Epidemiol Biomarkers Prev 2005;14(11 Pt 1):2481–6.
46. Ryan AM, Duong M, Healy L, et al. Obesity, metabolic syndrome and esophageal adenocarcinoma: epidemiology, etiology and new targets. Cancer Epidemiol 2011;35(4):309–19.
47. Akiyama T, Yoneda M, Inamori M, et al. Visceral obesity and the risk of Barrett's esophagus in Japanese patients with non-alcoholic fatty liver disease. BMC Gastroenterol 2009;9:56.

48. Vaughan TL, Kristal AR, Blount PL, et al. Nonsteroidal anti-inflammatory drug use, body mass index, and anthropometry in relation to genetic and flow cytometric abnormalities in Barrett's esophagus. Cancer Epidemiol Biomarkers Prev 2002;11(8):745–52.
49. Xu H, Barnes GT, Yang Q, et al. Chronic inflammation in fat plays a crucial role in the development of obesity-related insulin resistance. J Clin Invest 2003;112(12): 1821–30.
50. Cowey S, Hardy RW. The metabolic syndrome: a high-risk state for cancer? Am J Pathol 2006;169(5):1505–22.
51. Shoelson SE, Lee J, Goldfine AB. Inflammation and insulin resistance. J Clin Invest 2006;116(7):1793–801.
52. Ryan AM, Healy LA, Power DG, et al. Barrett esophagus: prevalence of central adiposity, metabolic syndrome, and a proinflammatory state. Ann Surg 2008; 247(6):909–15.
53. Flegal KM, Carroll MD, Ogden CL, et al. Prevalence and trends in obesity among US adults, 1999-2008. JAMA 2010;303(3):235–41.
54. Neovius M, Teixeira-Pinto A, Rasmussen F. Shift in the composition of obesity in young adult men in Sweden over a third of a century. Int J Obes (Lond) 2008; 32(5):832–6.
55. Pandeya N, Williams GM, Sadhegi S, et al. Associations of duration, intensity, and quantity of smoking with adenocarcinoma and squamous cell carcinoma of the esophagus. Am J Epidemiol 2008;168(1):105–14.
56. Cook MB, Kamangar F, Whiteman DC, et al. Cigarette smoking and adenocarcinomas of the esophagus and esophagogastric junction: a pooled analysis from the international BEACON consortium. J Natl Cancer Inst 2010;102(17): 1344–53.
57. Tramacere I, La Vecchia C, Negri E. Tobacco smoking and esophageal and gastric cardia adenocarcinoma: a meta-analysis. Epidemiology 2011;22(3): 344–9.
58. Desai TK, Krishnan K, Samala N, et al. The incidence of oesophageal adenocarcinoma in non-dysplastic Barrett's oesophagus: a meta-analysis. Gut 2012; 61(7):970–6.
59. Yang H, Sukocheva OA, Hussey DJ, et al. Estrogen, male dominance and esophageal adenocarcinoma: is there a link? World J Gastroenterol 2012; 18(5):393–400.
60. Baan R, Straif K, Grosse Y, et al. Carcinogenicity of alcoholic beverages. Lancet Oncol 2007;8(4):292–3.
61. Toh Y, Oki E, Ohgaki K, et al. Alcohol drinking, cigarette smoking, and the development of squamous cell carcinoma of the esophagus: molecular mechanisms of carcinogenesis. Int J Clin Oncol 2010;15(2):135–44.
62. Freedman ND, Murray LJ, Kamangar F, et al. Alcohol intake and risk of oesophageal adenocarcinoma: a pooled analysis from the BEACON Consortium. Gut 2011;60(8):1029–37.
63. Tramacere I, Pelucchi C, Bagnardi V, et al. A meta-analysis on alcohol drinking and esophageal and gastric cardia adenocarcinoma risk. Ann Oncol 2012; 23(2):287–97.
64. Polk DB, Peek RM Jr. Helicobacter pylori: gastric cancer and beyond. Nat Rev Cancer 2010;10(6):403–14.
65. Trikudanathan G, Philip A, Dasanu CA, et al. Association between Helicobacter pylori infection and pancreatic cancer. A cumulative meta-analysis. JOP 2011; 12(1):26–31.

66. Anderson LA, Murphy SJ, Johnston BT, et al. Relationship between *Helicobacter pylori* infection and gastric atrophy and the stages of the oesophageal inflammation, metaplasia, adenocarcinoma sequence: results from the FINBAR case-control study. Gut 2008;57(6):734–9.

67. Whiteman DC, Parmar P, Fahey P, et al. Association of *Helicobacter pylori* infection with reduced risk for esophageal cancer is independent of environmental and genetic modifiers. Gastroenterology 2010;139(1):73–83 [quiz: e11–2].

68. Islami F, Kamangar F. *Helicobacter pylori* and esophageal cancer risk: a meta-analysis. Cancer Prev Res (Phila) 2008;1(5):329–38.

69. Kubo A, Corley DA, Jensen CD, et al. Dietary factors and the risks of oesophageal adenocarcinoma and Barrett's oesophagus. Nutr Res Rev 2010;23(2):230–46.

70. Reid BJ, Li X, Galipeau PC, et al. Barrett's oesophagus and oesophageal adenocarcinoma: time for a new synthesis. Nat Rev Cancer 2010;10(2):87–101.

71. Shaheen NJ, Palmer LB. Improving screening practices for Barrett's esophagus. Surg Oncol Clin North Am 2009;18(3):423–37.

72. Donaldson L. A pathological concern understanding the rise in oesophageal cancer. CMO Annual Report. 2008:44–51. Available at: http://www.dh.gov.uk/prod_consum_dh/groups/dh_digitalassets/@dh/@en/documents/digitalasset/dh_086182.pdf. Accessed December 20, 2012.

73. Cook MB, Chow WH, Devesa SS. Oesophageal cancer incidence in the United States by race, sex, and histologic type, 1977-2005. Br J Cancer 2009;101(5):855–9.

74. Haffner SM. Relationship of metabolic risk factors and development of cardiovascular disease and diabetes. Obesity (Silver Spring) 2006;14(Suppl 3):121S–7S.

75. Ogden CL, Carroll MD, Curtin LR, et al. Prevalence of overweight and obesity in the United States, 1999-2004. JAMA 2006;295(13):1549–55.

76. Nguyen DM, El-Serag HB, Henderson L, et al. Medication usage and the risk of neoplasia in patients with Barrett's esophagus. Clin Gastroenterol Hepatol 2009;7(12):1299–304.

77. Liao LM, Vaughan TL, Corley DA, et al. Nonsteroidal anti-inflammatory drug use reduces risk of adenocarcinomas of the esophagus and esophagogastric junction in a pooled analysis. Gastroenterology 2012;142(3):442–452.e5 [quiz: e22–3].

78. CancerResearchUK. 2012. Available at: http://www.cancerresearchuk.org/cancer-info/cancerstats/types/oesophagus/?script=true. Accessed December 20, 2012.

79. Eloubeidi MA, Mason AC, Desmond RA, et al. Temporal trends (1973-1997) in survival of patients with esophageal adenocarcinoma in the United States: a glimmer of hope? Am J Gastroenterol 2003;98(7):1627–33.

80. Cooper GS, Kou TD, Chak A. Receipt of previous diagnoses and endoscopy and outcome from esophageal adenocarcinoma: a population-based study with temporal trends. Am J Gastroenterol 2009;104(6):1356–62.

81. Corley DA, Levin TR, Habel LA, et al. Surveillance and survival in Barrett's adenocarcinomas: a population-based study. Gastroenterology 2002;122(3):633–40.

82. Rubenstein JH, Sonnenberg A, Davis J, et al. Effect of a prior endoscopy on outcomes of esophageal adenocarcinoma among United States veterans. Gastrointest Endosc 2008;68(5):849–55.

83. Gerson LB, Groeneveld PW, Triadafilopoulos G. Cost-effectiveness model of endoscopic screening and surveillance in patients with gastroesophageal reflux disease. Clin Gastroenterol Hepatol 2004;2(10):868–79.

84. Gupta N, Bansal A, Wani SB, et al. Endoscopy for upper GI cancer screening in the general population: a cost-utility analysis. Gastrointest Endosc 2011;74(3): 610–624.e2.
85. Nietert PJ, Silverstein MD, Mokhashi MS, et al. Cost-effectiveness of screening a population with chronic gastroesophageal reflux. Gastrointest Endosc 2003; 57(3):311–8.
86. Shaheen NJ, Greenwald BD, Peery AF, et al. Safety and efficacy of endoscopic spray cryotherapy for Barrett's esophagus with high-grade dysplasia. Gastrointest Endosc 2010;71(4):680–5.
87. Shaheen NJ, Sharma P, Overholt BF, et al. Radiofrequency ablation in Barrett's esophagus with dysplasia. N Engl J Med 2009;360(22):2277–88.
88. Rex DK, Cummings OW, Shaw M, et al. Screening for Barrett's esophagus in colonoscopy patients with and without heartburn. Gastroenterology 2003; 125(6):1670–7.
89. Gerson LB, Shetler K, Triadafilopoulos G. Prevalence of Barrett's esophagus in asymptomatic individuals. Gastroenterology 2002;123(2):461–7.
90. Gerson LB, Banerjee S. Screening for Barrett's esophagus in asymptomatic women. Gastrointest Endosc 2009;70(5):867–73.
91. Barbiere JM, Lyratzopoulos G. Cost-effectiveness of endoscopic screening followed by surveillance for Barrett's esophagus: a review. Gastroenterology 2009; 137(6):1869–76.
92. Spechler SJ, Sharma P, Souza RF, et al. American Gastroenterological Association technical review on the management of Barrett's esophagus. Gastroenterology 2011;140(3):e18–52 [quiz: e13].
93. Wang KK, Sampliner RE. Updated guidelines 2008 for the diagnosis, surveillance and therapy of Barrett's esophagus. Am J Gastroenterol 2008;103(3): 788–97.
94. Saeian K, Staff DM, Vasilopoulos S, et al. Unsedated transnasal endoscopy accurately detects Barrett's metaplasia and dysplasia. Gastrointest Endosc 2002;56(4):472–8.
95. Shariff MK, Bird-Lieberman EL, O'Donovan M, et al. Randomized crossover study comparing efficacy of transnasal endoscopy with that of standard endoscopy to detect Barrett's esophagus. Gastrointest Endosc 2012;75(5): 954–61.
96. Jobe BA, Hunter JG, Chang EY, et al. Office-based unsedated small-caliber endoscopy is equivalent to conventional sedated endoscopy in screening and surveillance for Barrett's esophagus: a randomized and blinded comparison. Am J Gastroenterol 2006;101(12):2693–703.
97. Peery AF, Hoppo T, Garman KS, et al. Feasibility, safety, acceptability, and yield of office-based, screening transnasal esophagoscopy (with video). Gastrointest Endosc 2012;75(5):945–953.e2.
98. Galmiche JP, Sacher-Huvelin S, Coron E, et al. Screening for esophagitis and Barrett's esophagus with wireless esophageal capsule endoscopy: a multicenter prospective trial in patients with reflux symptoms. Am J Gastroenterol 2008; 103(3):538–45.
99. Lin OS, Schembre DB, Mergener K, et al. Blinded comparison of esophageal capsule endoscopy versus conventional endoscopy for a diagnosis of Barrett's esophagus in patients with chronic gastroesophageal reflux. Gastrointest Endosc 2007;65(4):577–83.
100. Sharma P, Wani S, Rastogi A, et al. The diagnostic accuracy of esophageal capsule endoscopy in patients with gastroesophageal reflux disease and

Barrett's esophagus: a blinded, prospective study. Am J Gastroenterol 2008; 103(3):525–32.

101. Gralnek IM, Adler SN, Yassin K, et al. Detecting esophageal disease with second-generation capsule endoscopy: initial evaluation of the PillCam ESO 2. Endoscopy 2008;40(4):275–9.

102. Ramirez FC, Akins R, Shaukat M. Screening of Barrett's esophagus with string-capsule endoscopy: a prospective blinded study of 100 consecutive patients using histology as the criterion standard. Gastrointest Endosc 2008;68(1):25–31.

103. Rubenstein JH, Inadomi JM, Brill JV, et al. Cost utility of screening for Barrett's esophagus with esophageal capsule endoscopy versus conventional upper endoscopy. Clin Gastroenterol Hepatol 2007;5(3):312–8.

104. Fennerty MB, DiTomasso J, Morales TG, et al. Screening for Barrett's esophagus by balloon cytology. Am J Gastroenterol 1995;90(8):1230–2.

105. Falk GW, Chittajallu R, Goldblum JR, et al. Surveillance of patients with Barrett's esophagus for dysplasia and cancer with balloon cytology. Gastroenterology 1997;112(6):1787–97.

106. Lao-Sirieix P, Boussioutas A, Kadri SR, et al. Non-endoscopic screening biomarkers for Barrett's oesophagus: from microarray analysis to the clinic. Gut 2009;58(11):1451–9.

107. Kadri S, Lao-Sirieix P, Fitzgerald RC. Developing a nonendoscopic screening test for Barrett's esophagus. Biomark Med 2011;5(3):397–404.

108. Benaglia T, Sharples LD, Fitzgerald RC, et al. Health benefits and cost-effectiveness of endoscopic and non-endoscopic Cytosponge screening for Barrett's esophagus. Gastroenterology 2012. [Epub ahead of print].

109. Qin DX, Wang GQ, Zuo JH, et al. Screening of esophageal and gastric cancer by occult blood bead detector. Cancer 1993;71(1):216–8.

110. Qin DX, Wang GQ, Yuan FL, et al. Screening for upper digestive tract cancer with an occult blood bead detector. Investigation of a normal north China population. Cancer 1988;62(5):1030–4.

111. Bennett C, Vakil N, Bergman J, et al. Consensus statements for management of Barrett's dysplasia and early-stage esophageal adenocarcinoma, based on a Delphi process. Gastroenterology 2012;143(2):336–46.

112. Choi SE, Hur C. Screening and surveillance for Barrett's esophagus: current issues and future directions. Curr Opin Gastroenterol 2012;28(4):377–81.

113. Somerville M, Garside R, Pitt M, et al. Surveillance of Barrett's oesophagus: is it worthwhile? Eur J Cancer 2008;44(4):588–99.

114. Strayer SM. Should we screen patients for Barrett's esophagus? Yes: men with long-standing reflux symptoms should be screened with endoscopy. Am Fam Physician 2011;83(10):1140, 2, 7.

115. Knox MA. Should we screen patients for Barrett's esophagus? No: the case against screening. Am Fam Physician 2011;83(10):1148, 50.

116. Hirst NG, Gordon LG, Whiteman DC, et al. Is endoscopic surveillance for non-dysplastic Barrett's esophagus cost-effective? Review of economic evaluations. J Gastroenterol Hepatol 2011;26(2):247–54.

117. Sharma P, Falk GW, Weston AP, et al. Dysplasia and cancer in a large multi-center cohort of patients with Barrett's esophagus. Clin Gastroenterol Hepatol 2006;4(5):566–72.

118. Weston AP, Badr AS, Hassanein RS. Prospective multivariate analysis of clinical, endoscopic, and histological factors predictive of the development of Barrett's multifocal high-grade dysplasia or adenocarcinoma. Am J Gastroenterol 1999; 94(12):3413–9.

119. O'Connor JB, Falk GW, Richter JE. The incidence of adenocarcinoma and dysplasia in Barrett's esophagus: report on the Cleveland Clinic Barrett's Esophagus Registry. Am J Gastroenterol 1999;94(8):2037–42.
120. Playford RJ. New British Society of Gastroenterology (BSG) guidelines for the diagnosis and management of Barrett's oesophagus. Gut 2006;55(4):442.
121. Spechler SJ, Sharma P, Souza RF, et al. American Gastroenterological Association medical position statement on the management of Barrett's esophagus. Gastroenterology 2011;140(3):1084–91.
122. Curvers WL, ten Kate FJ, Krishnadath KK, et al. Low-grade dysplasia in Barrett's esophagus: overdiagnosed and underestimated. Am J Gastroenterol 2010; 105(7):1523–30.
123. Wani S, Falk GW, Post J, et al. Risk factors for progression of low-grade dysplasia in patients with Barrett's esophagus. Gastroenterology 2011;141(4): 1179–86, 86.e1.
124. Cameron AJ, Carpenter HA. Barrett's esophagus, high-grade dysplasia, and early adenocarcinoma: a pathological study. Am J Gastroenterol 1997;92(4): 586–91.
125. Galipeau PC, Prevo LJ, Sanchez CA, et al. Clonal expansion and loss of heterozygosity at chromosomes 9p and 17p in premalignant esophageal (Barrett's) tissue. J Natl Cancer Inst 1999;91(24):2087–95.
126. Reid BJ, Haggitt RC, Rubin CE, et al. Barrett's esophagus. Correlation between flow cytometry and histology in detection of patients at risk for adenocarcinoma. Gastroenterology 1987;93(1):1–11.
127. Galipeau PC, Li X, Blount PL, et al. NSAIDs modulate CDKN2A, TP53, and DNA content risk for progression to esophageal adenocarcinoma. PLoS Med 2007; 4(2):e67.
128. Dunn JM, Mackenzie GD, Oukrif D, et al. Image cytometry accurately detects DNA ploidy abnormalities and predicts late relapse to high-grade dysplasia and adenocarcinoma in Barrett's oesophagus following photodynamic therapy. Br J Cancer 2010;102(11):1608–17.
129. Schulmann K, Sterian A, Berki A, et al. Inactivation of p16, RUNX3, and HPP1 occurs early in Barrett's-associated neoplastic progression and predicts progression risk. Oncogene 2005;24(25):4138–48.
130. Jin Z, Cheng Y, Gu W, et al. A multicenter, double-blinded validation study of methylation biomarkers for progression prediction in Barrett's esophagus. Cancer Res 2009;69(10):4112–5.
131. Chung SM, Kao J, Hyjek E, et al. p53 in esophageal adenocarcinoma: a critical reassessment of mutation frequency and identification of 72Arg as the dominant allele. Int J Oncol 2007;31(6):1351–5.
132. Jouret-Mourin A, Sempoux C, Duc KH, et al. Usefulness of histopathological markers in diagnosing Barrett's intraepithelial neoplasia (dysplasia). Acta Gastroenterol Belg 2009;72(4):425–32.
133. Kaye PV, Haider SA, Ilyas M, et al. Barrett's dysplasia and the Vienna classification: reproducibility, prediction of progression and impact of consensus reporting and p53 immunohistochemistry. Histopathology 2009;54(6):699–712.
134. Skacel M, Petras RE, Gramlich TL, et al. The diagnosis of low-grade dysplasia in Barrett's esophagus and its implications for disease progression. Am J Gastroenterol 2000;95(12):3383–7.
135. Murray L, Sedo A, Scott M, et al. TP53 and progression from Barrett's metaplasia to oesophageal adenocarcinoma in a UK population cohort. Gut 2006;55(10): 1390–7.

136. Lao-Sirieix P, Lovat L, Fitzgerald RC. Cyclin A immunocytology as a risk stratification tool for Barrett's esophagus surveillance. Clin Cancer Res 2007;13(2 Pt 1): 659–65.
137. Bird-Lieberman EL, Neves AA, Lao-Sirieix P, et al. Molecular imaging using fluorescent lectins permits rapid endoscopic identification of dysplasia in Barrett's esophagus. Nat Med 2012;18(2):315–21.
138. Bird-Lieberman EL, Dunn JM, Coleman HG, et al. Population-based study reveals new risk-stratification biomarker panel for Barrett's esophagus. Gastroenterology 2012;143(4):927–935.e3.

Endoscopic Therapy for Barrett's Esophagus and Early Esophageal Adenocarcinoma

Cadman L. Leggett, MD, Emmanuel C. Gorospe, MD, MPH,
Kenneth K. Wang, MD*

KEYWORDS

- Barrett's esophagus • Argon plasma coagulation • Radiofrequency ablation
- Multipolar electrocoagulation • Photodynamic therapy • Cryoablation
- Radiofrequency ablation • Endoscopic mucosal resection

KEY POINTS

- Endoscopic eradication therapy is considered a safe, effective, and durable treatment strategy for Barrett's esophagus complicated by high-grade dysplasia and early esophageal neoplasia.
- The endoscopist should be familiar with both mucosal resection and ablation techniques, and their respective indications.
- Patients should be enrolled in a comprehensive surveillance program that continues following endoscopic eradication therapy.
- Recurrent dysplasia can be approached endoscopically as long as appropriate staging is performed.

BACKGROUND

Endoscopic ablation therapy has evolved from being a possibility in patients who could not undergo esophagectomy to a standard of care for the treatment of early esophageal neoplasia (EAC). Its increasing efficacy and decreasing morbidity through the years have made this approach the preferred treatment for Barrett's esophagus (BE) with high-grade dysplasia (HGD) and early EAC.[1] Several treatment modalities are currently available, which can be broadly classified as mucosal resection and ablative techniques. These modalities are usually used in combination and as part of a treatment program that requires endoscopic surveillance.

Funding: The authors are supported by NIH U54 CA163004 and CA163004.
Barrett's Esophagus Unit, Division of Gastroenterology & Hepatology, Mayo Clinic, 200 First Street Southwest, Rochester, MN 55905, USA
* Corresponding author.
E-mail address: wang.kenneth@mayo.edu

Gastroenterol Clin N Am 42 (2013) 175–185
http://dx.doi.org/10.1016/j.gtc.2012.11.010

RISK STRATIFICATION OF BARRETT'S ESOPHAGUS

Risk stratification begins with a detailed examination of the Barrett's mucosa under white-light endoscopy. Irregularities in the mucosa are targeted with biopsies or endoscopic mucosal resection (EMR) because these sites are more likely to contain neoplasia. Tissue sampling is also performed at 4-quadrant intervals over the entire BE segment to detect dysplasia that may not be apparent under endoscopic evaluation. Advanced imaging technologies such as narrow-band imaging, confocal endomicroscopy, and optical coherence tomography can be used to enhance detection of dysplasia, but are currently not a substitute for thorough examination under high-resolution white-light endoscopy.

Endoscopic eradication therapy should be considered in patients with the highest risk of progression to invasive EAC whereby metastatic lymphadenopathy has been excluded.[2] Risk stratification is currently based on histopathologic evaluation for grade of dysplasia, which is unreliable because of the lack of agreement among pathologists regarding the exact degree of dysplasia. One indicator that low-grade dysplasia is more likely to progress is agreement between 2 or more pathologists.[3] The risk with nondysplastic BE is about 0.18% per year, less than half the risk estimated only 5 years ago. The decrease in cancer risk appears to be related to more reports from large population-based databases. The absolute risk of EAC increases in proportion to the grade of dysplasia with HGD, carrying a 30% 5-year cancer risk.[4] The risk of metastatic lymphadenopathy is proportional to the depth of invasion, and is low (<5%) for neoplasia confined to the mucosa (intramucosal adenocarcinoma, stage T1a).[2] Other risk factors for potential metastatic disease with early T1a cancer are evidence of lymphovascular invasion and high-grade malignancy. The most reliable technique to obtain this information is EMR, which can be used to diagnose, stage, and treat early cancer.

THEORY OF ABLATION

It is important to realize that it is unclear why ablation therapy results in squamous regeneration. The current belief is that intestinal metaplasia occurs because of chronic injury to the esophageal mucosa with the production of cytokines such as interleukin (IL)-1β, IL-6, and IL-8, which increase expression of transcription factors that promote intestinalization such as CDX2 and bone morphogenetic protein 4 (BMP4) (**Fig. 1**). These factors have been shown in animal models to act on gastric glandular stem cells to produce an intestinal phenotype that migrates proximally into the esophagus. These cytokines are also produced by adipocytes, and can be a partial biological explanation of how obesity promotes BE.

The elimination of BE caused by endoscopic injury and secondary production of squamous mucosa is unclear. Studies have found that the squamous mucosa that regenerates does not contain genetic abnormalities similar to the intestinal mucosa, indicating that there may well be a different cell of origin for these squamous stem cells. It is thought that, similar to keratinocytes in the cutaneous skin, the stem cells of origin of these squamous cells are the interpapillary basal cells. This assumption would imply that squamous regeneration should occur from neighboring squamous mucosa, and confirms early observations in ablation therapy that if 3 areas of squamous mucosa surrounded the area of treated columnar tissue, squamous regeneration was more likely than if the area was not in contact with any squamous mucosa. However, it has been observed that squamous islands appear to form if deep injury to the mucosa has occurred, as is seen with mucosal resection. It has also been found that bone marrow stem cells migrate to areas of deep tissue wounds throughout the

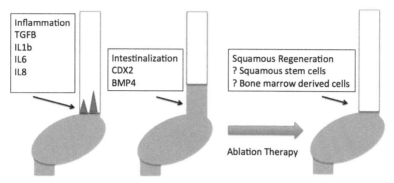

Fig. 1. Development of intestinal metaplasia, with the effects of cytokines on gastric stem cells causing intestinal metaplasia with cytokines that promote intestinal metaplasia. The intestinal phenotype is marked by expression of transcription factors such as BMP4 and CDX2. On ablation therapy, the intestinalized phenotype disappears and squamous regeneration appears to occur from neighboring squamous cells and bone marrow–derived stem cells. BMP, bone morphogenetic protein; IL, interleukin; TGFB, transforming growth factor β.

body, and it is possible that these isolated patches of squamous mucosa are the result of bone marrow–derived squamous stem cells. There is little clinical evidence that substantiates this hypothesis, and it would require a very unusual situation whereby a male patient undergoes ablation after a bone marrow transplant from a female to permit lineage tracing of the bone marrow donor.

ENDOSCOPIC MUCOSAL RESECTION

EMR refers to the use of a standard polypectomy technique in flat mucosa for the purposes of resecting suspicious and dysplastic lesions. Despite its designation as a "mucosal" resection technique, EMR actually extends into the submucosa. Hence, it is not uncommon that EMR is sometimes referred to as endoscopic resection (ER) (**Figs. 2** and **3**).

In the setting of appropriate risk stratification, patients with HGD and early EAC may be offered the choice to undergo EMR instead of esophagectomy. The risk of

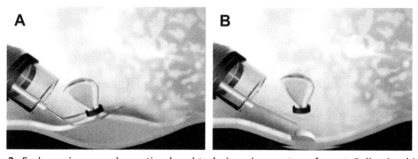

Fig. 2. Endoscopic mucosal resection band technique in a cartoon format. Following high-resolution white-light endoscopy, a nodular lesion is identified. The lesion is suctioned into the band-ligation device and a band is deployed, creating a pseudopolyp. (*A*) A hexagonal snare is placed over the pseudopolyp and (*B*) electrocautery is applied for resection.

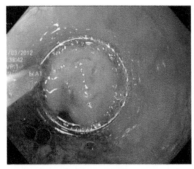

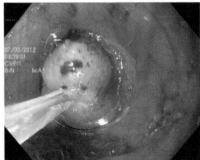
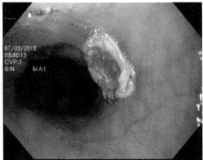

Fig. 3. This sequence represents initial placement of a snare in the resection cap. The snare is seen fitting around the lip of the cap. The second photo illustrates suctioning and snaring with the cap technique. The third shows the resulting defect in the mucosa after resection.

advanced malignancy depends on the depth of neoplastic luminal involvement. As such, EMR should only be attempted in patients with a low risk of locally advanced EAC or metastatic lymphadenopathy.[5,6] EMR has emerged as an indispensable tool in endoluminal therapy for dysplastic BE and early EAC. Its use has increased because it accomplishes the basic prerequisites of surgical therapy for malignancy in a mini-mally invasive manner. EMR also offers a dual advantage for tissue diagnosis aside from its therapeutic use. Studies have demonstrated that pathologists achieve improved interrater agreement and accuracy for detecting HGD and early EAC in comparison with traditional biopsies.[6,7]

In the United States there are 2 commercially available devices for esophageal EMR, either as a cap-type or multiband device. The cap technique uses a hard or soft plastic cap and snare for ligation of the target mucosa.[8] The cap also comes in flat and oblique configurations, with the oblique cap capable of removing more tissue. The cap technique requires a snare to be fitted on the end of the cap, and requires experience in placing it correctly. On the other hand, the multiband technique evolved as a modification of the variceal banding device. The banding device is available with 6 prefitted bands. With this kit the dysplastic mucosa is suctioned deep into the plastic cap, at which time the band is deployed (see **Fig. 2**). This band creates a pseudopolyp of tissue to prevent luminal perforation. Once the tissue of interest has been captured, a snare is used to resect the tissue.

The initial step of EMR is lifting the target mucosa with the use of a dilute epinephrine injection (1:200,000). The mucosal lift facilitates separation of the mucosa from the submucosa. This maneuver is crucial in preventing perforation during resection, especially when using the cap technique.[9] Once the resection is completed using of the snare, the EMR tissue should be retrieved for histopathologic evaluation to determine the grade of dysplasia and involvement of the margins.

Retrospective studies have shown that the efficacy of EMR is comparable with that of esophagectomy in the treatment of localized EAC. Complete eradication of dysplasia (CR-D) has been reported to be greater than 90% with or without subsequent ablation therapy.[10,11] EMR is well tolerated and has a low risk of complications under the hands of experienced endoscopists. Complications such as bleeding or perforation occur in fewer than 4% of cases, and these can be controlled with the use of hemoclips or stents.[12,13]

MUCOSAL ABLATIVE TECHNIQUES

Mucosal ablation refers to the induction of superficial tissue necrosis by thermal energy, freezing, mechanical debridement, or photochemical injury. The injured mucosa is replaced by normal squamous mucosa in the absence of acid reflux. A goal of mucosal ablation is to achieve CR-D as well as eradication of intestinal metaplasia (CR-IM) over the entire BE segment. CR-IM is thought to be necessary to further lower the risk of cancer development, as genetic abnormalities have been shown to persist after ablation.

Radiofrequency Ablation

Radiofrequency ablation (RFA) uses a bipolar electrode array to generate thermal energy (12 J/cm^2). Commercially available RFA devices include the HALO360, HALO90, HALO60, and HALO90Ultra (Covidien, Mansfield, MA, USA). The HALO360 is used for circumferential ablation of BE and consists of a 3-cm electrode array that encircles a 4-cm long balloon. A sizing balloon is used to preselect the treatment balloon size, which can range in diameter from 18 to 34 mm depending on the size of the esophagus (**Fig. 4**). The HALO90 consists of a flat array (20 × 13 mm) fitted on the tip the endoscope and used for focal ablation. The HALO60 device is 60% smaller that the HALO90 and is meant for individuals with smaller islands after circumferential treatment. The HALO90Flex is a HALO90 device with a 4-cm long treatment surface rather than the original 2-cm device. Direct contact of the electrode array with the esophageal mucosa is necessary for successful ablation.

The treatment consists of first carefully delineating the length of Barrett's segment to be treated followed by cleansing the surface with 1% *N*-acetylcysteine before RFA.

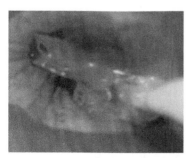 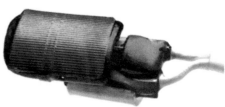

Fig. 4. (*Left*) The HALO360 circumferential balloon device is shown deflated after a single application of energy to the mucosa. The damaged mucosa is blanched, indicating thermal destruction of the mucosa. (*Right*) The HALO90 device, illustrating the presence of the electrode surface of the focal device that is typically mounted on an endoscope.

The treatment device is then applied to the surface at a dose of 12 J/cm^2 for the initial application. The surface of the mucosa is then cleaned and all the debris removed. Finally, the treatment is repeated at the same dose to the mucosa to complete the ablation. If low-grade dysplasia is treated, only 10 J/cm^2 is needed for the treatment energy.

RFA is an effective treatment modality for the eradication of dysplasia in BE. A randomized, multicenter, sham-controlled trial showed a rate of CR-D in 81% of participants with HGD compared with 19% in the sham arm.[14] The rate of development of EAC was reduced from 16% in the RFA group compared with 4% in the sham arm. A 6% rate of stricture formation was reported. The rate of CR-D at 2-year follow-up remained high, at 95%.[15] Failure to achieve CR-D with RFA can be due to the length of the segment of BE treated, the presence of genetic defects such as p16 loss, and the presence of a large diaphragmatic hernia, which could produce poor reflux control.[16]

Although RFA may be effective for nonnodular Barrett's lesions, it is recommended that patients with nodular Barrett's dysplasia have mucosal resection before RFA, as the treatment depth is fairly limited. As with other ablative devices, RFA does not allow tissue confirmation and leaves the patient and clinician the uncertainty of knowing the precise depth of invasion of any neoplastic lesion within the mucosa.

Argon Plasma Coagulation

Before RFA became widely available, argon plasma coagulation (APC) was the most widely available ablative therapy for BE. APC consists of a monopolar high-frequency probe that delivers thermal energy through ionized argon plasma, which can cause thermal injury to the mucosa. Its degree of injury is modulated by voltage, gas flow, and pressure from the probe (**Fig. 5**).

The application of APC in BE with HGD has been demonstrated in several open-label studies with reported high rates of CR-D (80%) after an average of 3 sessions.[17] Adverse events such as stricture formation may occur if applied over a wide area of thermal injury. APC is limited by its nonuniform, narrow field of application in comparison with RFA. Buried intestinal metaplasia in the post-APC neosquamous epithelium can occur in 20% to 30% of cases.[18,19] Previous studies have shown that APC is effective in patients with flat dysplastic BE lesions. The presence of mucosal

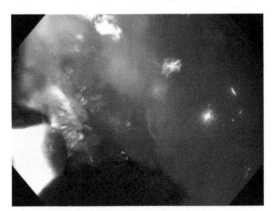

Fig. 5. Argon plasma coagulation of residual Barrett's mucosa. Electrical energy is conducted to the mucosa by a flow of ionized argon gas through a catheter, causing thermal damage by a noncontact method.

thickening and nodules will result in less effective outcomes. In these cases, EMR would be more appropriate. As such, APC can be an adjunct to EMR, with special application to the edges of the EMR lesion.

Multipolar Electrocoagulation

Multipolar electrocoagulation (MPEC) is another form of thermal ablative therapy. Similar to APC, it is widely available for hemostatic interventions in gastrointestinal endoscopy. In addition, it can be used for ablative therapy in BE complicated by dysplasia, but its application is mostly limited to nonnodular BE lesions. Given the small point of contact in the MPEC probe, ablation is usually accomplished with application of the probe to the mucosa tangentially in a back-and-forth motion.[20] The application time should be enough to produce a white coagulum similar to that produced with RFA. There have been 2 randomized studies comparing MPEC with other ablative techniques. In short-segment BE (<3 cm in length), complete ablation was achieved in 80% of patients despite the limited surface area of the probe.[21] No long-term follow-up studies are available.

Photodynamic Therapy

Photodynamic therapy (PDT) has one of the longest experiences as ablative therapy for BE. Its mechanism of action involves the use of a photosensitizer administered systemically and subsequently activated within the esophageal lumen by a light of appropriate wavelength. One of the advantages of PDT is its significant depth of penetration and ease of wide-field application as compared with APC, MPEC, and RFA. The drug is administered intravenously 2 days before photoradiation to allow adequate drug distribution at the time of photoradiation. The light dose is determined by the type of light delivery system, with a balloon catheter system requiring 130 J per centimeter fiber and a bare-fiber technique requiring 200 J per centimeter fiber. Light is applied at a power of 400 mW per centimeter fiber, with limitations attributable to thermal energy being pronounced at powers higher than this and the rate of photobleaching of the photosensitizer as the power of light is increased. Oral agents (aminolevulinic acid) that can be given to patients on the day of photoradiation have been used clinically in other countries, but such treatment has been associated with significant pain during photoradiation as well as vascular instability after drug ingestion. Other limitations to photodynamic therapy include costs, high rate of strictures, and cutaneous photosensitivity that can persist for 4 to 6 weeks after drug administration. Nevertheless, only PDT and RFA have been shown to have durable results in reducing the risks of EAC in BE complicated by dysplasia (CR-D 77% at 5 years for PDT).[22] Experience from the Mayo Clinic demonstrates that patients with HGD treated with PDT had long-term survival outcomes comparable even with esophagectomy.[1]

Cryoablation

Cryoablation is the application of extremely cold temperatures to induce tissue injury. It is the mainstay therapy for various applications in dermatologic, gynecologic, and other conditions in the nasopharyngeal tract. The mechanism of cryoablation entails rapid intense cooling followed by slow thawing, which results in injury (**Fig. 6**).[23] The final result is cell death by mostly inflammatory and apoptotic processes. There are 2 available cryogens, carbon dioxide and liquid nitrogen. The application of cryoablation for BE has been limited to very small studies. Most of these were studied in the setting of salvage therapy for persistent Barrett's dysplasia or palliative application in advanced esophageal cancer. The advantage of cryoablation is its low cost, simple technique, and low complication rates in comparison with other thermal ablative

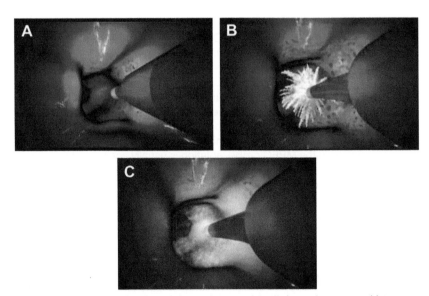

Fig. 6. Cryotherapy. (*A*) Following high-resolution white-light endoscopy and biopsy acquisition per standard protocol, the cryoablation catheter is advanced to the distal esophagus. (*B*) Cryotherapy is applied in repeated cycles of rapid freezing and slow thawing, to induce tissue necrosis (*C*).

devices. However, cryoablation still needs larger prospective clinical trials before it can be considered as a mainstay therapy for Barrett's dysplasia. Reported CR-D from a multicenter cohort study was 53% in patients with HGD.[24]

COMBINATION ENDOTHERAPY

The choice of endoscopic therapy starts with a detailed examination of the Barrett's mucosa under white-light high-resolution endoscopy (**Fig. 7**). Visible lesions can be targeted with EMR with diagnostic and therapeutic intent. Assessment of EMR margins is important in evaluating the completion of resection and depth of invasion. Once the EMR site heals (4–6 weeks), the remaining BE segment can be eliminated with mucosal ablative techniques.[25]

The choice of ablative therapy will depend on institutional practice and patient factors. RFA may be best suited for flat mucosa in a fairly straight esophagus where the ablation catheter can be in direct contact with the entire mucosa. Cryoablation can be considered for patients with scarring or an irregular esophageal contour, in whom the cryogen can be sprayed over the treatment area. This therapy may be the best in areas with prior stricture, as the stricture rates from this procedure are among the lowest reported. The use of photodynamic therapy has declined because of a higher rate of strictures compared with RFA.[22] APC and MPEC are used for local treatment of nonnodular BE. Comparative studies between ablative therapies are needed to evaluate long-term outcomes, including rate of recurrence.

Patients undergoing endoscopic eradication therapy should be enrolled in a comprehensive surveillance and staging program. The decision to pursue endoscopic therapy rather than surgery should involve discussion of the advantages and disadvantages of each approach. Institutional expertise in endoscopy, surgery, and pathology will likely influence the choice of therapy and outcomes.

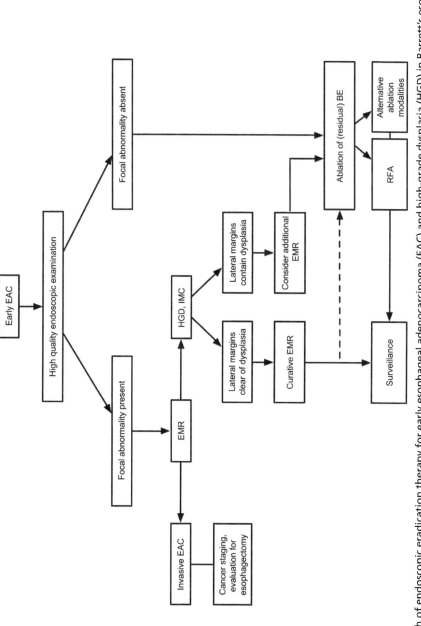

Fig. 7. Approach of endoscopic eradication therapy for early esophageal adenocarcinoma (EAC) and high-grade dysplasia (HGD) in Barrett's esophagus (BE). EMR, endoscopic mucosal resection; IMC, intramucosal adenocarcinoma; RFA, radiofrequency ablation.

RECURRENT DYSPLASIA

Recurrence of dysplasia and intestinal metaplasia following combination endotherapy with PDT and RFA ranges from 17% to 22% over a 1- to 3-year follow-up period.[15,26] Risk factors for recurrence include long-segment BE and piecemeal EMR.[27] Continued endoscopic surveillance following endotherapy is recommended, with intervals guided by prior histopathology and response to treatment. The treatment strategy for recurrent dysplasia is similar to primary dysplasia. EMR is used for the treatment and staging of areas highly suspicious for neoplasia, and ablative therapy is performed over recurrent BE. Whether switching to a different mucosal ablation modality has an added benefit in the eradication of recurrent dysplasia is unclear.

SUMMARY

Endoscopic eradication therapy is considered a safe, effective, and durable treatment strategy for BE complicated by HGD and early EAC. The endoscopist should be familiar with both mucosal resection and ablation techniques, and their respective indications. Patients should be enrolled in a comprehensive surveillance program that continues after endoscopic eradication therapy. Recurrent dysplasia can be approached endoscopically as long as appropriate staging is performed.

REFERENCES

1. Prasad GA, Wang KK, Buttar NS, et al. Long-term survival following endoscopic and surgical treatment of high-grade dysplasia in Barrett's esophagus. Gastroenterology 2007;132:1226.
2. Stein HJ, Feith M, Bruecher BL, et al. Early esophageal cancer: pattern of lymphatic spread and prognostic factors for long-term survival after surgical resection. Ann Surg 2005;242:566.
3. Prasad GA, Wang KK, Halling KC, et al. Utility of biomarkers in prediction of response to ablative therapy in Barrett's esophagus. Gastroenterology 2008; 135:370.
4. Rastogi A, Puli S, El-Serag HB, et al. Incidence of esophageal adenocarcinoma in patients with Barrett's esophagus and high-grade dysplasia: a meta-analysis. Gastrointest Endosc 2008;67:394.
5. Namasivayam V, Wang KK, Prasad GA. Endoscopic mucosal resection in the management of esophageal neoplasia: current status and future directions. Clin Gastroenterol Hepatol 2010;8:743.
6. Wani S, Mathur SC, Curvers WL, et al. Greater interobserver agreement by endoscopic mucosal resection than biopsy samples in Barrett's dysplasia. Clin Gastroenterol Hepatol 2010;8:783.
7. Mino-Kenudson M, Hull MJ, Brown I, et al. EMR for Barrett's esophagus-related superficial neoplasms offers better diagnostic reproducibility than mucosal biopsy. Gastrointest Endosc 2007;66:660.
8. Yamashita T, Zeniya A, Ishii H, et al. Endoscopic mucosal resection using a cap-fitted panendoscope and endoscopic submucosal dissection as optimal endoscopic procedures for superficial esophageal carcinoma. Surg Endosc 2011;25:2541.
9. Inoue H, Minami H, Kaga M, et al. Endoscopic mucosal resection and endoscopic submucosal dissection for esophageal dysplasia and carcinoma. Gastrointest Endosc Clin N Am 2010;20:25.

10. Ell C, May A, Pech O, et al. Curative endoscopic resection of early esophageal adenocarcinomas (Barrett's cancer). Gastrointest Endosc 2007;65:3.
11. May A, Gossner L, Pech O, et al. Local endoscopic therapy for intraepithelial high-grade neoplasia and early adenocarcinoma in Barrett's oesophagus: acute-phase and intermediate results of a new treatment approach. Eur J Gastroenterol Hepatol 2002;14:1085.
12. Leers JM, Vivaldi C, Schafer H, et al. Endoscopic therapy for esophageal perforation or anastomotic leak with a self-expandable metallic stent. Surg Endosc 2009;23:2258.
13. Shimizu Y, Kato M, Yamamoto J, et al. Endoscopic clip application for closure of esophageal perforations caused by EMR. Gastrointest Endosc 2004;60:636.
14. Shaheen NJ, Sharma P, Overholt BF, et al. Radiofrequency ablation in Barrett's esophagus with dysplasia. N Engl J Med 2009;360:2277.
15. Shaheen NJ, Overholt BF, Sampliner RE, et al. Durability of radiofrequency ablation in Barrett's esophagus with dysplasia. Gastroenterology 2011;141:460.
16. Krishnan K, Pandolfino JE, Kahrilas PJ, et al. Increased risk for persistent intestinal metaplasia in patients with Barrett's esophagus and uncontrolled reflux exposure before radiofrequency ablation. Gastroenterology 2012;143:576.
17. Attwood SE, Lewis CJ, Caplin S, et al. Argon beam plasma coagulation as therapy for high-grade dysplasia in Barrett's esophagus. Clin Gastroenterol Hepatol 2003;1:258.
18. Barham CP, Jones RL, Biddlestone LR, et al. Photothermal laser ablation of Barrett's oesophagus: endoscopic and histological evidence of squamous re-epithelialisation. Gut 1997;41:281.
19. Hornick JL, Mino-Kenudson M, Lauwers GY, et al. Buried Barrett's epithelium following photodynamic therapy shows reduced crypt proliferation and absence of DNA content abnormalities. Am J Gastroenterol 2008;103:38.
20. Dulai GS, Jensen DM, Cortina G, et al. Randomized trial of argon plasma coagulation vs. multipolar electrocoagulation for ablation of Barrett's esophagus. Gastrointest Endosc 2005;61:232.
21. Sampliner RE, Fennerty B, Garewal HS. Reversal of Barrett's esophagus with acid suppression and multipolar electrocoagulation: preliminary results. Gastrointest Endosc 1996;44:532.
22. Overholt BF, Panjehpour M, Halberg DL. Photodynamic therapy for Barrett's esophagus with dysplasia and/or early stage carcinoma: long-term results. Gastrointest Endosc 2003;58:183.
23. Johnston MH. Cryotherapy and other newer techniques. Gastrointest Endosc Clin N Am 2003;13:491.
24. Greenwald BD, Dumot JA, Horwhat JD, et al. Safety, tolerability, and efficacy of endoscopic low-pressure liquid nitrogen spray cryotherapy in the esophagus. Dis Esophagus 2010;23:13.
25. Okoro NI, Tomizawa Y, Dunagan KT, et al. Safety of prior endoscopic mucosal resection in patients receiving radiofrequency ablation of Barrett's esophagus. Clin Gastroenterol Hepatol 2012;10:150.
26. Badreddine RJ, Prasad GA, Wang KK, et al. Prevalence and predictors of recurrent neoplasia after ablation of Barrett's esophagus. Gastrointest Endosc 2010;71:697.
27. Esaki M, Matsumoto T, Hirakawa K, et al. Risk factors for local recurrence of superficial esophageal cancer after treatment by endoscopic mucosal resection. Endoscopy 2007;39:41.

Treatment Strategies for Esophageal Cancer

Dylan R. Nieman, MD, PhD, Jeffrey H. Peters, MD*

KEYWORDS

- Esophageal cancer • Treatment • Esophagectomy • Neoadjuvant • Chemoradiation
- Adenocarcinoma • Squamous cell carcinoma

KEY POINTS

- Esophageal cancer encompasses adenocarcinoma of the tubular esophageal and gastro-esophageal junction (cardia) as well as squamous cell carcinoma, two histologically and pathophysiologically distinct diseases.
- Biomarkers to aid in diagnosis, identifying at risk individuals, predicting response to therapy, and predicting overall prognosis are under development.
- Disease confined to the mucosa, without invasion of the muscularis mucosa, is amenable to endoscopic therapy, with a high cure rate.
- Patients with locoregional disease should receive multimodal neoadjuvant therapy before esophagectomy.
- Preoperative assessment should be performed, including cardiac and pulmonary evaluation as well as nutritional optimization and counseling.
- Curative esophagectomy can be performed with a variety of surgical approaches. Prognostic perioperative factors include complete R0 resection, the extent of lymphadenectomy, lack of blood transfusion, and absence of perioperative complications.
- Overall prognosis for patients with resectable locoregional disease depends on the pathologic depth of tumor invasion, degree of histologic differentiation, involvement of lymph nodes, and presence of distant metastasis. Five-year survival for surgery alone ranges from greater than 60% for stage 1B disease to ~15% for stage 3C disease.
- Overall 5-year survival for patients with resectable locoregional disease receiving neoadjuvant chemoradiation and esophagectomy is ~47%.

INTRODUCTION

Esophageal cancer is currently the sixth leading cause of cancer death worldwide.[1] In the last 40 years, the incidence of adenocarcinoma has increased by 600%.[2] The incidence increases steadily with age, with a median age at presentation of 68 years.[3]

Division of Thoracic and Foregut Surgery, Department of Surgery, University of Rochester Medical Center, 601 Elmwood Avenue, Rochester, NY 14642, USA
* Corresponding author. Department of Surgery, University of Rochester, 601 Elmwood Avenue, Box SURG, Rochester, NY 14642.
E-mail address: jeffrey_peters@urmc.rochester.edu

Gastroenterol Clin N Am 42 (2013) 187–197
http://dx.doi.org/10.1016/j.gtc.2012.11.007
0889-8553/13/$ – see front matter © 2013 Elsevier Inc. All rights reserved.

Esophageal cancer encompasses 2 distinct histologic diseases: esophageal squamous cell cancer (ESCC), which predominates in China, India, and central Asia, and esophageal adenocarcinoma (EAC), which predominates in Western countries.[4] Most esophageal tumors become symptomatic, usually heralded by dysphagia at late-stage disease. Understanding of the disease and its risk factors has improved in the last few decades but, despite significant advances in the oncologic and surgical care of these patients, overall survival is often poor.

BIOMARKERS

There is ample investigation into the identification and clinical development of diagnostic markers that indicate the presence of cancer, markers of progression predicting an increased risk of developing cancer, markers that indicate a response to or provide an avenue for chemotherapy and biological therapy, and prognostic markers that correlate with overall survival.[5] A 4-gene signature has been shown to predict survival in an independent validation cohort of patients with EAC. Those with none of the 4 gene markers had a 5-year survival of 58%; with 1 or 2 of the gene markers-year survival was 26%; and with 3 or 4 of the gene markers it was 14%. In a multivariate model adjusted for tumor-node-metastasis tumor staging, the 4-gene signature remained an independent predictor of mortality.[6]

As the number and variety of targeted chemotherapeutics increase, there is interest in assessing oncologic pathway susceptibility to treatment. Multiple trials of targeted therapies including Herceptin, gefitinib, and erlotinib are ongoing. Her2 is present in approximately 15% to 20% of patients with esophageal adenocarcinoma and in the presence of metastatic disease should now be routinely assessed. Limited data suggest a survival benefit of Herceptin therapy in patients with advanced adenocarcinoma who are Her2 positive.

TREATMENT
Mucosal Disease

As the accuracy of noninvasive determination of tumor depth and the sensitivity for detection of local lymph nodes has improved, pretreatment staging has allowed resection of mucosal cancers without removal of the esophagus. The threshold for consideration of endoscopic treatment is currently at the muscularis mucosa, above which lesions are classified as T1a and below which lesions are classified as T1b and there is submucosal involvement. Invasion into the submucosa substantially increases the likelihood of occult lymphovascular involvement, documented to be 15% to 25% in reports of en bloc surgical resections. Endoscopic mucosal resection is currently an excellent treatment option for mucosal cancers and is used increasingly with and without ablative techniques.[7–9]

Locoregional Disease

Neoadjuvant chemotherapy with radiation
Cisplatin-based chemotherapy in conjunction with radiation therapy has been shown to significantly improve survival compared with radiation therapy alone. The Radiation Therapy Oncology Group's randomized trial of 4 cycles of cisplatin and 5-fluorouracil (5-FU) with 50 Gy of external beam radiation versus 64 Gy of radiation alone was closed prematurely because of a median survival of 14 months in the chemoradiation group versus 9 months in the radiation alone group and 5-year survival of 27% versus 0%.[10] Approximately 85% of the study group had squamous cell cancer (SCC). Further, high-dose radiation does not seem to improve the outcomes of combined

chemoradiation: the American InterGroup study showed no benefit of 64.8 Gy versus 50.4 Gy in conjunction with chemotherapy.[11]

Multimodal neoadjuvant therapy before surgical resection has emerged as the optimal treatment of locoregional stage IIB to III cancers. Its role in submucosal clinically node-negative tumors remains to be defined, although a well-documented 15% to 25% prevalence of node metastases in the presence of submucosal lesions provides a rationale for its consideration. Several recent studies have shown survival benefits from preoperative neoadjuvant treatment. The Medical Research Council of the United Kingdom multicenter randomized control study of 2 cycles of cisplatin/5-FU separated by 3 weeks followed by surgery versus surgery alone showed an increase in median survival from 13.3 months to 16.8 months and 2-year survival from 34% to 43%.[12] The Fédération Nationale des Centres de Lutte contre le Cancer (FNCLCC) and the Fédération Francophone de Cancérologie Digestive (FFCD) multicenter Phase III trial found similar results with disease-free survival improved from 21% to 34% and overall survival improved from 24% to 38%.[13] The Medical Research Council Adjuvant Gastric Infusional Chemotherapy (MAGIC) trial went on to show that preoperative and postoperative chemotherapy with epirubicin, cisplatin, and 5-FU was associated with improved survival versus surgery alone (3% vs 23%).[14] Pennathur and colleagues[15] studied neoadjuvant chemotherapy with cisplatin, 5-FU, and paclitaxel, and found that patients who were downstaged as a result of treatment response showed significant survival benefit.

Studies of preoperative chemoradiation have mostly been underpowered, but have trended toward showing a survival advantage versus surgery alone. The most recent and best of these trials, known as the Chemoradiotherapy for Esophageal Cancer followed by Surgery Study (CROSS), studied 366 patients with esophageal or junctional cancers. The study randomized patients to surgery alone or preoperative treatment with carboplatin and paclitaxel for 5 weeks in conjunction with 41.4-Gy radiotherapy. Pathologic compete response (pCR) occurred in 29% of the chemoradiation group, with improvement in median survival from 24 to 49 months, and 5-year survival from 34% to 47%.[16]

Two recent studies have evaluated the value of chemoradiation compared with chemotherapy alone. A phase III trial comparing cisplatin, 5-FU, and leucovorin with or without 30-Gy induction radiotherapy for 126 patients with EAC showed that rates of pCR increased from 2% to 15%, rates of pN0 resection improved from 36% to 64%, and median survival improved from 21 to 33 months.[17] A phase II trial of cisplatin and 5-FU with or without 35-Gy induction therapy for 75 patients with EAC showed that rates of pCR improved from 8% to 31% and median survival improved from 36% to 45%.[18] Both studies were underpowered to show a significant survival advantage, but they suggested the usefulness of multimodal induction therapy.

It has been recognized that 10% to 15% of esophageal adenocarcinomas express HER2, and, to a lesser extent, other potentially targetable markers including epidermal growth factor receptor. Numerous trials are underway to evaluate the use of targeted biological therapies including cetuximab, trastuzumab, erlotinib, and gefitinib in conjunction with chemoradiotherapy.

Preoperative assessment and counseling

Esophagectomy is a potentially morbid procedure. Although it provides the best locoregional control and potential for cure, the risks of surgery are weighed against its benefit compared with alternate therapies. To ensure the selection of patients who would benefit most from esophagectomy, every effort must be made to assess the preoperative physiologic status of the patient. Several instruments have been developed for predicting perioperative mortality, identifying risk factors including age, preoperative weight loss; pulmonary, vascular, or cardiac disease; and both hospital and surgeon volume of esophageal resection.[19–22]

In all patients, preoperative risk factor modification should include smoking cessation, blood pressure and blood sugar control, perioperative β-blockade if indicated, and optimization of nutritional status.[23] Perhaps the most important modifiable risk factor, nutritional status can be difficult to augment for patients with esophageal disorders. Preoperative dilation, stenting, or feeding tube placement may facilitate caloric intake. The value of immunonutrition before surgery in reducing the risk of perioperative infections has been suggested and is currently under investigation.[24]

Evaluation of cardiac (stress echocardiogram) and pulmonary function tests (PFTs) is necessary to identify the occasional patient with severe organ dysfunction. Preoperative nutrition counseling can be useful in easing the transition to the postsurgical period.[25] Following esophagectomy, most patients experience a 1-month to 2-month adaptation toward full caloric intake. Patient education and participation are essential to optimizing long-term outcomes and quality of life.

Surgical approach

There are a variety of surgical approaches to esophageal resection, each with specific advantages and disadvantages. Factors important in selecting the optimal approach include the location of the tumor, extent of lymph node dissection, body habitus, prior chemoradiation therapy, comorbidities, and surgeon experience.

Ivor Lewis esophagectomy Used for tumors of the midesophagus, distal esophagus, or gastroesophageal junction (GEJ), the Ivor Lewis esophagectomy involves a laparotomy and right thoracotomy, with intrathoracic esophagogastric anastomosis. The procedure begins with an upper midline laparotomy to examine for metastatic disease and confirm resectability. The triangular ligament is divided, the left lateral segment of the liver retracted medially, the gastrohepatic ligament divided, and the dissection carried down to the right crus. The phrenoesophageal membrane is divided along the right crus and over the esophagus, and then circumferential dissection of the esophagus is performed at the hiatus. The gastrocolic omentum is opened along the greater curvature of the stomach leaving a safe margin for the gastroepiploic artery and vein. The stomach is reflected anteromedially and the short and posterior gastric vessels are divided. The left gastric artery and vein are divided and all lymphatic tissue is swept with the esophagogastric specimen. The right gastric artery is carefully preserved as a component of the blood supply for the gastric conduit. A pyloromyotomy or pyloroplasty is performed to augment gastric emptying and the stomach is divided vertically with serial firings of a GIA stapler, maintaining a margin of 4 to 5 cm from the tumor. The stomach is commonly tethered to the esophagogastric specimen with sutures and the hiatus is enlarged to allow passage of conduit into the mediastinum. The distal esophagus is dissected slightly through the hiatus and the abdomen closed. The patient is then repositioned into the left lateral decubitus position for a right posterolateral thoracotomy.

For the thoracic portion of the procedure, the right lung is isolated and retracted, the thoracic esophagus mobilized, and the azygous vein divided. The esophageal dissection can be done either with or without a specific en bloc dissection of mediastinal lymph nodes. Periesophageal, subcarinal, and available paratracheal lymph nodes are dissected with the esophagus. Many surgeons prefer to specifically ligate the thoracic duct as it enters the thorax to minimize the potential for chyle leak. The esophagogastric specimen and conduit are delivered into the chest without torsion and the proximal esophagus is transected above the level of the azygous vein. An end-to-side esophagogastric anastomosis is then performed in the upper chest and the thoracotomy is closed.

A 3-incision esophagectomy A 3-incision esophagectomy is similar to an Ivor Lewis procedure except that it usually begins with the thoracotomy portion of the procedure and the chest incision is closed without anastomosis to allow gastric pull-up to the neck for reconstruction. It is preferred in patients with tumors above the carina in which a transhiatal dissection may prove difficult or dangerous and in which a shorter esophageal remnant is necessary to provide adequate margins. The addition of a left-sided cervical esophagogastric anastomosis allows for wider resection margins for tumors of the upper and middle thirds of the esophagus.[26] Rather than beginning in the abdomen, it is common to start in left lateral decubitus position with a right posterolateral thoracotomy. The esophagus is first mobilized from the thoracic inlet to the diaphragm, allowing definitive assessment of intrathoracic resectability before the abdominal portion of the operation. After the chest is closed, the patient is placed in the supine position and the abdominal portion is performed as described earlier for the Ivor Lewis esophagectomy.

A left cervical incision along the anterior border of the sternocleidomastoid muscle is created and the dissection is carried posteriorly with careful attention to the recurrent laryngeal nerve. The esophagus is divided and the specimen removed via the laparotomy incision. The gastric conduit is then pulled through the posterior mediastinum and an end-to-side or end-to-end cervical anastomosis performed. From the abdomen, the conduit is gently retracted to avoid redundancy and tacked to the diaphragm at the hiatus to prevent herniation.

En Bloc esophagectomy En Bloc esophagectomy can be performed with either a cervical or intrathoracic anastomosis and requires a right thoracotomy. The procedure entails a specific effort to widely dissect all mediastinal and upper abdominal tissue from the carina to the celiac axis. The thoracic dissection plane begins outside the azygous venous system and includes resection of the thoracic duct and left pleura.

Transhiatal esophagectomy Transhiatal esophagectomy relies on dissection of the thoracic esophagus primarily through the abdominal incision (**Fig. 1**). The distal third of the esophagus can usually be dissected under direct vision, whereas the proximal two-thirds are mobilized bluntly via the surgeon's hand through the esophageal hiatus. The patient is placed in the supine position with the neck extended to the right, and the operation begins in a similar fashion to the procedure, with upper midline incision, exploration of the abdomen, exposure of the hiatus, mobilization of the stomach with preservation of the gastroepiploic arcade, mobilization of the esophagus to the hiatus, and ligation of the left gastric artery. A modified pyloroplasty is performed approximately and the diaphragm is incised anteriorly to widen the hiatus. The blunt dissection is first performed posteriorly along the aorta and spine, then anteriorly below the pericardium and trachea. Anterior and posterior dissection is usually straightforward. The lateral aspects of the esophagus including small vessels and the branches of the vagus nerves to the tracheobronchial tree is more difficult but can be accomplished with careful finger and hand dissection. An incision is made along the anterior border of the left sternocleidomastoid muscle, the platysma is divided, and the internal jugular vein and carotid sheath retracted laterally. Dissection of the cervical esophagus down the prevertebral fascia is performed. Blunt finger dissection is performed posteriorly and the tracheoesophageal groove is developed with concern for the recurrent laryngeal nerve. Mediastinal mobilization is then performed by blunt dissection with one hand entering the mediastinum via the cervical

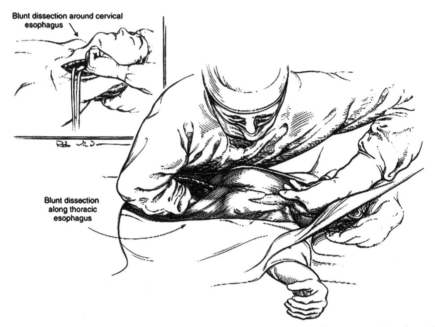

Fig. 1. Transhiatal esophagectomy. (*From* McCarron E, Doty JR, Heitmiller RF. Transhiatal esoph-agectomy. CTSNet: The Cardiothoracic Surgery Network. Available at: http://www.ctsnet.org/sections/clinicalresources/thoracic/expert_tech-22.html?CFID=55168496&CFTOKEN=76076481. Accessed January 12, 2013. Copyright © 2013, CTSNet.org. All rights reserved; used with permission.)

incision and the other via the abdominal incision and through the hiatus. This blunt dissection is continued with consideration for the posterior membranous trachea and the azygous vein until the operator's fingers meet and circumferential mobilization of the esophagus is achieved. The esophagus is divided cervically, delivered into the abdomen, the stomach divided, and the specimen is removed. The gastric conduit is then prepared in the usual manner, pulled up through the mediastinum into the chest, and a cervical anastomosis is performed near the thoracic inlet. The gastric conduit is gently retracted to avoid redundancy and the hiatus repaired.

Left thoracoabdominal esophagectomy Left thoracoabdominal esophagectomy provides simultaneous exposure of the thoracic and abdominal fields via a left thoracoabdominal approach. It has the advantage of a single incision and single surgical positioning. The patient is placed in the right lateral decubitus position and an incision is made along the left sixth or seventh intercostal spaces. After exploring the abdomen and confirming resectability, the chest is entered and the diaphragm is taken down along the chest wall leaving a cuff of muscle circumferentially to facilitate closure. The conduit preparation and mediastinal anastomosis take place in a manner similar to the Ivor Lewis esophagectomy, with reapproximation of the diaphragm at the close of the case.

Minimally invasive esophagectomy Minimally invasive esophagectomy is currently offered at a limited number of high-volume centers and generally follows the procedural flow of either 3-incision or Ivor Lewis esophagectomy. It is accomplished via thoracoscopic and laparoscopic access into the chest and abdomen. In the Ivor Lewis variant, a stapled anastomosis is performed thoracoscopically, whereas in the

3-incision variant a cervical anastomosis is performed in a stapled or hand-sewn manner.[27,28] With a capable surgeon, it may offer the benefits of more traditional approaches with reduced incisional morbidity, but it is technically challenging and not widely practiced.

Other technical considerations

Each of these surgical approaches has a slightly different balance of operative time, facility for lymph node dissection, and potential complications. The Ivor Lewis and left thoracoabdominal approaches avoid the cervical incision, but are most appropriate for tumors of the mid and distal thirds of the esophagus and GEJ. The left thoracoabdominal approach offers access to both surgical fields simultaneously without the need for repositioning, but the incision may be associated with more postoperative morbidity. A 3-incision approach includes a neck incision but may avoid the mediastinal and intrathoracic consequences of an intrathoracic anastomotic leak. Transhiatal esophagectomy leaves the thoracic pleura intact, and may have the benefit of limiting anastomotic complications to the mediastinum and preserving the thoracic space, but involves blind and blunt mobilization of the thoracic esophagus and limited dissection of the periesophageal lymphatics. En bloc resection is designed to keep the specimen with all surrounding lymphatic tissue intact without violating any paraesophageal planes, but requires extensive exposure and generally longer operative times to achieve a more oncologically sound resection.

Other considerations include the routine placement of a feeding tube and surgical drains. A jejunal feeding tube is commonly placed for postoperative enteral nutrition during recovery, which can be done in both open and laparoscopic procedures and is usually placed 30 cm or so from the ligament of Treitz. The colon or jejunum may be used as the reconstructive conduit if the stomach is not possible. The left colon is preferred because of its more predictable blood supply and smaller diameter, although the right colon is also a suitable conduit.[29] An important consideration with colonic or jejunal interposition is the involvement of 2 additional anastomoses: the enteroentero anastomosis and anastomoses at the proximal esophageal and distal gastric resection margins, each subject to potential complications.

Tumor location Cervical esophageal tumors are uncommon, almost universally squamous in histology, and commonly invade surrounding cervical structures including the trachea, thyroid, and larynx. They are treated more like head and neck cancers. Adequate surgical resection may involve the larynx, pharynx, thyroid, and a radical neck dissection. Although not an established standard of care, primary chemoradiation without surgery may provide long-term survival equivalent to surgery, with less morbidity. Upper thoracic esophageal cancers are also commonly squamous, and are usually approached via a 3-incision approach with a cervical incision and anastomosis to obtain an adequate proximal margin. Midthoracic esophageal tumors may involve the carina or descending thoracic aorta and, if resectability remains in question despite thorough preoperative radiographic assessment, a right-sided video-assisted thoracoscopic approach may be used to assess the extent of the tumor. In these cases, a transthoracic approach, either Ivor Lewis or 3 incision, provides optimal exposure for safe dissection.

Postoperative care After surgery, most patients are monitored in an intensive care unit or step-down unit for 24 to 72 hours. Enteral nutrition usually begins on the third postoperative day. An assessment of the anastomosis is often performed 5 to 7 days after surgery and before oral feeds are initiated. The authors prefer to do this via upper endoscopy, which allows an accurate assessment of both the integrity of the anastomosis and blood supply of the conduit. The typical hospital stay is 7 to 14 days.

Systemic or Unresectable Disease

Between 25% and 40% of patients with esophageal cancer still present with either metastases to lung, liver, bone, or, less commonly, widespread nodal metastases precluding an R0 resection. Treatment in this setting largely consists of palliative systemic chemotherapy, which has been shown to provide a survival benefit compared with no treatment. Radiation therapy is usually not included, although it may be of benefit in select patients with obstruction caused by large intraluminal tumors or bone pain. Endoscopic placement of an intraluminal expanding metal esophageal stent may allow continued oral intake of liquids and soft solids and palliate dysphagia.

Recurrent Disease

The most common failure of esophagectomy in the treatment of esophageal cancer is recurrent disease, 80% of which occurs in the first 2 years. Roughly one-third is local and two-thirds systemic recurrence. Treatment options include chemotherapy, further radiation when possible, and palliative interventions as described earlier. There are few specific data on the benefit of palliative chemotherapy or radiation once the cancer has recurred, but numerous reports suggest that they are generally well tolerated and may carry a modest survival benefit.

Outcomes and Prognosis

Perioperative morbidity and mortality following esophagectomy has historically been high. A review of 46,492 esophagectomies performed in the 1980s showed a 30-day mortality of 13% and a 5-year survival of 20%.[30] Since that time there have been significant advances in anesthesia and analgesia, critical care, nutrition, staging, patient selection, and operative techniques. Recent series from high-volume centers report perioperative mortalities of 5% or less.[31,32] Morbidity following esophagectomy is common, occurring in 30% and 60% of patients. The most common complications include respiratory issues (pneumonia and respiratory failure), arrhythmia (atrial fibrillation), and anastomotic leak. Other less common complications include chylothorax and left recurrent nerve palsy.

Overall, survival for patients with resectable esophageal cancer has improved significantly over the last 30 years.[33] Prognosis is largely stage dependent and, for patients with early esophageal cancer limited to the mucosa, cure is expected. The most recent American Joint Committee on Cancer/International Union against Cancer Staging system (seventh edition), is based on data from 3 continents and 4627 patients who underwent esophagectomy alone without chemotherapy or radiation. Five-year, risk-adjusted survival was ~80% for stage 0 and stage 1A cancers. Survival was slightly better for adenocarcinoma than for SCC (**Fig. 2**).[34] Most reports of patients with early adenocarcinoma treated with endoscopic resection and ablation show equally promising outcomes.[7,9,35,36] Long-term survival data are forthcoming.

For patients with stage 1B disease, the 5-year survival with surgery alone decreases to 64% for EAC and 62% ESCC. For stage 2A disease, still without nodal involvement at the time of surgery, 5-year survival is 50% for EAC and 55% for ESCC with surgery alone. With nodal involvement, this decreases to 40% for stage 2B disease, 25% for stage 3A disease, and 15% to 17% for stage 3B to 3C disease.[34] The use of preoperative chemoradiation in these groups probably improves these outcomes, as noted earlier. Patients in the CROSS trial, most of whom were T3 and N1 clinical stage before neoadjuvant treatment, had an overall 5-year survival of 47%.[16] Important prognostic factors include a complete R0 resection, extent of lymphadenectomy, lack of perioperative blood transfusion, and absence of perioperative complications. In patients

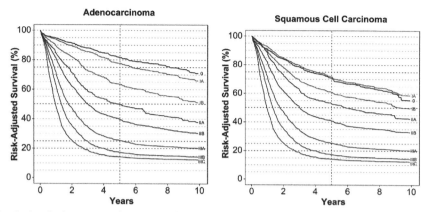

Fig. 2. Survival curves with surgical therapy alone. (*From* Rice TW, Rusch VW, Ishwaran H, et al. Cancer of the esophagus and esophagogastric junction: data-driven staging for the seventh edition of the American Joint Committee on Cancer/International Union Against Cancer Cancer Staging Manuals. Cancer 2010;116:3763–73; with permission.)

with metastatic or unresectable disease at the time of diagnosis, the prognosis is grim, with 1-year survival of less than 20%.

SUMMARY

- Esophageal cancer encompasses adenocarcinoma of the esophagus and cardia and squamous cell carcinoma, two histologically and pathophysiologically distinct diseases.
- Biomarkers to aid in diagnosis, identification of at-risk individuals, prediction of response to therapy, and prediction of overall prognosis are under development.
- Disease confined to the mucosa, without invasion of the muscularis mucosa, is amenable to endoscopic therapy with a high cure rate.
- Patients with locoregional disease should receive multimodal neoadjuvant therapy before esophagectomy.
- Preoperative assessment should be performed, including cardiac and pulmonary evaluation as well as nutritional optimization and counseling.
- Curative esophagectomy can be performed with a variety of surgical approaches. Prognostic perioperative factors include complete R0 resection, the extent of lymphadenectomy, lack of blood transfusion, and absence of perioperative complications.
- Overall prognosis for patients with resectable locoregional disease depends on the pathologic depth of tumor invasion, degree of histologic differentiation, involvement of lymph nodes, and presence of distant metastasis. Five-year survival for surgery alone ranges from greater than 60% for stage 1B disease to ~15% for stage 3C disease.
- Overall 5-year survival for patients with resectable locoregional disease receiving neoadjuvant chemoradiation and esophagectomy is ~47%.

REFERENCES

1. Kamangar F, Dores GM, Anderson WF. Patterns of cancer incidence, mortality, and prevalence across five continents: defining priorities to reduce cancer disparities in different geographic regions of the world. J Clin Oncol 2006;24:2137–50.

2. Eslick GD. Epidemiology of esophageal cancer. Gastroenterol Clin North Am 2009;38:17–25, vii.
3. Eloubeidi MA, Desmond R, Arguedas MR, et al. Prognostic factors for the survival of patients with esophageal carcinoma in the U.S.: the importance of tumor length and lymph node status. Cancer 2002;95:1434–43.
4. Devesa SS, Blot WJ, Fraumeni JF Jr. Changing patterns in the incidence of esophageal and gastric carcinoma in the United States. Cancer 1998;83: 2049–53.
5. Varghese S, Lao-Sirieix P, Fitzgerald RC. Identification and clinical implementation of biomarkers for Barrett's esophagus. Gastroenterology 2012;142:435–441.e2.
6. Peters CJ, Rees JR, Hardwick RH, et al. A 4-gene signature predicts survival of patients with resected adenocarcinoma of the esophagus, junction, and gastric cardia. Gastroenterology 2010;139:1995–2004.e15.
7. Ell C, May A, Pech O, et al. Curative endoscopic resection of early esophageal adenocarcinomas (Barrett's cancer). Gastrointest Endosc 2007;65:3–10.
8. Lopes CV, Hela M, Pesenti C, et al. Circumferential endoscopic resection of Barrett's esophagus with high-grade dysplasia or early adenocarcinoma. Surg Endosc 2007;21:820–4.
9. Galey KM, Wilshire CL, Watson TJ, et al. Endoscopic management of early esophageal neoplasia: an emerging standard. J Gastrointest Surg 2011;15: 1728–35.
10. Herskovic A, Martz K, al-Sarraf M, et al. Combined chemotherapy and radiotherapy compared with radiotherapy alone in patients with cancer of the esophagus. N Engl J Med 1992;326:1593–8.
11. Minsky BD, Pajak TF, Ginsberg RJ, et al. INT 0123 (Radiation Therapy Oncology Group 94-05) phase III trial of combined-modality therapy for esophageal cancer: high-dose versus standard-dose radiation therapy. J Clin Oncol 2002;20: 1167–74.
12. Medical Research Council Oesophageal Cancer Working Group. Surgical resection with or without preoperative chemotherapy in oesophageal cancer: a randomised controlled trial. Lancet 2002;359:1727–33.
13. Ychou M, Boige V, Pignon JP, et al. Perioperative chemotherapy compared with surgery alone for resectable gastroesophageal adenocarcinoma: an FNCLCC and FFCD multicenter phase III trial. J Clin Oncol 2011;29:1715–21.
14. Cunningham D, Allum WH, Stenning SP, et al. Perioperative chemotherapy versus surgery alone for resectable gastroesophageal cancer. N Engl J Med 2006;355: 11–20.
15. Pennathur A, Luketich JD, Landreneau RJ, et al. Long-term results of a phase II trial of neoadjuvant chemotherapy followed by esophagectomy for locally advanced esophageal neoplasm. Ann Thorac Surg 2008;85:1930–6 [discussion: 6–7].
16. van Hagen P, Hulshof MC, van Lanschot JJ, et al. Preoperative chemoradiotherapy for esophageal or junctional cancer. N Engl J Med 2012;366:2074–84.
17. Stahl M, Walz MK, Stuschke M, et al. Phase III comparison of preoperative chemotherapy compared with chemoradiotherapy in patients with locally advanced adenocarcinoma of the esophagogastric junction. J Clin Oncol 2009;27:851–6.
18. Burmeister BH, Thomas JM, Burmeister EA, et al. Is concurrent radiation therapy required in patients receiving preoperative chemotherapy for adenocarcinoma of the oesophagus? A randomised phase II trial. Eur J Cancer 2011;47:354–60.
19. Charlson ME, Pompei P, Ales KL, et al. A new method of classifying prognostic comorbidity in longitudinal studies: development and validation. J Chronic Dis 1987;40:373–83.

20. Ra J, Paulson EC, Kucharczuk J, et al. Postoperative mortality after esophagectomy for cancer: development of a preoperative risk prediction model. Ann Surg Oncol 2008;15:1577–84.

21. Kozower BD, Stukenborg GJ. Hospital esophageal cancer resection volume does not predict patient mortality risk. Ann Thorac Surg 2012;93:1690–6 [discussion: 6–8].

22. Grotenhuis BA, Wijnhoven BP, Grune F, et al. Preoperative risk assessment and prevention of complications in patients with esophageal cancer. J Surg Oncol 2010;101:270–8.

23. Ryan AM, Hearty A, Prichard RS, et al. Association of hypoalbuminemia on the first postoperative day and complications following esophagectomy. J Gastrointest Surg 2007;11:1355–60.

24. Mudge L, Isenring E, Jamieson GG. Immunonutrition in patients undergoing esophageal cancer resection. Dis Esophagus 2011;24:160–5.

25. Kight CE. Nutrition considerations in esophagectomy patients. Nutr Clin Pract 2008;23:521–8.

26. McKeown KC. Total three-stage oesophagectomy for cancer of the oesophagus. Br J Surg 1976;63:259–62.

27. Luketich JD, Schauer PR, Christie NA, et al. Minimally invasive esophagectomy. Ann Thorac Surg 2000;70:906–11 [discussion: 11–2].

28. Fernando HC, Christie NA, Luketich JD. Thoracoscopic and laparoscopic esophagectomy. Semin Thorac Cardiovasc Surg 2000;12:195–200.

29. Postlethwait RW. Colonic interposition for esophageal substitution. Surg Gynecol Obstet 1983;156:377–83.

30. Muller JM, Erasmi H, Stelzner M, et al. Surgical therapy of oesophageal carcinoma. Br J Surg 1990;77:845–57.

31. Casson AG, van Lanschot JJ. Improving outcomes after esophagectomy: the impact of operative volume. J Surg Oncol 2005;92:262–6.

32. Schuchert MJ, Luketich JD, Fernando HC. Complications of minimally invasive esophagectomy. Semin Thorac Cardiovasc Surg 2004;16:133–41.

33. Siegel R, DeSantis C, Virgo K, et al. Cancer treatment and survivorship statistics, 2012. CA Cancer J Clin 2012;62:220–41.

34. Rice TW, Rusch VW, Ishwaran H, et al. Cancer of the esophagus and esophagogastric junction: data-driven staging for the seventh edition of the American Joint Committee on Cancer/International Union Against Cancer Cancer Staging Manuals. Cancer 2010;116:3763–73.

35. May A, Gossner L, Pech O, et al. Local endoscopic therapy for intraepithelial high-grade neoplasia and early adenocarcinoma in Barrett's oesophagus: acute-phase and intermediate results of a new treatment approach. Eur J Gastroenterol Hepatol 2002;14:1085–91.

36. Buttar NS, Wang KK, Lutzke LS, et al. Combined endoscopic mucosal resection and photodynamic therapy for esophageal neoplasia within Barrett's esophagus. Gastrointest Endosc 2001;54:682–8.

Index

Note: Page numbers of article titles are in **boldface** type.

Gastroenterol Clin N Am 42 (2013) 199–209
http://dx.doi.org/10.1016/S0889-8553(13)00009-5
0889-8553/13/$ – see front matter © 2013 Elsevier Inc. All rights reserved.

gastro.theclinics.com

recurrent, 194
systemic, 193–194
unresectable, 193–194
Cannabinoid receptor agonists, for GERD, 108
Cap-device, for mucosal resection, 178
Capsule endoscopy, for adenocarcinoma screening, 161
Chemoradiotherapy for Esophageal Cancer followed by Surgery Study (CROSS), 189, 194
Chemotherapy, for cancer, 188–189
Chest pain, in spastic disorders, 32
Chicago classification
    of motility disorders, 2
    of spastic disorders, 28
Cholestyramine, for GERD, 96
Cholinergic activity, in spastic disorders, 31
Ciclesonide, for eosinophilic esophagitis, 140
Cisapride, for GERD, 108
Cisplatin, for cancer, 188–189
Clouse plots, 2, 7
Compartmentalized pressure, in manometry, 6–7
Computed tomography, for spastic disorder, 33–34
Continuous positive airway pressure, for GERD, 62
Contractile deceleration point, 4–5, 29
Contractile front velocity, 5, 29
Contractile vigor, 5–6
Corkscrew esophagus, 32, 36
Corticosteroids, for eosinophilic esophagitis, 139–140
Cough
    impedance-pH testing in, 23–24
    in GERD, 74–77
Crêpe-paper mucosa, in eosinophilic esophagitis, 135–136
Cromolyn, for eosinophilic esophagitis, 141
CROSS (Chemoradiotherapy for Esophageal Cancer followed by Surgery Study), 189, 194
Cryoablation, for Barrett's esophagus and adenocarcinoma, 181–182
Cyclin A, in adenocarcinoma, 164–165
Cytology, for adenocarcinoma screening, 162
Cytosponge, for adenocarcinoma screening, 162

D

Dexlansoprazole, for GERD, 64, 98–99, 101
Dexrabeprazole, for GERD, 99
Diet
    adenocarcinoma due to, 158–159
    for eosinophilic esophagitis, 141–142
Diffuse spasm, esophageal, 9
Dilation
    for achalasia, 48–50
    for eosinophilic esophagitis, 142–143
    for spastic disorders, 38
Distal contractile integral, 5–6, 29
Distal contractile latency, 30

Printed and bound by CPI Group (UK) Ltd, Croydon, CR0 4YY

03/10/2024

01040443-0002